Cancer Immunotherapy: Current Advancements and Future Perspectives

Cancer Immunotherapy: Current Advancements and Future Perspectives

Guest Editors

Stefano Forte

Gianluca Ferini

MDPI

Basel • Beijing • Wuhan • Barcelona • Belgrade • Novi Sad • Cluj • Manchester

Guest Editors

Stefano Forte
Genomics and Molecular Oncology Unit
Istituto Oncologico del Mediterraneo
Viagrande
Italy

Gianluca Ferini
Radiotherapy Unit
REM Radioterapia
Viagrande
Italy

Editorial Office
MDPI AG
Grosspeteranlage 5
4052 Basel, Switzerland

This is a reprint of the Special Issue, published open access by the journal *Journal of Personalized Medicine* (ISSN 2075-4426), freely accessible at: https://www.mdpi.com/journal/jpm/special_issues/62U2ZJFVX1.

For citation purposes, cite each article independently as indicated on the article page online and as indicated below:

Lastname, A.A.; Lastname, B.B. Article Title. *Journal Name* **Year**, *Volume Number*, Page Range.

ISBN 978-3-7258-8087-4 (Hbk)
ISBN 978-3-7258-8088-1 (PDF)
https://doi.org/10.3390/books978-3-7258-8088-1

Contents

Preface

This Special Issue focuses on the evolving landscape of cancer treatment strategies that involve the activation and modulation of the immune system, including the integration of radiotherapy, immunotherapy, and other systemic approaches. The aim of this reprint is to provide a concise yet comprehensive overview of current clinical and translational advances, highlighting how these approaches can be optimized through a deeper understanding of tumor biology and immune dynamics.

The contributions gathered in this reprint explore key aspects such as treatment response, disease control, and safety across different tumor types, while also addressing the modulation of the tumor microenvironment and anti-tumor immune responses induced by therapeutic interventions. In addition, emerging evidence on predictive biomarkers is presented, supporting more informed and individualized therapeutic strategies.

This reprint is intended for clinicians, researchers, and healthcare professionals involved in oncology, radiation oncology, and cancer immunology. The motivation behind this collection is to provide a focused resource that reflects current practice and ongoing developments, while also fostering further research and collaboration in the field.

Stefano Forte and Gianluca Ferini
Guest Editors

Journal of
Personalized Medicine

MDPI

Editorial

Radiotherapy and Immunotherapy at a Crossroads: Mechanistic Foundations, Emerging Evidence, and a New Horizon for Precision Oncology

Gianluca Ferini [1,2,*] and Stefano Forte [3]

1 REM Radioterapia srl, 95029 Catania, Italy
2 Department of Medicine and Surgery, University Kore of Enna, 94100 Enna, Italy
3 Mediterranean Institute of Oncology, 95029 Catania, Italy; stefano.forte@grupposamed.com
* Correspondence: gianluca.ferini@unikore.it; Tel.: +39-095-78-94-581

The trajectory of modern oncology is increasingly defined by the convergence of two therapeutic paradigms that were once considered only marginally related: radiotherapy and immunotherapy. For decades, radiotherapy (RT) was perceived primarily as a local treatment, its systemic consequences regarded as incidental rather than intentional. Immunotherapy, by contrast, has been heralded as the modality capable of harnessing or reawakening the body's own defenses, offering the tantalizing possibility of long-term disease control or even eradication. Yet, the clinical reality has proven more nuanced. Despite the remarkable successes of immune checkpoint inhibitors, adoptive cellular immunotherapy, and various emerging forms of immune-based modulation, the proportion of patients achieving durable responses remains limited. The immune system, even when pharmacologically stimulated, is frequently thwarted by the complexity of tumor microenvironments, by heterogeneity within metastatic lesions, and by the emergence of localized immune escape.

This Special Issue was conceived to illuminate how radiotherapy, particularly when thoughtfully integrated into multimodal strategies, can act as a biological amplifier of antitumor immunity. The contributions assembled here span tumor types that differ profoundly in histology, immune landscape, and clinical behavior, yet collectively reveal a consistent and compelling narrative: radiation has the capacity to reshape the tumor microenvironment, restore immune competence, eliminate resistant clones, and ultimately extend or deepen the therapeutic reach of immunotherapy. The present manuscript collection explores this principle across a spectrum of clinical scenarios, from rare tumors such as Merkel cell carcinoma (MCC), mucosal vaginal melanoma, and glioblastoma, to more common malignancies like renal cell carcinoma (RCC) and squamous cell skin cancers. They also examine how radiotherapy's immunomodulatory effects may potentiate not only checkpoint inhibitors but also more advanced strategies, including CAR-T cells and next-generation spatially fractionated techniques such as lattice therapy.

What emerges, across this heterogeneous landscape, is a unifying mechanistic foundation that positions radiotherapy as an indispensable partner in the future of immuno-oncology. This editorial aims to integrate and interpret these findings within a narrative framework that captures both the complexity and the translational potential of the field, while also addressing recent advances in cancer vaccines, T-cell lymphomas, and nanoparticle-based theranostic approaches.

Radiotherapy as a Corrective Force in Immunotherapy Resistance

One of the clearest themes derived from the contributions of this Special Issue is the crucial role of radiotherapy in addressing oligoprogression during immunotherapy. Oligoprogression, defined as the emergence of limited sites of disease growth while systemic therapy continues to control the broader metastatic burden, has become an increasingly recognized phenomenon as immune checkpoint inhibitors (ICIs) and immune checkpoint inhibitor–tyrosine kinase inhibitor (ICI–TKI) combinations gain prominence. Rather than signaling systemic therapeutic failure, oligoprogression frequently represents the emergence of subclones that have acquired or maintained localized resistance mechanisms [1]. In this context, radiotherapy serves as a corrective force that suppresses these foci of resistance, thereby prolonging the systemic benefit of immunotherapy [2].

The experience reported by Ferini et al. in metastatic MCC illustrates this principle with striking clarity. Their retrospective cohort describes patients experiencing oligoprogression while undergoing treatment with avelumab, a PD-L1 inhibitor that has transformed the management of advanced MCC. Radiotherapy was directed to all sites of progressive disease and was delivered in palliative-dose schedules, most commonly 30 Gy in 10 fractions. The results demonstrate a remarkably high objective response rate of 75%, with 100% local control and survival outcomes that surpass historical expectations in this highly aggressive tumor type. Post-radiotherapy progression-free survival reached 60% at both 6 and 12 months, and overall survival exceeded 85% at one year and more than 64% at two years [3]. These numbers underscore not only the radiosensitivity of MCC but also the profound immunologic collaboration between RT and checkpoint inhibition.

The biological underpinnings of this synergy are multifaceted and well established in the literature. In general, radiation induces immunogenic cell death, increases the availability of tumor antigens, enhances major histocompatibility complex expression, and stimulates dendritic cell maturation, thereby reprogramming the irradiated tumor into an active immunological node that promotes systemic antitumor immunity [4,5]. Yet, the study also expands the conceptual framework of oligoprogression itself. MCC frequently presents with subclinical in-transit metastases and extensive, interconnected cutaneous disease targets that extend beyond conventional oligoprogression definitions based solely on lesion volume and count. Notably, despite the irradiation of very large target volumes (one exceeding 3700 cubic centimeters), the investigators achieved excellent tumor control with minimal toxicity, thereby questioning the adequacy of simple numerical and volumetric parameters as determinants of radiotherapy feasibility [3]. These findings reinforce the notion that radiotherapy can meaningfully extend the efficacy of immunotherapy, even when disease extent complicates traditional clinical decision-making.

A complementary narrative emerges in the work of Lo Greco et al., who analyze the outcomes of patients with advanced or metastatic cutaneous squamous cell carcinoma (CSCC) treated with cemiplimab in combination with radiotherapy. The results here are compelling as well. Across twenty treated lesions, the investigators report an 85% rate of complete or partial response, with no cases of disease progression during follow-up periods extending beyond twenty months. What makes these findings particularly noteworthy is their consistency across different radiation regimens: hypofractionated courses were deployed for frail patients or small-volume disease, while conventionally fractionated schedules were used for larger or more anatomically constrained regions. Regardless of fractionation, the integration of radiotherapy and cemiplimab resulted in consistently favorable clinical outcomes [6].

CSCC is characterized by high tumor mutational burden due to cumulative ultraviolet damage. This biological profile renders the disease intrinsically responsive to immune checkpoint blockade [7]; however, even within this favorable immunogenic context, radiotherapy proved capable of further amplifying treatment response. The combination enabled rapid and sustained tumor regression without introducing additional toxicity; only grade I and II adverse events were observed, reinforcing the feasibility and safety of this synergistic

https://doi.org/10.3390/jpm16050256

approach [6]. These findings suggest that radiotherapy is not merely a fallback strategy for local control but an active immunologic co-factor capable of intensifying systemic treatment effects.

The study by La Vecchia et al. in metastatic RCC further deepens this argument by examining the role of stereotactic body radiation therapy (SBRT) in patients treated with combination ICI–TKI therapy. RCC has traditionally been considered radioresistant; however, the safe delivery of ultra-hypofractionated high-radiation doses made possible by the development of stereotactic techniques has fundamentally altered this perception. In the setting of oligoprogression, SBRT achieved excellent local control (100% at six months and 70% at one year), while enabling a median next-line systemic treatment-free survival of twenty months.

This metric is especially meaningful, as delaying the need for further systemic therapy reduces both cumulative toxicity and financial burden, extending the period during which patients can maintain a stable quality of life. The investigators emphasize that RT enhances tumor immunogenicity by releasing damage-associated molecular patterns and reducing inter-metastatic seeding, thereby reinforcing the systemic activity of ICIs and TKIs. Their findings consolidate the concept that RT, even in anatomically or biologically challenging tumors, can function as a strategic extension of targeted systemic therapies [8].

Radiotherapy and Immune Modulation in Rare and Treatment-Resistant Tumors

Beyond scenarios of oligoprogressive disease, this Special Issue also addresses the interaction between radiotherapy and immune modulation in tumors traditionally regarded as refractory to immunotherapy. Glioblastoma and mucosal vaginal melanoma exemplify malignancies characterized by profound immune suppression, marked intratumoral heterogeneity, and historically limited responsiveness to immune-based treatments. Within this challenging landscape, the contributions collected here do not propose universal solutions but instead delineate the biological boundaries and conditional opportunities through which immune engagement may occur.

Within this spectrum, glioblastoma represents a critical biological limit for radiotherapy-mediated immune modulation. The disease is defined by immune exclusion, dominant myeloid suppression, dysfunctional T-cell trafficking, and a stromal architecture that actively impairs effective immune surveillance [9]. The glioblastoma case included in this Special Issue is therefore informative, not because it establishes a reproducible therapeutic strategy, but because it clarifies the constraints under which radiotherapy operates in this setting. The patient experienced an unexpected and durable regression of a non-resected lesion in the context of prolonged intravesical bacillus Calmette–Guérin (BCG) therapy administered for bladder cancer. As emphasized by the authors, the observed clinical course primarily supports a role for BCG-induced systemic immune activation rather than for radiotherapy itself, which was delivered as part of standard chemoradiotherapy. This observation suggests that, in tumors such as glioblastoma, radiotherapy alone may be insufficient to overcome intrinsic immune resistance and that only exceptionally strong, non-tumor-specific immune stimuli may transiently alter the expected disease trajectory. Importantly, this case does not undermine the rationale for combining radiotherapy with immunotherapy; rather, it suggests that in tumors such as glioblastoma, radiotherapy alone may be insufficient and that achieving therapeutic efficacy likely depends on the presence of additional immune-activating factors [10].

A complementary perspective emerges from the review of mucosal vaginal melanoma, a rare and biologically aggressive malignancy with limited therapeutic options. In contrast to cutaneous melanoma, mucosal variants typically exhibit lower tumor mutational burden, reduced immunogenicity, and inferior responsiveness to immune checkpoint inhibitors [11]. Surgical management is frequently constrained by anatomical considerations, and local recurrence rates remain high [12]. In this context, radiotherapy assumes a central role, not only in achieving local control but also in modulating tumor antigenicity and shaping a microenvironment more permissive to immune infiltration. The reviewed evidence suggests that radiotherapy may synergize with anti-PD-1 therapies, expanding the subset of patients who derive benefit from immunotherapy in a disease historically considered poorly immunogenic. Although high-level prospective data remain limited, these observations support continued investigation into how radiotherapy may recalibrate immune visibility in rare tumors with adverse biological features [13].

Rewriting the Biology of Solid Tumors: Radiotherapy and CAR-T Cell Therapy

Among the contributions of this Special Issue, the narrative review on CAR-T cells offers one of the most profound mechanistic insights into the future of immuno-oncology. While CAR-T therapy has achieved transformative success in hematologic malignancies, its application in solid tumors has been consistently limited by a dense and immunosuppressive tumor microenvironment, characterized by heterogeneous and unstable antigen expression [14,15]. Radiotherapy presents a unique opportunity to overcome these challenges, and the review articulates multiple layers of synergy that may ultimately enable the extension of CAR-T therapy into solid tumor settings.

Radiotherapy, depending on dose and fractionation, exerts heterogeneous immunomodulatory forces. High-dose radiation induces immunogenic cell death, increases antigen release, and stimulates the maturation of dendritic cells, creating an inflammatory milieu capable of improving CAR-T cell recognition. Low-dose radiation, by contrast, remodels the tumor stroma, normalizes aberrant vasculature, polarizes macrophages toward an antitumor phenotype, and promotes T-cell infiltration. Both radiation modalities converge on the shared goal of overcoming the barriers that prevent CAR-T cells from trafficking into, persisting within, and effectively destroying solid tumor masses.

The review also highlights the problem of intratumoral hypoxia, a major impediment to CAR-T infiltration and persistence. By modulating vascular flow and reducing hypoxic niches, RT may create a more permissive microenvironment for CAR-T activity. Moreover, the development of hypoxia-responsive CAR constructs represents an elegant example of how synthetic biology may align with radiobiology to refine treatment specificity and enhance safety.

Perhaps the most intriguing element of the review is the exploration of LATTICE radiotherapy, an innovative form of spatially fractionated radiation that delivers high-dose "peaks" to metabolically active tumor areas while maintaining low-dose "valleys" in the surrounding tissue [16,17]. This design preserves vascular integrity, enhances immune trafficking, and generates a rich supply of antigens via immunogenic cell death in the peaks. Early evidence suggests that LATTICE RT can significantly amplify not only CAR-T cell activity but also the efficacy of checkpoint inhibitors, potentially inducing robust systemic immune responses that extend beyond the irradiated field. The authors introduce the concept of "radscopal effects," wherein the combination of high-dose and low-dose irradiation potentiates immune activation in distant tumor sites, adding a new layer of nuance to the classical abscopal phenomenon.

Collectively, these insights position radiotherapy as an architect of immune permissiveness in solid tumors, capable of dismantling physical and biological barriers that have historically thwarted CAR-T approaches. The implications for future clinical research are profound [18].

Personalizing DNA Cancer Vaccines

In this evolving landscape of precision immuno-oncology, the review by Wu et al. provides a comprehensive framework for understanding how personalized DNA cancer vaccines are reshaping antigen-specific immune priming. Moving beyond vac-

https://doi.org/10.3390/jpm16050256

cine strategies based on uniform antigen selection, the authors describe a paradigm in which patient-specific neoantigens, derived from somatic mutations, aberrant splicing events, cryptic translation products, or extrachromosomal DNA, become central drivers of therapeutic specificity. Advances in next-generation sequencing, immunopeptidomics, ribosome profiling, and computational prediction of MHC binding and T-cell receptor recognition are progressively transforming neoantigen discovery from a largely theoretical concept into an increasingly clinically actionable pipeline. Within this framework, DNA-based vaccines emerge as a particularly versatile platform. Compared with RNA-based approaches, they offer molecular stability, favorable safety profiles, prolonged intracellular persistence, and manufacturing flexibility, all of which are critical in the personalized setting. Wu et al. illustrate how advances in vector design and delivery strategies are overcoming historical limitations in nuclear delivery and immunogenicity, while emphasizing that personalized DNA vaccines are most effective when deployed as part of rational combination strategies with immune checkpoint inhibitors, cytokine adjuvants, chemotherapy, and radiotherapy. From the perspective of this Special Issue, this contribution addresses a distinct and essential dimension of precision immunotherapy. Radiotherapy, as discussed throughout this editorial, plays a complementary role by supporting antigen release, enhancing MHC expression, remodeling suppressive tumor microenvironments, and facilitating immune cell infiltration. In this context, Wu et al. note that combining radiotherapy with DNA cancer vaccines can promote antigen presentation and create more permissive conditions for vaccine-induced T-cell responses, while personalized neoantigen selection may help counteract immune escape driven by tumor heterogeneity and clonal evolution. In this sense, personalized DNA vaccines and radiotherapy converge on a shared biological objective, broadening and sustaining antitumor immune pressure across spatially and temporally evolving disease.

Clinical evidence from early-phase studies in triple-negative breast cancer [19], hepatocellular carcinoma [20], glioblastoma [21], melanoma [22], and other solid tumors highlights both the promise and the current limitations of personalized DNA cancer vaccines. The induction of neoantigen-specific T-cell responses, signals of recurrence-free survival benefit in the adjuvant setting, and favorable safety profiles suggest particular relevance in early-stage disease or maintenance strategies. At the same time, Wu et al. critically examine biological barriers, such as immune tolerance, MHC downregulation, T-cell exhaustion, and the immunosuppressive tumor microenvironment, that constrain efficacy in advanced disease and motivate rational combination approaches, including integration with radiotherapy and other immune-modulating interventions.

Overall, precision immunotherapy will increasingly depend on strategies that combine molecular personalization with biological contextualization. Personalized DNA cancer vaccines exemplify this shift, particularly when integrated into multimodal approaches capable of reshaping the tumor microenvironment and sustaining patient-specific immune control [23].

Personalized Immunotherapy for T-Cell Lymphomas: From Immune Escape to Precision Therapeutics

In the context of precision immuno-oncology, T-cell lymphomas represent a unique and particularly challenging paradigm. Unlike most solid tumors and B-cell malignancies, these diseases arise from cells that are themselves integral components of the immune system. As comprehensively discussed by Casan et al., this biological paradox profoundly reshapes the conceptual and practical foundations of immunotherapy, transforming immune escape from a secondary resistance mechanism into an intrinsic feature of disease biology.

The review delineates how T-cell lymphomas exploit multiple layers of immune dysfunction, including antigenic ambiguity, phenotypic plasticity, and immune mimicry, to

https://doi.org/10.3390/jpm16050256

evade therapeutic pressure. Malignant T-cells may downregulate or alter target antigen expression, adopt regulatory or exhausted phenotypes, and interfere with normal immune surveillance, thereby limiting the efficacy of immune-based interventions that rely on intact antitumor immunity. Under these conditions, conventional immunotherapeutic strategies designed to amplify immune responses can paradoxically exacerbate immunosuppression or lead to off-target toxicity, underscoring the need for disease-specific therapeutic logic. From this perspective, the concept of personalization extends well beyond molecular profiling alone. As emphasized by the authors, effective immunotherapy for T-cell lymphomas requires an integrated understanding of tumor subtype, cellular origin, differentiation state, and microenvironmental context. The review highlights how distinct entities, such as cutaneous versus peripheral T-cell lymphomas, exhibit divergent patterns of immune interaction and therapeutic vulnerability, precluding uniform treatment approaches. Personalization therefore emerges as an adaptive process, informed by dynamic tumor–immune interactions rather than static biomarkers.

Casan et al. further examine how contemporary therapeutic strategies attempt to navigate this complexity through rational target selection and combination approaches. Rather than providing an exhaustive catalog of agents, the review focuses on underlying principles guiding the use of immune checkpoint modulation, monoclonal antibodies, epigenetic therapies, and emerging cellular strategies. These interventions are discussed, not as isolated solutions, but as context-dependent tools whose efficacy is shaped by immune escape mechanisms, treatment sequencing, and patient-specific disease characteristics.

Clinical evidence summarized in the review reflects both the promise and the limitations of personalized immunotherapy in T-cell lymphomas. While selected approaches have demonstrated meaningful activity in defined patient subsets, durable responses remain inconsistent, and therapeutic resistance frequently emerges. The authors critically address the biological and immunologic constraints that underlie these outcomes, including T-cell exhaustion, immune tolerance, and the profoundly immunosuppressive tumor microenvironment that characterizes advanced disease. These insights reinforce the notion that therapeutic success in T-cell lymphomas depends less on intensifying immune activation and more on precisely modulating immune context.

From the perspective of this Special Issue, this contribution occupies a distinct and essential thematic space. By interrogating immunotherapy in a setting where the immune system itself is the site of malignant transformation, the review underscores the limits of generalized immunotherapeutic paradigms and highlights the necessity of precision strategies grounded in disease biology. In doing so, it complements the broader narrative of this Special Issue by illustrating that durable immunologic control cannot be achieved through amplification alone, but requires a nuanced understanding of immune escape, adaptability, and context-specific intervention [24].

Radiolabeled Vitamins and Nanosystems as Potential Agents in Oncology Theranostics

As precision oncology continues to diversify beyond immunomodulatory approaches, increasing attention has been directed toward theranostic strategies that couple molecular imaging with targeted radionuclide therapy. In this context, the review by Basirinia et al. addresses the development of radiolabeled vitamins and nanosystems as biologically inspired platforms for oncology theranostics, emphasizing their ability to integrate diagnosis, treatment, and response monitoring within a single molecular construct, and to inform treatment personalization in immunologically heterogeneous tumors. The authors focus on vitamins such as folate (vitamin B9) and cobalamin (vitamin B12) as targeting vectors, exploiting physiological uptake mechanisms that are frequently upregulated in cancer cells and within components of the tumor microenvironment. By exploiting receptor-mediated internalization, radiolabeled vitamins offer a rational strategy for tu-

https://doi.org/10.3390/jpm16050256

mor selectivity, combining favorable safety profiles with broad applicability across tumor types. Importantly, the review highlights how these targeting strategies may complement immunotherapeutic approaches by refining tumor localization, improving patient stratification, and enabling image-guided combination regimens. Preclinical evidence supporting the use of vitamin-based conjugates paired with diagnostic and therapeutic radionuclides is discussed, illustrating coherent theranostic workflows that can support treatment planning and response assessment. Nanosystems are presented as key technological enablers that extend this concept. Nanoparticles and related carriers provide structural versatility, improved pharmacokinetics, and opportunities for multivalent targeting, including the co-delivery of radionuclides and immunomodulatory agents. Functionalization with vitamins supports active tumor uptake while allowing the incorporation of radionuclides or additional payloads, offering modular solutions to challenges such as tumor heterogeneity, suboptimal biodistribution, and immune-excluded disease niches. Importantly, the review adopts a measured and critical translational perspective. Despite encouraging in vitro and in vivo data, most vitamin- and nanoparticle-based radioconjugates remain in the preclinical domain. Persistent challenges related to radiochemical stability, dosimetry, renal accumulation, and scalable manufacturing are clearly identified as limiting factors for clinical implementation [25,26]. Rather than overstating near-term applicability, the authors delineate realistic development pathways for radiotheranostic platforms, including their potential role within multimodal strategies that integrate targeted radiation delivery with systemic immunotherapy. From the perspective of this Special Issue, this contribution highlights a complementary dimension of precision oncology that intersects with immunotherapy at the level of tumor targeting, microenvironmental modulation, and image-guided treatment adaptation. Radiolabeled vitamins and nanosystems exemplify how advances in nuclear medicine and nanotechnology may converge with immuno-oncology to support patient-specific treatment planning, adaptive therapeutic strategies, and real-time assessment of therapeutic efficacy, reinforcing the notion that precision oncology increasingly relies on the integration of biological insight with technological innovation [27].

A Convergent Vision for the Future of Immuno-Radiotherapy

Taken together, the contributions in this Special Issue articulate a coherent vision of radiotherapy not as an ancillary component of cancer treatment but as a central pillar of modern immuno-oncology. Across highly diverse tumors, patient populations, and therapeutic strategies, radiotherapy consistently demonstrates its capacity to deepen and prolong immune responses. In MCC, CSCC, and RCC, RT suppresses escape lesions and extends the lifespan of systemic therapies. In glioblastoma and mucosal vaginal melanoma, it reconfigures profoundly hostile microenvironments, enabling immune interventions that would otherwise be futile. In the realm of adoptive immunotherapy, RT becomes a biological enabler, shaping the conditions in which CAR-T cells might finally realize their potential in solid tumors.

The future of oncologic care will increasingly depend on such integrated strategies. As immunotherapy evolves into ever more personalized and complex modalities, ranging from vaccines and cellular therapies to nanoparticle-guided theranostics, radiotherapy stands as the versatile partner capable of shaping the biological terrain in ways no drug alone can achieve. This Special Issue captures the early contours of this transformation, pointing toward a future in which the boundaries between local and systemic therapy are replaced by a unified therapeutic philosophy grounded in biology, precision, and synergy.

Conflicts of Interest: Dr. Gianluca Ferini is employed by REM RADIOTERAPIA S.R.L. This research received no external funding. This institution was not involved in the study design, data collection, analysis, interpretation of data, the writing of this article, or the decision to submit it for publication.

https://doi.org/10.3390/jpm16050256

All authors declare that the research was conducted in the absence of any commercial or financial relationships that could be construed as a potential conflict of interest.

References

1. Sharma, P.; Hu-Lieskovan, S.; Wargo, J.A.; Ribas, A. Primary, Adaptive, and Acquired Resistance to Cancer Immunotherapy. *Cell* **2017**, *168*, 707–723. [CrossRef]
2. Zagardo, V.; Martorana, E.; Harikar, M.; Pergolizzi, S.; Ferini, G. Effectiveness of radiotherapy in delaying treatment changes in primary or secondary immunorefractory oligoprogressive patients: Preliminary results from a single-center study. *Discov. Oncol.* **2024**, *15*, 531. [CrossRef] [PubMed]
3. Ferini, G.; Zagardo, V.; Critelli, P.; Santacaterina, A.; Sava, S.; Harikar, M.M.; Venkataram, T.; Umana, G.E.; Viola, A.; Valenti, V.; et al. Introducing Radiotherapy in Metastatic Merkel Cell Carcinoma Patients with Limited Progression on Avelumab: An Effective Step against Primary and Secondary Immune Resistance? *J. Pers. Med.* **2023**, *13*, 841. [CrossRef] [PubMed]
4. Golden, E.B.; Apetoh, L. Radiotherapy and immunogenic cell death. *Semin. Radiat. Oncol.* **2015**, *25*, 11–17. [CrossRef] [PubMed]
5. Zhu, S.; Wang, Y.; Tang, J.; Cao, M. Radiotherapy induced immunogenic cell death by remodeling tumor immune microenvironment. *Front Immunol.* **2022**, *13*, 1074477. [CrossRef]
6. Greco, M.C.L.; Marano, G.; Milazzotto, R.; Liardo, R.L.E.; Finocchiaro, I.; La Rocca, M.; Basile, A.; Foti, P.V.; Palmucci, S.; David, E.; et al. The Immunomodulatory Potential of Concurrent High-Dose Radiotherapy and Immune Checkpoint Inhibitor Cemiplimab in Advanced Cutaneous Squamous Cell Carcinoma: Initial Results. *J. Pers. Med.* **2024**, *14*, 581. [CrossRef]
7. Ferini, G.; Palmisciano, P.; Forte, S.; Viola, A.; Martorana, E.; Parisi, S.; Valenti, V.; Fichera, C.; Umana, G.E.; Pergolizzi, S. Advanced or Metastatic Cutaneous Squamous Cell Carcinoma: The Current and Future Role of Radiation Therapy in the Era of Immunotherapy. *Cancers* **2022**, *14*, 1871. [CrossRef]
8. La Vecchia, M.; Federico, M.; Aiello, D.; Zagardo, V.; Mazzonello, A.; Testa, L.; La Paglia, L.; Bruno, T.; Fazio, I. The Role of Stereotactic Body Radiotherapy (SBRT) in Oligoprogressive Renal Cell Carcinoma (RCC) Treated with ICIs–TKIs: A Retrospective Multicentric Study. *J. Pers. Med.* **2024**, *14*, 1030. [CrossRef]
9. Lim, M.; Xia, Y.; Bettegowda, C.; Weller, M. Current state of immunotherapy for glioblastoma. *Nat. Rev. Clin. Oncol.* **2018**, *15*, 422–442. [CrossRef]
10. Scalia, G.; Ferini, G.; Marrone, S.; Salvati, M.; Yamamoto, V.; Kateb, B.; Schulte, R.; Forte, S.; Umana, G.E. Unexpected Transient Glioblastoma Regression in a Patient Previously Treated with Bacillus Calmette–Guérin Therapy: A Case Report and Immunomodulatory Effects Hypothesis. *J. Pers. Med.* **2023**, *13*, 1661. [CrossRef]
11. Nassar, K.W.; Tan, A.C. The mutational landscape of mucosal melanoma. *Semin. Cancer Biol.* **2020**, *61*, 139–148. [CrossRef]
12. Li, J.; Kan, H.; Zhao, L.; Sun, Z.; Bai, C. Immune checkpoint inhibitors in advanced or metastatic mucosal melanoma: A systematic review. *Ther. Adv. Med. Oncol.* **2020**, *12*, 1758835920922028. [CrossRef] [PubMed]
13. Cuccia, F.; D'Alessandro, S.; Blasi, L.; Chiantera, V.; Ferrera, G. The Role of Radiotherapy in the Management of Vaginal Melanoma: A Literature Review with a Focus on the Potential Synergistic Role of Immunotherapy. *J. Pers. Med.* **2023**, *13*, 1142. [CrossRef] [PubMed]
14. Newick, K.; O'Brien, S.; Moon, E.; Albelda, S.M. CAR T Cell Therapy for Solid Tumors. *Annu. Rev. Med.* **2017**, *68*, 139–152. [CrossRef]
15. Escobar, G.; Berger, T.R.; Maus, M.V. CAR-T therapy in solid tumors: Challenges and breakthroughs. *Cell Rep. Med.* **2025**, *6*, 102353. [CrossRef]
16. Wu, X.; Perez, N.C.; Zheng, Y.; Li, X.; Jiang, L.; Amendola, B.E.; Xu, B.; Mayr, N.A.; Lu, J.J.; Hatoum, G.F.; et al. The Technical and Clinical Implementation of LATTICE Radiation Therapy (LRT). *Radiat. Res.* **2020**, *194*, 737–746. [CrossRef]
17. Ahmed, M.M.; Wu, X.; Mohiuddin, M.; Perez, N.C.; Zhang, H.; Amendola, B.E.; Malachowska, B.; Mohiuddin, M.; Guha, C. Optimizing GRID and Lattice Spatially Fractionated Radiation Therapy: Innovative Strategies for Radioresistant and Bulky Tumor Management. *Semin. Radiat. Oncol.* **2024**, *34*, 310–322. [CrossRef] [PubMed]
18. Pontoriero, A.; Critelli, P.; Chillari, F.; Ferrantelli, G.; Sciacca, M.; Brogna, A.; Parisi, S.; Pergolizzi, S. Modulation of Radiation Doses and Chimeric Antigen Receptor T Cells: A Promising New Weapon in Solid Tumors—A Narrative Review. *J. Pers. Med.* **2023**, *13*, 1261. [CrossRef]
19. Zhang, X.; Goedegebuure, S.P.; Chen, M.Y.; Mishra, R.; Zhang, F.; Yu, Y.Y.; Singhal, K.; Li, L.; Gao, F.; Myers, N.B.; et al. Neoantigen DNA vaccines are safe, feasible, and induce neoantigen-specific immune responses in triple-negative breast cancer patients. *Genome Med.* **2024**, *16*, 131. [CrossRef]
20. Yarchoan, M.; Gane, E.J.; Marron, T.U.; Perales-Linares, R.; Yan, J.; Cooch, N.; Shu, D.H.; Fertig, E.J.; Kagohara, L.T.; Bartha, G.; et al. Personalized neoantigen vaccine and pembrolizumab in advanced hepatocellular carcinoma: A phase 1/2 trial. *Nat. Med.* **2024**, *30*, 1044–1053. [CrossRef]

21. Garfinkle, E.A.; Miller, K.E.; Livingstone, A.J.; Perales-Linares, R.; Cooch, N.; Perales-Puchalt, A.; Rochestie, S.; Peters, J.; Sardesai, N.Y.; Gillanders, W.E.; et al. Abstract 1174: Incorporation of multisector analysis into the design of personalized DNA vaccines for patients with newly diagnosed glioblastoma. *Cancer Res.* **2024**, *84*, 1174. [CrossRef]
22. Kleine-Kohlbrecher, D.; Viborg, N.; Pavlidis, M.A.; Lausen, M.; Trolle, T.; Thuesen, N.H.; Garde, C.; Jespersen, A.; Jepsen, T.S.; Lauenborg, B.W.; et al. 623 AI-designed personalized neoantigen vaccine, EVX-02, induces robust T-cell responses in melanoma patients. *J. Immunother. Cancer* **2023**, *11*, A1–A1731. [CrossRef]
23. Wu, A.A.; Peng, K.; Vukovich, M.; Zhu, M.; Lin, Y.; Bagga, A.; Wu, T.; Hung, C.-F. Personalizing DNA Cancer Vaccines. *J. Pers. Med.* **2025**, *15*, 474. [CrossRef]
24. Casan, J.M.L.; Ong, X.J.; van der Weyden, C.; Yannakou, C.K.; Zhu, J.; D'Souza, C.; Neeson, P.; Prince, H.M. Personalized Immunotherapy for T Cell Lymphomas: From Immune Escape to Precision Therapeutics. *J. Pers. Med.* **2025**, *15*, 560. [CrossRef] [PubMed]
25. Tran, H.H.; Yamaguchi, A.; Manning, H.C. Radiotheranostic landscape: A review of clinical and preclinical development. *Eur. J. Nucl. Med. Mol. Imaging* **2025**, *52*, 2685–2709. [CrossRef]
26. Ninatti, G.; Lee, S.T.; Scott, A.M. Radioligand Therapy in Cancer Management: A Global Perspective. *Cancers* **2025**, *17*, 3412. [CrossRef] [PubMed]
27. Basirinia, G.; Comelli, A.; Alongi, P.; Ali, M.; Salvaggio, G.; Longo, C.; Di Raimondo, D.; Tuttolomondo, A.; Benfante, V. Radiolabeled Vitamins and Nanosystems as Potential Agents in Oncology Theranostics: Developed Approaches and Future Perspectives. *J. Pers. Med.* **2026**, *16*, 36. [CrossRef]

https://doi.org/10.3390/jpm16050256

Journal of
Personalized Medicine

MDPI

Review

Radiolabeled Vitamins and Nanosystems as Potential Agents in Oncology Theranostics: Developed Approaches and Future Perspectives

Ghazal Basirinia [1,2], Albert Comelli [2,3,*,†], Pierpaolo Alongi [4,5], Muhammad Ali [2,3], Giuseppe Salvaggio [5], Costanza Longo [6], Domenico Di Raimondo [1], Antonino Tuttolomondo [1] and Viviana Benfante [1,4,*,†]

1 Department of Health Promotion, Mother and Child Care, Internal Medicine and Medical Specialties, Molecular and Clinical Medicine, University of Palermo, 90127 Palermo, Italy; gbasirinia@fondazionerimed.com (G.B.); domenico.diraimondo@unipa.it (D.D.R.); bruno.tuttolomondo@unipa.it (A.T.)
2 Ri.MED Foundation, Via Bandiera 11, 90133 Palermo, Italy; amuhammad@fondazionerimed.com
3 NBFC—National Biodiversity Future Center, 90133 Palermo, Italy
4 Advanced Diagnostic Imaging-INNOVA Project, Department of Radiological Sciences, A.R.N.A.S. Civico Di Cristina e Benfratelli Hospitals, P.zza N. Leotta 4, 90127 Palermo, Italy; pierpaolo.alongi@unipa.it
5 Department of Biomedicine, Neuroscience and Advanced Diagnostics (BiND), University of Palermo, 90127 Palermo, Italy; giuseppe.salvaggio@policlinico.pa.it
6 Nuclear Medicine Unit, A.R.N.A.S. Civico Di Cristina e Benfratelli Hospitals, P.zza N. Leotta 4, 90127 Palermo, Italy; costanza.longo@arnascivico.it
* Correspondence: acomelli@fondazionerimed.com (A.C.); viviana.benfante@arnascivico.it (V.B.)
† These authors contributed equally to this work.

Abstract

Theranostic approaches employing radioactive materials have emerged as innovative strategies that integrate molecular imaging with targeted therapy using nanosystems, thereby advancing the paradigm of precision medicine in oncology. Each year, substantial research efforts are dedicated to developing molecular probes capable of detecting early-stage tumors, with improved efficacy and reduced toxicity to the surrounding healthy tissues. Radiopharmaceuticals based on vitamins and nanoparticles are among the most promising developments in this field, as they possess a high level of specificity and low toxicity. Vitamin B9 and vitamin B12 represent notable examples, as their targeting properties exploit the overexpression of corresponding receptors in tumor cells. In this context, future directions may include the radiolabeling of nanoparticles functionalized with these vitamins using isotopes such as [^{68}Ga] and [^{177}Lu], thereby enabling both diagnostic imaging and therapeutic applications. Despite the encouraging preclinical evidence, many in vitro and in vivo studies employing these strategies do not sufficiently address their translational applicability to radiotheranostics. This review highlights the most promising advances in the diagnostic and therapeutic potential of vitamin and nanoparticle-based systems. It aims to critically evaluate current findings and propose hypotheses for further study in the emerging field of radiopharmaceutical theranostics.

Keywords: targeted radionuclide therapy (TRT); vitamin-related radiopharmaceuticals; vitamin; B9; folate; B12; theranostics; nanoparticles

1. Introduction

Precision oncology theranostics combines diagnostic imaging with targeted therapies. This approach relies on nuclear medicine to identify and target tumor-specific biomarkers using positron emission tomography (PET) and single-photon emission computed tomography (SPECT) [1].

PET and SPECT are functional imaging techniques that utilize radioactive tracers. PET employes positron-emitting isotopes such as (^{18}F, ^{15}O, and ^{11}C), whereas SPECT uses gamma emitters including (^{123}I and ^{99m}Tc). Superior resolution and sensitivity offer with PET, but it is more expensive, while SPECT is more affordable and widely available [2,3].

Targeted radionuclide therapy (TRT) is a nuclear medicine approach that delivers ionizing radiation directly to cancer cells by exploiting the specific accumulation of radiolabeled compounds at the tumor site [4].

Radiopharmaceuticals are designed using selected radionuclides and [4,5] biomolecules to achieve effective tumor targeting, optimizing factors such as half-life and energy to enhance tumor destruction while minimizing resistance [6]. Each radiopharmaceutical consists of two key components: a carrier molecule or ligand, which facilitates targeted delivery, and a radionuclide, whose nuclear properties determine its diagnostic or therapeutic function [7]. Carriers play a pivotal role in the precise delivery of radionuclides to specific biological targets. Chelators are essential for stabilizing metallic radionuclides such as ^{99m}Tc and $^{66/68}Ga$, while linkers may be incorporated to improve pharmacokinetics and binding affinity [8,9]. The proper selection of these elements is critical for maximizing therapeutic efficacy while minimizing biological damage [10].

Radionuclides, as inherently unstable atoms, undergo radioactive decay during which they emit alpha particles, beta particles, Auger electrons, or gamma rays. Because of their energy and ionizing properties, these emissions can induce irreversible DNA damage in cancer cells, ultimately triggering apoptosis (Figure 1) [11]. Beta and alpha emitters are the primary components of radionuclide-based treatments, while Auger emitters are used less commonly. The development of carrier molecules has expanded the clinical use of beta emitters, such as yttrium-90 [^{90}Y] and lutetium-177 [^{177}Lu]. Although alpha emitters have been utilized for several decades, their short tissue penetration and highly localized radiation delivery have recently increased their appeal for treating small tumors [12]. Therefore, careful selection of the appropriate radionuclide is essential to maximize therapeutic benefits while ensuring radiation safety [13].

Molecular imaging has emerged as a transformative diagnostic modality, offering superior sensitivity and spatial resolution compared with conventional imaging techniques. The integration of molecular imaging with highly specific and biologically active tracers enables the visualization and quantification of pathological processes at the cellular and molecular levels. This allows for detection of small or otherwise indiscernible lesions. This capability holds significant implications for oncology, where early identification of malignant changes, accurate tumor staging, and real-time assessment of therapeutic response are crucial for optimizing patient outcomes [14]. The key advantages of using vitamins in radiopharmaceutical design are their low cost, non-toxicity, accessibility, and proven anti-cancer properties [15]. In cancer diagnosis, targeted radionuclide imaging has shown promising results. Radiolabeled vitamins for cancer SPECT and PET represent a flexible approach in both preclinical and clinical research [16,17]. Notably, they have demonstrated effective results in the diagnosis of various cancers, including breast, ovarian, lung, and colon cancers. A major challenge in this approach is the synthesis of suitable vitamin-metal conjugates to minimize unintended radiotracer accumulation in non-target tissues and reduce adverse effects. Additional challenges involve achieving efficient transport, specific uptake, and retention of radiolabeled vitamins in tumor tissues. Thus, Vitamin based radiopharmaceuticals are expected to play a key role in cancer diagnosis and therapy, becoming indispensable tools in nuclear medicine [18].

https://doi.org/10.3390/jpm16010036

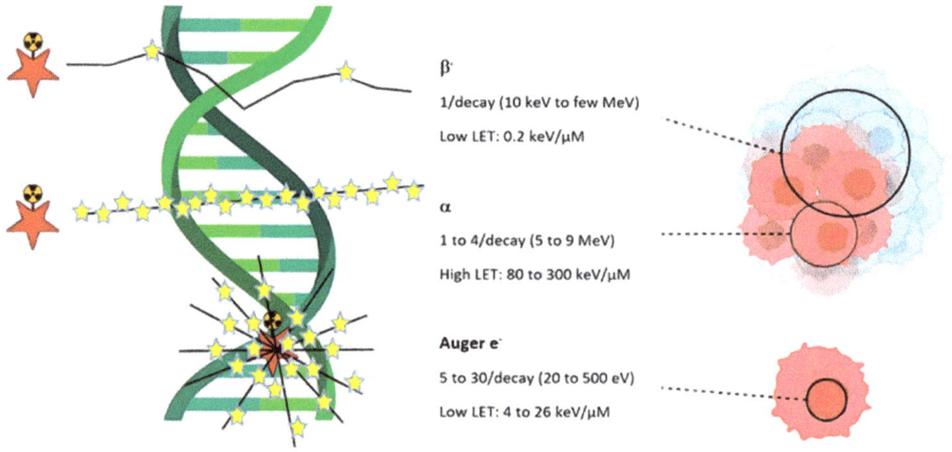

Figure 1. Linear Energy Transfer (LET) for various particle types, including beta-minus (β^-) particles, alpha (α) particles, and Auger electrons. Red stars are the radiation source and yellow stars show disintegrations. This figure depicts the effects of these types of radiation on DNA and biological structures highlighting differences in their energy and ionization patterns. β^- radiation, has low linear energy transfer (LET ~0.2 keV/µm), causes widespread but relatively mild damage. α radiation, with high LET (80–300 keV/µm), creates dense, localized ionization due to significant damage to DNA and cells. Despite the low energy of Auger electrons with (20–500 eV), produce highly concentrated ionization with severe damage in areas near their emission, particularly, around DNA. Thus, when the LET increases, the intensity of damage becomes greater, while the affected area decreases. Reprinted from Ref. [11], Copyright 2023, Pharmaceutics. This article is an open access article distributed under the terms and conditions of the Creative Commons Attribution (CC BY) license.

Monoclonal antibodies, small peptides, and nanoparticles smaller than 100 nanometers can be radiolabeled with specialized radionuclide for theranostic applications. Prostate-specific membrane antigen (PSMA) is one of the most widely used biomarkers in radiotheranostics; However, since it is also overexpressed in other tumors, radioprotective strategies for healthy organs are essential [19,20]. Given that vitamins are physiological components of the human body, it is interesting to explore their potential involvement in the development and testing of new radiolabeled compounds for both diagnosis and therapy, from a radiotheranostic perspective. The idea is to collect state-of-the-art materials to convey information regarding the use of therapeutic radionuclides, such as Lutetium-177, and diagnostics such as Gallium-68, tumor biomarkers, along with tumor biomarkers and vitamins employed in nanoscale formulations for precision oncology.

Current cancer treatments include chemotherapy, radiation therapy, immunotherapy, surgery, and various combinations of these approaches. Despite their benefits, conventional chemotherapeutics are non-selective and can damage healthy tissue, leading to unwanted side effects. This can contribute to multidrug resistance, further limiting in therapeutic options for most aggressive forms of cancer, such as metastatic cancer [21].

Nanotechnology-based compounds exploit nanocarriers designed to encapsulate therapeutic agents, such as chemotherapeutics or radionuclides. Their structure allows for extremely precise targeting of tumor cells and, thanks to their biocompatibility, protection of the surrounding tissues. Passive targeting exploits the permeability of blood vessels in the tumor microenvironment to promote nanocarrier accumulation on the lesion. Active targeting involves decorating nanocarrier surfaces with specific biological ligands that attach to tumor cells, enhancing specific treatment [22].

https://doi.org/10.3390/jpm16010036

Nanotechnology scaffolds hold promise for improving therapeutic efficacy, reducing side effects in healthy tissues, and thereby enhancing patient safety. However, despite the experimental evidence, only a few nanocarriers tested in animal models advance to clinical trials. This could be due to challenges in conversion of data from the in vitro and preclinical phase into clinical dosimetry and cytotoxicity assessments [23].

In healthy tissues, folate receptors are minimally expressed and primarily localized to cells involved in embryonic development and folate homeostasis. In contrast, under certain pathological conditions, folate receptors are overexpressed in specific tissues, presenting opportunities for targeted therapeutic intervention. Folate receptors can be targeted by folic acid or other high-affinity folate receptor (FR) ligands and anti-FR monoclonal antibodies [24].

In addition to being the cost-effective strategy, folic acid is conjugated to the surface of drugs or nanoparticles, usually via a linker such as polyethylene glycol [25]. The use of nanoformulations containing anti-FR monoclonal antibodies has also been extensively studied in oncology, allowing FR to be targeted more specifically to sites of inflammation or macrophages within the tumor microenvironment [26]. A promising application of folate receptor targeting is in ovarian cancer treatment and imaging, as the majority of epithelial ovarian carcinomas overexpress folate receptors, accounting for nearly 95% of ovarian cancer deaths [27]. Increasing vitamin B12 values can be indicative of the presence of malignancies, in particular hematological diseases, reflecting the presence of proliferating cells and immune responses associated with cancer [28].

Folate and vitamin B12 are partially associated with the same pathway, specifically the methyl trap hypothesis and thus low levels of methionine synthase. This pathway could be targeted to increase the binding and activation of therapeutic agents in tumors characterized by folate and vitamin B12 [29]. In the near future, it would be interesting to radiolabeling nanoparticles based on these vitamins with [^{68}Ga] and [^{177}Lu] for diagnosing and treating patients. However, many preclinical in vitro and in vivo studies employ these approaches without addressing their applicability in radiotheranostics.

This review highlights the most promising results in diagnostics and therapy of these systems, critically trying to outline hypotheses that can be investigated in the near future in the field of radiopharmaceutical theranostics.

2. Methods

This review was conducted in order to provide a critical assessment of the current state of preclinical research on vitamin-based radiopharmaceuticals in oncology. To ensure a comprehensive, transparent, and unbiased synthesis of the evidence, a systematic approach was employed, guided by the PRISMA-ScR (Preferred Reporting Items for Systematic reviews and Meta-Analyses extension for Scoping Reviews) [30] framework where applicable. The protocol for this scoping review was not registered in a publicly accessible database.

2.1. Search Strategy and Information Sources

A systematic literature search was performed across three major electronic databases: PubMed, Scopus, and Google Scholar. The search strategy was designed to encompass the core concepts of the review: cancer types, radionuclide therapy, theranostics, vitamins, and nanotechnology. The following search string was adapted for each database: ("Gastric Cancer" OR "Breast Cancer" OR "Colorectal Cancer" OR "Brain Cancer" OR "Prostate Cancer" OR "Ovarian Cancer") AND ("Targeted Radionuclide Therapy" OR TRT OR Theranostic) AND ("Vitamin B9" OR Folate OR "Folic Acid" OR "Vitamin B12" OR Cobalamin) AND (Radiopharmaceutical OR Radionuclide OR Nanoparticle). The search was limited to studies published in English between 1 January 2000 and 31 October 2025.

https://doi.org/10.3390/jpm16010036

2.2. Eligibility and Exclusion Criteria

Studies were included if they met the following criteria: (1) original research articles or reviews investigating vitamin-based radiopharmaceuticals; (2) included in vitro and/or in vivo preclinical models; (3) focused on diagnostic or therapeutic applications in oncology. Exclusion criteria were: (1) non-English publications; (2) conference abstracts, editorials, or patents; (3) studies not involving a radiolabeled vitamin or vitamin-conjugated nanosystem; and (4) studies focused solely on clinical case reports without novel preclinical data.

2.3. Study Selection and Data Extraction

The study selection process is summarized in a PRISMA-style flow diagram (Figure 2). After removing duplicates, titles and abstracts were screened for relevance. Full-text articles that met the initial criteria were then retrieved and evaluated against the predefined inclusion and exclusion criteria. Any differences in study selection were resolved through discussion, with additional input sought when necessary. Data from the eligible studies were extracted into a standardized spreadsheet, capturing information such as the first author, publication year, cancer model, radionuclide, targeted agent (vitamin conjugate), key findings (including uptake values, imaging performance, and therapeutic outcomes), and the vitamin utilized. For more information, please refer to the Supplementary Materials.

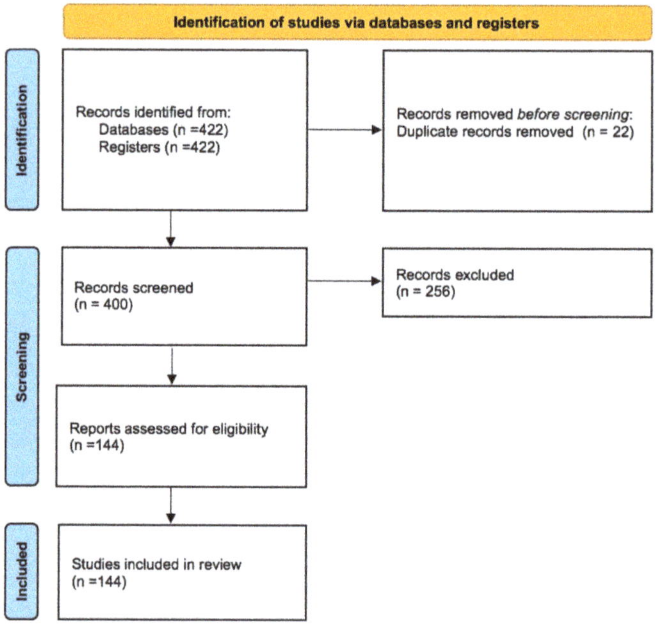

Figure 2. PRISMA Flow Diagram of the Study Selection Process.

- Identification: Records identified from databases (n = 422).
- Screening: Records screened after duplicates removed (n = 400).
- Eligibility: Full-text articles assessed for eligibility (n = 144).
- Included: Studies included in the qualitative synthesis (n = 144)

3. Gastric Cancer-Targeted Vitamin-Based Radionuclide Agents

Gastric cancer (GC) represents the fourth leading cause of cancer-related mortality worldwide and continues to be among the most prevalent malignancies, with an estimated

https://doi.org/10.3390/jpm16010036

400,000 new cases diagnosed annually [31,32]. GC constitutes a major global health challenge, with its burden being especially pronounced in East Asian populations. The disease is characterized by both a high incidence rate and an overall poor prognosis, outcomes that are largely attributable to the fact that the majority of cases are diagnosed at advanced stages when therapeutic options are limited and curative treatment is less feasible. Consequently, the late detection of GC not only worsens survival outcomes but also amplifies its impact as a critical public health concern in the region [33,34]. While WHO classifications exist, an effective biological classification for clinical use is still lacking [35]. Primary treatments, such as surgery and chemotherapy, as well as other therapies, including radiotherapy, immunotherapy, and targeted therapy, are investigated. Despite these options, the survival rate is low, less than 42% for metastatic cancers [36]. Therefore, the urgent need for novel therapeutic strategies is crucial to reducing GC-related mortality. GC is characterized by a heterogeneous cell population that drives malignancy through dysregulated growth, differentiation, angiogenesis, migration, and metastasis in a highly complex carcinogenic process [37,38]. GC pathogenesis is strongly influenced by environmental factors, with Helicobacter pylori infection, diet, and smoking being significant risk factors [39]. Analysis of genomic data of GC tissues indicating four molecular subtypes: EBV, MSI, GS, and CIN which each one has shown different features like extreme DNA hypermethylation for EBV, high mutation rates for MSI, low fewer genomic alterations for GS and marked aneuploidy also receptor tyrosine kinase amplifications in CIN subtype, which this may guide the personalized treatment potential regarding these features impacted on the therapeutic strategies [40]. Additionally, Epstein–Barr virus (EBV) infection has been identified as a potential etiological agent in 5–10% of GC cases [41]. The use of biomarkers in GC diagnosis and treatment, particularly those targeted integrin receptors, HER2, Claudin 18, and glutathione-responsive systems, has driven significant advancements in targeted therapies and nanotechnology. The future of GC management is expected to advance toward personalized medicine, wherein biomarker-based strategies with their potential to enhance the optimization of targeted radionuclide therapies, offer hope for improved treatment outcomes [42].

Takashima et al. investigated a ^{211}At-labeled anti-TF monoclonal antibody (clone 1084) in both in vitro (MKN-1, MKN-45, NUGC-3 cell lines) and in vivo (xenograft mouse) gastric cancer models. Tissue Factor specifically targets Clone 1084, with the therapeutic efficacy of the ^{211}At–anti-TF conjugate through precise accumulation in TF-positive tumors and localized delivery of high-LET α-radiation. They showed that sodium ascorbate, a free radical scavenger, prevented ^{211}At-induced antibody denaturation, preserving its antitumor activity. Though vitamin-derived, sodium ascorbate served as a stabilizer, not a targeting agent, enhancing therapeutic safety and efficacy [43].

Moreover, Muller et al. presented [^{177}Lu]-labeled folate conjugates incorporating an albumin-binding component, known as cm09, to increase blood circulation and optimize the rate of tumor-to-kidney uptake. High radiolabeling efficiency (>98%) and strong plasma protein binding (91%) were demonstrated by [^{177}Lu]Lu-cm09. Additionally, it showed specific tumor uptake (17.56% ID/g at four h) with reduced kidney accumulation. Biologically, the albumin-binding component extends systemic circulation through reversible interaction with serum albumin, which reduced renal filtration and folate receptor, effectively lowering kidney accumulation without compromising tumor-specific uptake. SPECT imaging displayed significant tumor-to-background ratios in mice with KB tumors. Specifically, these conjugates exhibited a tumor-to-kidney ratio that was 5 to 6 times higher than those without the albumin binder, which resulted in extended survival [44].

Si and colleagues evaluated three different bioactive molecules labeled with [^{68}Ga], namely [^{68}Ga]Ga-DOTA-RGD, [^{68}Ga]Ga-DOTA-FA, and [^{68}Ga]Ga-DOTA-BSA, which were prepared using new approaches under mild conditions. The preclinical studies were conducted using human gastric cancer (MGC-803) and ovarian carcinoma (SKOV-3) cell lines, as well as tumor-bearing mice, as animal models. Synthesizing these radiotracers using new strategies has shown great biological and chemical functions, also demonstrating high affinity and stability. Thus, all labeling processes, such as chelation, linking, and purification, were performed in under 40 min to maintain molecular bioactivity; due to this efficient and significant approach, they approved the promising potential of [^{68}Ga]-DOTA-Mal in providing novel PET tracers and advancing PET imaging technologies [45].

The development of [^{68}Ga]Ga-DOTA-folate, [^{68}Ga]Ga-NODAGA-folate, and [^{68}Ga]Ga-NOTA-folate displayed significant advancement in creating PET radiotracers targeting FR-positive tumors. Each compound was designed to enhance tumor specificity, stability, and imaging performance using specific chelators (DOTA, NODAGA, and NOTA) to complex gallium-68. Preclinical studies highlighted their strong affinity for FRs and effective tumor uptake, with PET imaging showing high imaging contrast and biodistribution profiles. Importantly, competitive blocking with excess folic acid or EC20 was utilized in multiple models, which confirmed target specificity and temporary receptor saturation in normal tissues, particularly renal FR-α, can reduce retention of the kidney without significantly tumor accumulation effect. These findings emphasize their potential as diagnostic agents for FR-positive cancers and provide valuable tools in non-invasive imaging and precision medicine, also highlighting the clinical relevance of co-infusion approaches and informing organ-at-risk dosimetry considerations for future therapeutic folate conjugates [46–48].

Additionally, a new [^{68}Ga]Ga-NOTA-folic acid conjugate developed by Jain et al. is used for PET imaging of tumors that overexpress folate receptors and for evaluating its potential in human nasopharyngeal carcinoma cell lines with overexpressed folate receptors, as well as for preliminary biodistribution studies in normal Swiss mice. The synthesis was successful, and radiolabeling was performed with an efficiency of over 95% and a binding affinity to cells. It showed specific uptake by KB cells, which was blocked by cold folic acid, and holds potential applicability in other FR-positive cancers, such as gastric cancer. The biodistribution study of the [^{68}Ga]Ga-NOTA-folic acid conjugate in normal mice showed a strong correlation between the tracer and kidneys. Additional studies in tumor models are required to validate its imaging potential with future optimization focused on reducing renal dosimetry risk to enhance its clinical applicability [49].

Lu et al. reported an in vitro and in vivo evaluation of newly synthesized folate conjugates, HYNIC-NHHN-FA, radiolabeled with [^{99m}Tc], which used different coligand systems. They analyzed the biological profile of these radiotracers in KB tumor cells, which are folate receptor (FR)-positive. The biodistribution study in mice models demonstrated that the radiocomplex [^{99m}Tc]Tc-(HYNIC-NHHN-FA) (tricine/TPPMS) was primarily absorbed in the stomach and intestines, indicating rapid elimination of radioactivity through the gastrointestinal system due to low tumor uptake, suggesting that optimizing coligand chemistry significantly influences both pharmacokinetics and tumor-to-background contrast. As a result, [^{99m}Tc]Tc-(HYNIC-NHHN-FA) (tricine/TPPTS) indicates a promising candidate for FR imaging [50]. Another experiment by Xie et al. focused on FR-positive KB tumors as the target and developed [^{99m}Tc]Tc-labeled folate-based SPECT radiotracer. To optimize binding affinity, they utilized HYNIC as a chelator and polyethylene glycol (PEG) as a linker. The radiotracer [^{99m}Tc]Tc-(HYNIC-PEG2-FA) (EDDA) exhibited moderate uptake in the gastrointestinal tract, suggesting its involvement in excretion. Additionally, a significant accumulation of [^{99m}Tc]Tc-folate was observed in the kidney. The administration of excess folic acid significantly reduced radiotracer uptake in both tumors and kidneys,

https://doi.org/10.3390/jpm16010036

confirming receptor-specific targeting and showing the biological basis of competitive receptor saturation as a blocking strategy to reduce renal exposure [51].

Kim et al. designed a novel [^{99m}Tc]Tc-ECG-EDA (Glu-Cys-Gly-ethylenediamine)-folate as an FR-positive KB tumor imaging agent, utilizing a mouse tumor model for in vivo studies. ECG-EDA-folate was radiolabeled with [^{99m}Tc], exhibiting high efficiency and stability (>96%), which demonstrated specific targeting of FR-positive tumors, as confirmed by micro-SPECT/CT imaging and reduced uptake with excess folate. These findings provide valuable insights for developing advanced folate-peptide conjugates for tumor imaging applications [52].

Boss et al. synthesized and compared three pairs of α- and γ-conjugated fluorinated folate derivatives, which were radiolabeled with fluorine-18 [^{18}F]. The process of radiolabeling yielded high purities of radiochemicals (>95%) and a range of significant activities from 25 to 196 GBq/µmol. The in vitro assay demonstrated a strong FR-α binding affinity in all derivatives, with IC50 values ranging from 1.4 to 2.2 nM. In vivo studies in FR-positive tumor-bearing mice, regressing to PET imaging and biodistribution assays, demonstrated that sites of conjugation impacted biodistribution due to non-specific liver uptake of α-regioisomers compared to γ-regioisomers, which exhibited reduced kidney uptake of up to 50%. Thus, the results underscore the critical role of radiolabeling site selection in designing [^{18}F]-based radiofolates as a novel way for advanced folate-based radiotracer designs [53].

Betzel et al. investigated a new radiotracer, 3-aza-2-[^{18}F]F-fluorofolic acid, for imaging FR-positive tumors. In vitro testing demonstrated strong FR-α binding affinity ($IC_{50} \approx 0.8$ nM). In vivo PET imaging of FR-positive KB tumor-bearing mice revealed substantial tumor uptake ($\approx$12.6% ID/g at 90 min post-injection). High accumulation was also observed in the kidneys ($\approx$57% ID/g) and salivary glands ($\approx$14% ID/g), both of which are organs known to express physiological levels of FR. Additionally, minor non-specific uptake occurred in the liver. Thus, the tracer demonstrated favorable in vitro and in vivo properties and enabled high contrast and minimal off-target accumulation, which showed notable advantages with its efficient synthesis process and clinical potential [54]. Additionally, a new radiolabeled folic acid derivative (2′-[^{18}F]F-fluorofolic acid) has been developed in a preclinical study by Ross et al. that showed high affinity and specificity for folate receptors. This radioligand outperforms previous [^{18}F]-labeled radiofolates in terms of receptor selectivity and, to date, is considered to be the most promising [^{18}F] radioligand for imaging folate receptor-positive tumors, due to integrating synthetic efficiency, minimal off-target accumulation, and favorable organ dosimetry, which are essential attributes for the future clinical translation of FR-targeted cancer imaging [55]. The other radiotracer, [^{18}F]F-fluorodeoxyglucose-folate, was synthesized by Fisher and colleagues, who used a glucose-based radiolabeled prosthetic group to enhance hydrophilicity. High affinity and specificity for folate receptors due to in vitro and in vivo studies, demonstrated the potential of this radiotracer for PET imaging of FR-positive cancers and inflammation [56] and its efficient use for clinical translation [57].

4. Breast Cancer-Targeted Vitamin-Based Radionuclide Agents

Breast cancer (BC) is a malignant disorder that remains a major global health concern for women due to its high incidence and mortality. Its development is influenced by several risk factors, including genetic and hereditary predispositions. Advances in treatment strategies have increasingly focused on molecular characteristics, such as HER2 activation, estrogen receptor (ER) and progesterone receptor (PR) expression, gene mutations, and tumor microenvironment markers [58]. Early diagnosis of breast cancer significantly improves prognosis and patient survival. However, conventional imaging techniques often lack the sensitivity to detect tumors before morphological changes become apparent. In

https://doi.org/10.3390/jpm16010036

contrast, radionuclide-based molecular imaging modalities, such as positron emission tomography (PET) and single-photon emission computed tomography (SPECT), provide functional insights into breast cancer. These approaches enable non-invasive visualization of tumors and molecular markers, thereby enhancing early detection and improving treatment precision. Furthermore, the development of radionuclide probes targeting specific receptors and biomarkers has greatly advanced breast cancer theranostics [59].

Guzik et al. explored the use of [^{177}Lu]Lu-DOTA-folate as an immune stimulus to enhance the efficacy of anti-CTLA-4 immunotherapy in a syngeneic mouse model of breast tumors. Experiments demonstrated specific targeting of NF9006 tumor cells by the radiolabeled folate in vitro and in vivo. Although [^{177}Lu]Lu-DOTA-folate or anti-CTLA-4 therapy alone had a minimal impact on tumor growth and survival, which did not significantly enhance survival time in mice compared to control groups, their combination resulted in marked tumor growth inhibition and prolonged survival beyond 70 days without noticeable side effects. This synergistic effect is due to immunogenic cell death being inhibited by [^{177}Lu]Lu-DOTA-folate-induced radiation, which makes tumor microenvironments more responsive to immune checkpoint blockade. These results showed the potential of folate-based radioconjugates to enhance immunotherapy strategies and hold promise for further clinical research [60].

Aranda-Lara et al. developed [^{177}Lu]Lu-Folate-Bombesin ([^{177}Lu]Lu-Folate-BN) for the imaging and therapy of FR and GRPR-positive breast tumors. Preclinical studies on the T47D human breast cancer cell line and T47D tumor-bearing mice, which delivered 23.97 $\pm$ 2.1 Gy after 74 MBq injection, with precise Micro-SPECT/CT imaging, demonstrating the promising potential of [^{177}Lu]Lu-Folate-BN as a theranostic radiopharmaceutical due to their concomitant identification of GRPR and FRα. The results obtained warrant a further clinical study specifically aimed at evaluating in vivo tumor uptake, quantifying radiation dose delivered, and assessing therapeutic efficacy [61]. Furthermore, in another study, they synthesized the Lys1 (α,γ-Folate)-Lys3 (EDDA/HYNIC)-Bombesin (1–14) conjugate ([^{99m}Tc] Tc-Bombesin–Folate) to target FRα and GRPR, and analyzed its potential in vitro and in vivo. The purity of [^{99m}Tc]-labeling was 96 $\pm$ 2.1%, which was achieved via High-performance liquid chromatography (HPLC), and the preclinical results showed strong uptake (5.43% ID/g), inhibited by cold FA/Bombesin and confirming dual FRα/GRPR targeting for imaging improvement [62].

In addition, Mendoza-Nava et al. performed a preclinical study on the development of a ^{177}Lu-labeled dendrimer (PAMAM-G4) conjugated with folate and bombesin, incorporating gold nanoparticles (AuNPs) for the targeted imaging and therapy of breast tumors overexpressing FR and GRPR. Actually, AuNPs were synthesized within the internal cavity and functionalized with folate and bombesin for FR and GRPR co-targeting, also DOTA chelators for dual-receptor targeting and radiolabeling. Comprehensive physicochemical characterization of AuNPs showed enhanced luminescent properties suitable for optical imaging. The formulation achieved high radiochemical purity (>95%) and 41.15% tumor cell uptake, highlighting its potential for dual optical and nuclear imaging not only in breast tumors overexpressing GRPRs and FRs, but also for targeted radiotherapy [63]. In other experiments performed by Gupta et al. they synthesized [^{177}Lu] Lu-IONP-Folate for the treatment of folate receptor-positive cancers, aiming to reduce renal radiation exposure. Using SPECT/CT voxel-based dosimetry and results showed a ~50% lower kidney dose than [^{177}Lu]Lu-Folate, making it a safer, personalized TRT option for breast cancer, which showed their potential for clinical application when using the voxel-based dosimetry method. Additionally, IONP integration enables improved safety and supports the development of individualized therapeutic planning [64].

https://doi.org/10.3390/jpm16010036

Kuda-Wedagedara et al. reported the synthesis of 89Zirconium-labeled cobalamin ([^{89}Zr]Zr-Cbl), which was modified with desferrioxamine and proved successful and suitable for tumor imaging. The studies were conducted in both in vitro and in vivo settings on a positive breast cancer cell line and mice. Additionally, they evaluated the uptake and pharmacokinetics of the CD320-positive MDA-MB-453 breast cancer cells and xenografted mice that confirmed targeting the CD320 receptor which mediates vitamin B_{12} internalization via receptor-mediated endocytosis. However, under sustained therapeutic pressure, may lead to tumor adaptation or altering receptor trafficking, thereby limiting tracer uptake and long-term efficacy. The in vitro test showed a 6–10-fold higher uptake of [^{89}Zr]Zr-Cbl rather than uptake in the presence of an excess of cyano-Cbl (CN-Cbl), also PET imaging and biodistribution study in nude mice exhibited a clear visualization of the tumor and high accumulation in kidneys and liver after 48-hr post-injection respectively (Figure 3). The results showed the feasibility of synthesizing a Cbl-based tracer that can be utilized for both in vivo and ex vivo studies of Cbl trafficking. This tracer has the potential to visualize tumors expressing transcobalamin (TC) receptors, such as CD320. Thus, monitoring receptor expression heterogeneity is important to overcome potential resistance mechanisms in transcobalamin receptor–based therapies [65].

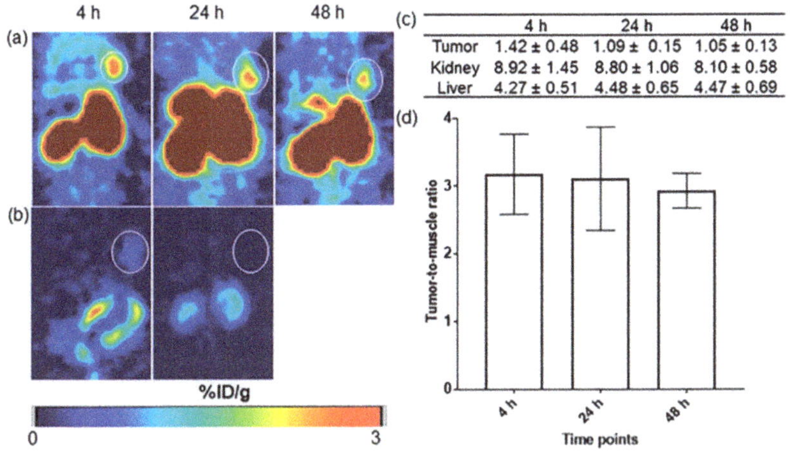

Figure 3. PET images of mice with MDA-MB-453 tumors show (**a**) uptake of ([^{89}Zr]Zr-Cbl at 4, 24, and 48 h post-injection (p.i.), with (**b**) reduced tumor uptake when co-injected with excess unlabeled Cbl. Quantitative analysis includes (**c**)%ID/g values for key organs and (**d**) tumor-to-muscle ratios, with tumors which marked by white circles. Reprinted with permission from Ref. [65], Copyright 2017, ACS Omega.

Ucar et al. developed folate-targeted nanostructured lipid carriers (NLCs) for delivering paclitaxel (PTX) to folate receptor (FR)-overexpressing tumors. In vitro studies using MCF-7, HeLa, and A549 cell lines, and in vivo rat models, demonstrated enhanced cellular uptake and cytotoxicity in FR-positive cells. The NLCs were modified with folate-PEG-CHEMS to improve targeting and circulation, then radiolabeled with [^{99m}Tc(CO)$_3$]$^+$. Radiolabeling was efficient, and biodistribution studies confirmed higher uptake in FR-positive tissues. These results support [^{99m}Tc]Tc-(CO)$_3$-PTX-NLCs as promising candidates for FR-targeted theranostic applications, highlighting the potential of radiolabeled lipid-based nanoparticles in precision oncology [66].

The study by Temma et al. focused on radiolabeling anti-MT1-mAb with [^{99m}Tc] to detect MT1-MMP, an enzyme with high expression on the surface of malignant tumor cells, which is suitable for a diagnostic target. HYNIC was used as a chelating agent,

https://doi.org/10.3390/jpm16010036

and the probe synthesis was performed with significant immunoactivity (84%) and high radiochemical purity (>92%). Western blotting confirmed the expression of MT1-MMP in breast tumor models, and the biodistribution study revealed a specific accumulation of the tumor over time, with tumor-to-blood ratios exceeding 1.3 after 48 h. Also, the dose effecting was 5.0 mSv/MBq. The results suggested [^{99m}Tc]Tc-anti-MT1-MMP mAb as an imaging agent that has the potential for breast cancer diagnosis in nuclear medicine for future translational imaging clinically [67].

Silindir-Gunay et al. designed liposomal imaging agents for SPECT and SPECT/CT to assess their effectiveness. Folate-conjugated, PEGylated, [^{99m}Tc]-radiolabeled liposomes (Folate-PE:DMPC: DTPA-PE) demonstrated prolonged circulation, high tumor uptake, and specific targeting of folate receptors in 4T1 cells. Thus, these liposomes suggested promising alternatives to [^{99m}Tc]Tc-Sestamibi, while further in vivo studies are required for validation [68]. Mollarazi et al. focused on developing biocompatible, water-soluble [^{153}Sm]-labeled chitosan nanoparticles (NPs) with folate and polyethyleneimine for targeted cancer therapy. The spherical NPs (~250 nm) were stable and exhibited significant uptake in MCF-7 and 4T1 cells with specific FR targeting. In vivo studies exhibited renal excretion and minor tumor accumulation up to 96 h, suggesting that folic acid-functionalized chitosan NPs could be promising for FR-targeted therapy also due to their rapid removal from the kidneys in comparison with other presented liver-accumulating agents [69].

In another study, Guo et al. introduced a new FR-targeting agent for SPECT imaging, focusing on improving contrast through multimerization and PEGylation. [^{99m}Tc]-labeled folate derivatives displayed high tumor uptake in KB cells, specific targeting, and significant biodistribution via micro-SPECT/CT imaging. Alongside, the PEGylated monomeric [^{99m}Tc]Tc-HYNFA showed the most considerable tumor uptake and imaging contrast, which suggested more effectiveness for designing the radio-folates that could be promising agents for breast cancer diagnosis and treatment monitoring [70].

5. Colorectal Cancer-Targeted Vitamin-Based Radionuclide Agents

Colorectal cancer is the second most common cause of cancer-related deaths and the third most common cancer globally. Exposure to risk factors, demographic differences, genetic susceptibility, and genetic mutations impacts its treatment response and prognosis [71]. The development of therapeutic strategies that integrate multiple drugs has gained significant attention in addressing multidrug resistance (MDR). Combination therapies, such as chemotherapy combined with immunotherapy, have demonstrated promising efficacy in targeting key proteins, including the epidermal growth factor receptor (EGFR) and the vascular endothelial growth factor receptor (VEGFR). Furthermore, the identification and validation of critical biomarkers play a crucial role in advancing personalized medicine, enabling a deeper understanding of MDR mechanisms and associated toxicities. These approaches enhance treatment efficacy and also contribute to tailored therapy, leading to improved clinical outcomes [72]. Currently, the increased understanding of radiochemistry, bioengineering, and cancer biology has significantly enhanced the potential of targeted radionuclide therapy to address the efficient treatment of solid tumors [73].

Kotun et al. developed the first PET imaging agent based on a vitamin B12-derivative, [^{64}Cu]Cu-B12-en-Bn-NOTA, to assess tumor-associated nutritional demand. Preclinical studies in various human and murine cancer models (HCT116, SKOV-3, B16-F10) showed notable tumor uptake (2.20–4.84% ID/g at 6 h), mediated by transcobalamin II (TCII) receptors. These mechanisms facilitate the cellular internalization of vitamin B_{12} via receptor-mediated endocytosis. Tumor specificity was confirmed by a 95% reduction in uptake following co-injection with native B12. However, high renal accumulation remains a limitation for clinical translation. These findings support vitamin B12-based radiotracers

https://doi.org/10.3390/jpm16010036

as promising PET probes for imaging tumor metabolism, while emphasizing the need for receptor-expression monitoring with future optimization needed to reduce off-target kidney uptake and validation in higher-species models before clinical application [74].

Above that, the use of folate-conjugated shell-cross-linked nanoparticles (SCKs) for targeted tumor imaging and therapy, highlighted by Rossin et al. illustrated a specific FR interaction and [^{64}Cu] radiolabeling for biodistribution studies. The SCKs showed significant RES uptake, long circulation, and passive tumor accumulation. Additionally, folate-specific binding was observed in smaller tumors, indicating the potential of SCKs for early-stage cancer treatment and suggesting a promising approach for targeted imaging and therapy in colorectal cancer [75].

Cheal et al. conducted in vitro and in vivo experiments on colorectal cancer cell lines and mouse models. They introduced a glycodendrimer-based clearing agent (CCAα16-DOTA-Y^{3+}) for pre-targeted radioimmunotherapy (DOTA-PRIT) using [^{177}Lu] Lu-DOTA-B. The agent effectively delivered radiation to tumors (468 cGy/MBq) and favorable tumor-to-normal tissue dose ratios, with the highest ratio (~550) for the stomach. The radiolabeling with [^{177}Lu] ensured precise imaging and therapeutic targeting, indicating strong selectivity and minimal off-target effects. These findings highlight the potential of high-therapeutic index (high-TI) DOTA-PRIT for targeted treatment of stomach tumors, ensuring effective tumor treatment while minimizing the risk of damage to normal stomach tissues [76].

In other preclinical studies, Smit. Jones et al. characterized and radiolabeled monoclonal antibody MORAb-003 which targeted folate receptor alpha (FRA). MORAb-003 was conjugated with DOTA and labeled with [^{111}In] and [^{131}I]. Cellular retention was assessed in human ovarian adenocarcinoma (IGROV1) and colon adenocarcinoma (SW620) cell lines, which demonstrated high FRA affinity and significant internalization, with [^{111}In] exhibiting intracellular retention. At the same time, [^{131}I] was released as iodide that showed low intercellular retention (Figure 4). In vivo, biodistribution studies in tumor-bearing mice showed that [^{111}In]In-DOTA-MORAb-003 had significant tumor uptake ($32 \pm 5\%$ ID/g at 4 days) and a 110-h blood clearance rate. Organ clearance followed the same pattern, showing low retention after 8 days. In addition, clinical trials in a small group of patients validated effective tumor targeting and favorable biodistribution of MORAb-003, supporting its potential for radioimmunoscintigraphy, radioimmunotherapy, and targeted treatment of FRA-expressing cancers [77].

Kim et al. examined tumor targeting using triphenylphosphonium (TPP) cations (membrane potential-based) and FA (FR-targeting) with FDA-approved silica nanoparticles (SNPs) as carriers. The radiochemical purity of [^{89}Zr]-labeled SNPs was >99%. PET imaging and cellular uptake analysis revealed that TPP-modified SNPs (SFT-5) exhibited a significant tumor affinity in CT-26 cancer cells, confirming that targeting membrane potential via TPP is more effective compared to FA receptor-based targeting [78]. The other study, conducted by Kim et al., showed significant potential of micro-scale silica wires (SMWs) as a drug carrier for targeting FR, which was conjugated with FA and labeled with [^{89}Zr] for PET imaging in preclinical assays. They confirmed that the FA-conjugated sample stayed at the tumor site for a longer period and reported the unique in vivo behavior of [^{89}Zr]Zr-FA-SMWs [79].

Choi et al. conducted a study on synthesizing the HBED-CC-EDBE-folate precursor (HCEF) and labeling it with [^{68}Ga], which was assessed by HPLC and TLC regarding radiochemical yield and purity. The study showed efficient radiolabeling with a 98% yield at room temperature. Preclinical studies showed strong binding of the probe in folate receptor-positive cancer cells and selective accumulation in tumors, confirming [^{68}Ga]Ga-HCEF as a promising tool for cancer diagnosis using PET imaging [80].

https://doi.org/10.3390/jpm16010036

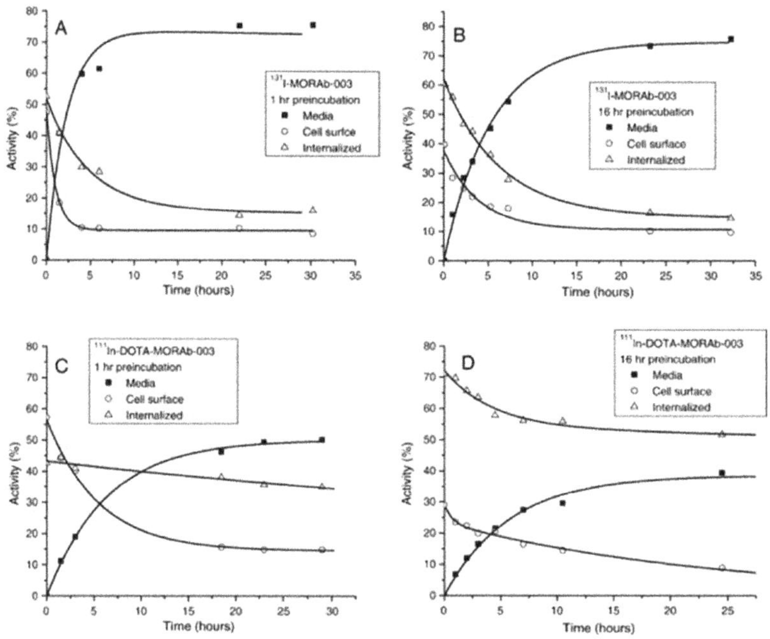

Figure 4. Radioactivity distribution in IGROV1 cells after incubation at 37 °C with either [^{131}I]I-MORAb-003 ((**A**): 1 h; (**B**): 16 h) or [^{111}In]In-DOTA–MORAb-003 ((**C**): 1 h; (**D**): 16 h). Reprinted with permission from Ref. [77]. Copyright 2008, Elsevier.

Khatik et al. developed a novel oral drug delivery system for the targeted treatment of colorectal cancer using curcumin-loaded gliadin nanoparticles (Gd NPs), surface-functionalized with folic acid (FA) and coated with Eudragit S-100 (ES) for colon-specific release. This folate-targeted nanocarrier was designed to exploit the overexpression of folate receptors in tumor cells. In vitro studies confirmed its ability to induce apoptosis in cancer cells, while in vivo gamma scintigraphy demonstrated efficient tumor localization and sustained release of the therapeutic agent. The results highlight the potential of this system as a safe and effective strategy for prolonged oral therapy in colorectal cancer [81].

Additionally, [^{99m}Tc]Tc-PAMA-cobalamin, a novel radiolabeled vitamin B12 derivative synthesized by Sah et al., targets tumors by avoiding normal tissue uptake through transcobalamin. It binds to a protein expressed in many tumors, like haptocorrin. In a study involving 10 metastatic cancer patients, 6 showed positive tumor uptake in lung, colon, breast, and hypopharyngeal cancers, indicating tumor-specific uptake via haptocorrin-mediated binding. Administering cold cobalamin before scanning enhanced tumor uptake and improved imaging quality while maintaining low renal uptake, that showed long-term dosimetry considerations needed for clinical translation. Overall, this research confirms [^{99m}Tc]Tc-PAMA-cobalamin could be a promising tool for cancer imaging [82].

6. Brain Cancer-Targeted Vitamin-Based Radionuclide Agents

Brain tumors, or brain cancer, are characterized by the uncontrolled proliferation of abnormal or malignant cells within the brain or its surrounding tissues, leading to the formation of pathological masses. Patients diagnosed with malignant brain tumors frequently face severe clinical challenges, substantial morbidity, and poor prognosis [83], with an average survival of about 14 months with aggressive treatment. A key challenge that needs to be addressed is the ability of these compounds to cross the blood–brain barrier

https://doi.org/10.3390/jpm16010036

(BBB), which limits the entry of many chemotherapeutic agents into the brain. Despite conventional therapies, receptor-mediated transcytosis remains a problem with limited efficacy and difficulty. As vitamins A and C, for example, are showing promise in this regard, it would be worthwhile to explore how other vitamins or nanoconstructs based on them could be used to enhance the targeting related to BBB crossing [84,85]. However, recent advancements in nanotechnology make an innovation route in cancer therapy [86]. Moreover, progress in nuclear medicine has introduced promising innovative strategies for glioblastoma treatment, particularly through radioimmunotherapy, radiopeptide therapy, and radionanoparticles. Additionally, radiopharmaceuticals have shown the ability to enhance stabilizing or improving neurological conditions with minimal side effects, highlighting their potential as an effective tool for glioblastoma therapy [87].

Miner et al. highlighted [^{18}F]F-FOL as a folate-based PET imaging agent that targets overexpressed folate receptors (FRs) for detecting gliomas in a rat model and assesses FR expression in human glioblastoma samples. PET imaging of glioma-bearing rats demonstrated a significantly higher tumor-to-brain uptake ratio (TBR) over time for [^{18}F]F-FOL compared to [^{18}F]F-FDG. Ex vivo studies confirmed the superior TBR of [^{18}F]F-FOL, supported by immunostaining, which revealed upregulated FR-α in glioma regions and FR-β at the tumor periphery. Moreover, in human glioblastoma samples, similar FR expression patterns were observed. These results suggest the potential of FR-targeted agents like [^{18}F]F-FOL for the detection and treatment of gliomas in both preclinical and clinical settings [88].

In addition, Liang et al. introduced [^{18}F]F-AlF-NOTA-Asp2-PEG2-Folate, a PET tracer designed with a hydrophilic linker to improve pharmacokinetics. The tracer was created efficiently within 30 min, and FR in KB cells showed high specificity and affinity. In KB tumor-bearing mice, [^{18}F]F-AlF-NOTA-Asp2-PEG2-Folate indicated good tumor uptake (1.7% ID/g), reduced accumulation in the kidney and liver, and rapid clearance from normal tissues in comparison with [^{18}F]F-AlF-NOTA-Folate. The folate receptor via high-affinity endocytosis facilitates ligand internalization which make selective tumor accumulation of folate-conjugated tracers. However, variable FR expression and disruptions in receptor transport or recycling can diminish tracer accumulation, particularly in more aggressive or resistant tumors. Thus, these findings hold the [^{18}F]F-AlF-NOTA-Asp2-PEG2-Folate, a promising option for PET imaging in FR-positive tumors and a critical improvement for clinical translation [89].

Shi et al. performed an experiment using a folate-receptor-targeted imaging probe, [^{64}Cu]Cu-DOTA-FA-ICG, NIR-II fluorescence imaging of glioblastoma (GBM). The probe formed nanoparticles and accumulated specifically in GBM tumors, which enabled real-time tumor visualization during surgery. Nonetheless, intratumoral heterogeneity and microenvironment-driven modulation of FR levels may limit complete tumor delineation and contribute to residual disease, so safe translation of DOTA-FA-ICG and ^{64}Cu-DOTA-FA-ICG is crucial. This innovation improves tumor differentiation and surgical accuracy [90].

Korany et al. developed a direct synthesis method for amorphous selenium nanoparticles (SeNPs) coated with vitamin C and radiolabeled with [^{99m}Tc] for in vivo imaging studies in both healthy and tumor-bearing mice. The resulting nano complex demonstrated optimal particle size, high colloidal stability, and a radiolabeling yield of 96 $\pm$ 2%, maintaining stability for over six hours. Biodistribution analysis revealed favorable target-to-non-target ratios in tumor-bearing models. While vitamin C was primarily employed as a stabilizing and coating agent, its presence may also contribute indirectly to the radiolabeling efficiency and biocompatibility of the system. These findings support the potential of [^{99m}Tc]Tc-VitC-SeNPs as promising agents for solid tumor imaging [91].

https://doi.org/10.3390/jpm16010036

A radiolabeled folate-loaded micelles or non-invasive intranasal delivery, developed by Upadhaya et al., to target brain tumors by exploiting folate receptor overexpression in glioma cells, the micelles were efficiently labeled with [^{99m}Tc] (>95% yield). Their nanoscale size and mucoadhesive properties facilitated direct brain delivery. In vivo studies showed high brain uptake, and SPECT imaging confirmed effective targeting, highlighting the potential for diagnosing brain and other cancers [92].

Nosrati et al. introduced [^{99m}Tc]Tc-BPTG-1 and [^{99m}Tc]Tc-BPTG-2 for glioblastoma imaging as potential radiotracers. In vitro tests showed strong uptake in U87-MG cells, with tumor accumulation exceeding muscle and brain levels in mice. The radiotracers were cleared via the liver and kidneys, which showed the greatest activity, highlighting their potential for GBM diagnosis [93].

Another radiopharmaceutical targeted the folate receptor (Ga-DF-Folate) was developed by Mathias and colleagues using [^{66}Ga] and [^{68}Ga] radionuclides for PET imaging. In mice with folate-receptor-positive tumors, [^{66}Ga] imaging was successful despite its high positron energy. Dual-isotope autoradiography with [^{18}F]F-FDG and [^{111}In]In-DTPA-Folate revealed tumor heterogeneity and regional tracer variations. Given the prominent role of kidneys in folate tracer clearance, precise renal dosimetry remains a major consideration for implementing FR-targeted Ga-labeled agents in clinical imaging [94].

In addition, Zhang et al. designed a novel [^{68}Ga]-labeled PET tracer targeting FRs, such as Pteroyl-Lys-DOTA and Pteroyl-Lys-DAV-DOTA. These compounds were successfully synthesized, radiolabeled with [^{68}Ga], and evaluated in FR-positive KB cells and tumor-bearing mice. Both showed high tumor specificity, with tumor uptake values of 10.06% ID/g and 11.05% ID/g at 2 h post-injection and clear tumor visualization in Micro-PET imaging, which supported their potential as FR-targeted PET probes for applications in cancer diagnosis and therapy [95].

7. Prostate Cancer-Targeted Vitamin-Based Radionuclide Agents

Prostate cancer represents a major global health challenge and is among the leading causes of cancer-related mortality in men. A substantial proportion of patients are diagnosed with advanced-stage disease. Clinical diagnosis primarily relies on the digital rectal examination and measurement of prostate-specific antigen (PSA) levels, with confirmation obtained through histopathological analysis of biopsy tissue. Current therapeutic interventions for localized disease include radical prostatectomy and radiotherapy, while advanced or metastatic disease is managed with systemic therapies such as androgen deprivation therapy and chemotherapy. To overcome challenges including drug resistance and dose-limiting toxicities, emerging strategies such as combination therapies and nanoparticle-based drug delivery systems are under investigation to improve therapeutic efficacy and reduce adverse effects [96].

Ak et al. introduced [^{99m}Tc]Tc-folate–PEG–doxorubicin, a radiolabeled nanoconjugate for imaging prostate cancer and localizing the drug. Based on biodistribution studies performed in rats, folate ligands have a higher affinity for folate receptors than control groups. With a high specificity for tumor tissue, this radiolabeled conjugate suggests strong potential for prostate cancer diagnosis and real-time tracking of drug distribution [97]. Also, L. Dhas et al. created folic acid-conjugated chitosan-coated PLGA nanoparticles for targeted prostate cancer therapy. Bicalutamide-loaded NPs demonstrated efficient drug encapsulation, controlled release, and in vitro cytotoxicity in DU145 human prostate cancer cell lines. They exhibited higher cytotoxic effects compared to the uncoated nanoparticles (UPN) and the pure drug. Stability and hemolysis studies validated its safety and potential for prostate cancer treatment with further in vivo investigations [98].

https://doi.org/10.3390/jpm16010036

A new peptide derivative of folic acid known as EC20, identified by P Leamon et al., to coordinate with [^{99m}Tc] for potential cancer imaging applications. EC20 illustrated a high affinity for FR-positive tumor cells. In vitro study confirmed that EC20 could compete effectively with 3H-folic acid for cell binding, either alone or as a metal chelate. Upon intravenous injection into Balb/c mice, [^{99m}Tc]Tc-EC20 exhibited rapid clearance from circulation (plasma half-life ~4 min) and was excreted via urine. [^{99m}Tc]Tc-EC20 predominantly accumulated in FR-positive tumors and kidneys, were confirmed by Gamma scintigraphy and biodistribution studies. These results suggest a significant potential of [^{99m}Tc]Tc-EC20 as a non-invasive imaging agent for detecting FR-positive human cancers [99].

Guo et al. designed [^{99m}Tc]Tc-HYNIC-D1-FA2, a radiolabeled dimeric folate-based tracer, for targeted imaging of FR-overexpressing tumors. The tracer was synthesized via click chemistry and exhibited strong tumor binding (IC50 = 19.06 nM) and high hydrophilicity (log P = −2.52). In KB tumor-bearing mice, a biodistribution study demonstrated high tumor and kidney uptake, which was notably reduced when free folic acid was used for blocking, as observed upon pre-saturation with excess folic acid, confirming high receptor specificity of the ^{99m}Tc-labeled folate derivatives. Micro-SPECT/CT imaging showed effective tumor visualization, suggesting that [^{99m}Tc]Tc-HYNIC-D1-FA2 could be a promising FR-targeted imaging agent for cancer treatment [100].

In addition, two folate derivatives, CN5FA and CNPFA, were synthesized by Feng et al. and radiolabeled with [^{99m}Tc] to create [^{99m}Tc]Tc-CN5FA and [^{99m}Tc]Tc-CNPFA complexes. These complexes demonstrated high radiochemical purity (>95%), hydrophilicity, and good in vitro stability. Competitive binding assays in KB cells confirmed the specificity of this receptor for folate. In vivo, studies in KB tumor-bearing mice revealed selective tumor uptake, with [^{99m}Tc]Tc-CNPFA exhibiting higher tumor-to-muscle ratios than [^{99m}Tc]Tc-CN5FA due to its superior SPECT/CT imaging. These findings indicate that the [^{99m}Tc]-labeled complexes could be promising agents for prostate cancer imaging [101].

Ross et al. developed a PET imaging tracer targeting FR, [^{18}F]F-click folate, for tumors that utilize click chemistry. They synthesized in high radiochemical yield and strong binding FR affinity with the 25–35% and (Ki = 9.76 nM), respectively, in in vitro study. PET imaging in mice demonstrated significant tumor uptake (3.13% ID/g), but high liver excretion resulted in a background signal. While exhibiting good in vitro binding for FR-positive tumors, further optimization is necessary to enhance in vivo imaging quality [102].

Yigit et al. used a radiolabeled form of ascorbic acid with [^{99m}Tc] and evaluated its radiopharmaceutical potential in vivo in rats. They successfully labeled the [^{99m}Tc] ascorbic acid ([^{99m}Tc]Tc-AA) using the stannous chloride method, achieving a 93% yield under optimal conditions. After injection into Wistar rats, a biodistribution study showed the [^{99m}Tc] Tc-AA accumulated in the prostate and kidneys at 60 min. Given the prominent kidney accumulation, renal dosimetry is a key consideration should ^{99m}Tc-AA advance, which is suggested as a promising imaging agent for these organs in future diagnostic applications [103].

Schibli et al. developed a novel [^{99m}Tc] radiolabeled vitamin B12 derivative (PAMA-4-B12) to enhance tumor targeting and diagnostic imaging while minimizing non-specific binding to transport proteins, such as TC, which often leads to unwanted accumulation in the liver, kidneys, and glands. Tumor localization occurs through vitamin B_{12} receptor–associated endocytosis. The radiochemical purity of PAMA-4-B12 was >95%, and targeted tumors efficiently in various animal models, including prostate carcinoma, showed fast renal elimination and minimal liver uptake. In a clinical pilot study with patients with different cancers, including prostate carcinoma, PAMA-4-B12 showed fast renal elimination, but there was unexpectedly high liver uptake indicating species-dependent pharmacokinetics. These findings suggest that PAMA-4-B12 holds promise as a diagnostic and therapeutic

https://doi.org/10.3390/jpm16010036

agent for certain carcinomas, with ongoing investigations needed to address liver uptake, especially for clinical prostate cancer applications [104].

Waibel et al. investigated modified vitamin B12 derivatives for targeted imaging of hyperproliferative cancer cells. Using colon (LS 147T) and prostate (LNCaP) carcinoma cell lines, as well as in vivo mouse models, they assessed biodistribution and tumor specificity. By altering B12 to bypass the transcobalamin II pathway, off-target uptake in normal tissues was minimized and enhancing tumor accumulation. Transcobalamin I was proposed as a tumor-specific receptor. TCI-mediated endocytosis enhanced tumor uptake and improved tumor-to-blood ratios while reducing renal and hepatic exposure, which highlighting the clinical potential of B12-based radiopharmaceuticals with consideration to heterogeneity in TCI expression across tumor types that warrants further investigation [105].

8. Ovarian Cancer-Targeted Vitamin-Based Radionuclide Agents

Ovarian cancer (OC) is a heterogeneous disease with multiple subtypes, each requiring different treatment approaches. Due to the lack of effective screening, it is often diagnosed late, and standard treatments such as surgery and platinum-based chemotherapy are performed. High-grade serous carcinoma (HGSC), the most prevalent type, initially responds well to treatment but often develops resistance to treatment [106]. For this reason, early detection of cancer is crucial for effective treatment and better survival outcomes. Nuclear medicine plays a significant role in cancer diagnosis and therapy. Advancing SPECT and PET-based theranostic tools for ovarian cancer highlights their advantages for diagnosis and treatment [107–109].

Reber et al. designed a radioiodinated folate conjugate to selectively target FR-positive tumors while minimizing kidney toxicity. This addressed the issue of high kidney uptake as a key limitation of traditional radiofolates, which created a risk of renal radiation damage during therapy. Two variants, [^{125}I]I-2 and [$^{125/131}$I]I-4, showed high stability, FR-specific binding and strong tumor accumulation. In vitro studies displayed [^{131}I]I-4 reduced FR-positive tumor cell viability. Pre-injection with pemetrexed improved tumor imaging via SPECT/CT, suggesting these conjugates are promising for the diagnosis and therapy of FR-positive cancers like ovarian cancers [110].

Moreover, Aljammaz et al. developed [^{124}I]I-SIB-folate and [^{124}I]I-SIP-folate conjugates for enhancing the imaging of folate receptor-positive cancers. They employed a rapid two-step process, achieving high radiochemical yields (>90% and >60%) and purity (>98%). In vitro and in vivo studies demonstrated effective tumor targeting, particularly for [^{124}I]I-SIP-folate, with good biodistribution and receptor-specific uptake. All the results showed the potential of [^{124}I]I-SIP-folate as a PET imaging prob for ovarian cancer diagnosis, staging, and treatment monitoring [111].

Aljammaz et al. synthesized novel [^{18}F]F-fluorobenzene and pyridinecarbohydrazide-folate/methotrexate conjugates and used nucleophilic displacement reactions. They achieved high radiochemical yields and purity with (>80%) and (>97%), respectively, without requiring HPLC purification, allowing for quick and efficient methods for folate derivative radiofluorination. Various experiments confirmed significant receptor-mediated uptake, while animal experiments demonstrated fast blood clearance and significant tumor accumulation, particularly for [^{18}F]F-2-folate. Micro-PET imaging validated these results, highlighting [^{18}F]F-2-folate could be a promising molecular probe for detecting and monitoring folate receptor-positive cancers, such as ovarian cancer and its metastases [112]. In another experiment, Aljammaz et al. improved PET Imaging of folate receptor-positive tumors by developing [^{18}F]F-FDG-folate and methotrexate conjugates ([^{18}F]F-5 and [^{18}F]F-8). These were produced rapidly and in a one-step process with high yields (>80%) and purities (>98%). In vivo studies in mice showed rapid clearance and significant tumor

https://doi.org/10.3390/jpm16010036

uptake, particularly for [^{18}F]F-5. Receptor-blocking experiments via excess folic acid confirm specific FR-mediated internalization via high-affinity endocytosis. While, receptor overexpression favors tumor targeting, resistance may occur through downregulation of FR or altered folate transport pathways but suggested [^{18}F]F-5, a potential imaging probe for ovarian and other cancers [113].

Siwowska et al. evaluated [^{47}Sc]Sc-labeled DOTA-folate as a potential for targeted radionuclide therapy in folate receptor-positive ovarian cancer, compared to [^{177}Lu]Lu-folate and [^{90}Y]Y-folate. In vitro studies showed effective reduction in tumor cell viability in [^{47}Sc]Sc-folate, which was the same for [^{177}Lu]Lu-folate, while the [^{90}Y]Y-folate, due to higher energy emission, was more potent. In vivo experiments in mice demonstrated comparable tumor growth inhibition and prolonged survival (39–43 days vs. 26 days in controls) with no severe side effects for all three radiofolates. Therefore, the results indicate [^{47}Sc] as a promising alternative to [^{177}Lu] and a promising candidate for clinical use and theranostic applications [114].

Guo et al. investigated a novel therapeutic approach for ovarian cancer by developing [^{177}Lu]Lu-FA-DOTA-PEG-PLGA nanoparticles. These nanoparticles integrate FR-mediated targeting, PEG-PLGA for biodegradability and DOTA for radiolabeling, achieving high labeling efficiency (97–98%) and, minimal kidney accumulation. Micro-SPECT/CT imaging in OC tumor-bearing mice confirmed tumor localization, and treatment significantly inhibited tumor growth and, reduced ascitic fluid also, no major toxicity was shown through histological analysis. These findings suggest that [^{177}Lu]Lu-FA-DOTA-PEG-PLGA nanoparticles could serve as a promising strategy for OC treatment [115].

To enhance DDS by overcoming challenges related to safety, efficacy, and tumor penetration, Wu et al. developed EC112002, an ultrasmall FRα-targeted silica nanoparticle drug conjugate (CDC); this nanoplatforms demonstrated high specificity for FRα, efficient tumor penetration, rapid systemic clearance, and minimal off-target effects following an extensive screening of over 500 formulations. In preclinical studies comparing EC112002 with traditional antibody–drug conjugates (ADCs), EC112002 showed enhanced tumor penetration into 3D tumor models and significant targeted cytotoxicity. These attributes position EC112002 as a promising clinically translatable DDS with potential applications in targeted cancer therapies, including ovarian cancer [116].

Tang and Chen et al., explored a folate-targeted albumin nanoparticle system, specifically [^{188}Re]Re-folate-CDDP/HAS MNP, for evaluating the therapeutic efficacy in ovarian cancer treatment. Preclinical studies were assessed in SKOV3 cells and tumor-bearing mice using various combinations of chemotherapy, radiotherapy, and hyperthermia. The therapeutic mechanism induced DNA damage and folate receptor–mediated targeting of tumor cells by delivering rhenium-188 for $\beta-$ radiation, cisplatin enhances cytotoxicity through DNA cross-linking and magnetic hyperthermia to enhance radiosensitivity and drug penetration for synergistic antitumor effects. All treatments groups included (B) chemotherapy; (C) radiotherapy; (D) hyperthermia; (E) chemotherapy and radiotherapy; (F) chemotherapy and hyperthermia; (G) radiotherapy and hyperthermia; (H) chemotherapy, radiotherapy and hyperthermia, significantly suppressed tumor growth and the strongest effect achieved by triple combination (H) with ($p < 0.05$). Apoptosis rates increased across groups, reaching 57.16% in group H. In vivo studies further confirmed a significant reduction in tumor mass among treated groups, specifically in group H ($p < 0.05$). Thus, all findings highlight the effect of multimodal therapy for ovarian cancer [117].

A novel system presented by Oumzil et al. named [^{99m}Tc]Tc-labeled cisplatin nanoparticles ([^{99m}Tc]Tc-NP-PEGFA), is functionalized with folic acid for targeted drug delivery. The researchers synthesized PEG-based nucleolipids for stable nanoparticle formation and efficient radiolabeling with [^{99m}Tc]. In vitro studies of these NPs on two ovarian cancer cell

https://doi.org/10.3390/jpm16010036

lines (IGROV1 and SKOV3) showed high stability and cellular uptake, whereas prolonged blood circulation and enhanced tumor accumulation were observed in vivo, supporting their potential as targeted drug delivery systems in theranostic applications for cancer therapy [118].

9. Meta-Analysis of Tumor Uptake Ratios

A comparative analysis of the tumor uptake data, expressed as percentage injected dose per gram (% ID/g) from the preclinical studies reviewed, reveals distinct patterns in the targeting efficacy of different vitamin-based radiopharmaceuticals across various cancer types. This meta-analysis highlights the most promising agents and identifies trends in performance.

The compiled data, primarily from Tables 1 and 2, and in-text results, indicate that folate-based radioconjugates consistently demonstrate high and specific tumor accumulation. For instance, folate-targeted agents showed a wide range of tumor uptake, from moderate levels of ~1.7–5.4% ID/g to exceptionally high values exceeding 10–17% ID/g in optimized systems. Notably, Muller et al. reported a remarkable 17.56% ID/g at 4 h for the albumin-binding folate conjugate [44]. Similarly, Zhang et al. demonstrated high uptake with [^{68}Ga] Ga−Pteroyl−Lys conjugates, achieving 10.06% ID/g and 11.05% ID/g [95]. These high values are often attributed to strategies that enhance circulation time, such as albumin binders or PEGylation, which promote the Enhanced Permeability and Retention (EPR) effect and improve receptor-mediated uptake.

Table 1. Comparison of Vitamin-Based and Conventional Radiopharmaceuticals.

Aspect	Vitamin-Based Radiopharmaceuticals	Conventional Radiopharmaceuticals
Targeting Mechanism	Exploits overexpression of vitamin receptors (e.g., Folate Receptor α, Transcobalamin receptor) or vitamin transport systems on tumor cells [65].	Targets specific biomarkers like PSMA, Somatostatin Receptors (SSTR), or antigens (e.g., CD20, CEA) [119,120].
Representative Agents	[^{68}Ga]Ga-DOTA-Folate, [^{177}Lu]Lu-DOTA-Folate, [^{99m}Tc]Tc-PAMA-Cobalamin [82]	[^{68}Ga]Ga-PSMA-11, [^{177}Lu]Lu-PSMA-617, [^{177}Lu]Lu-DOTATATE, [^{131}I]I-MIBG [121–124]
Key Advantages	High Biocompatibility & Low Immunogenicity: Vitamins are endogenous, naturally processed molecules. Low Cost & Accessibility: Vitamins are inexpensive and readily available. Proven Safety Profile: Generally non-toxic at physiological doses. Potential for Multimodality: Can be integrated with nanosystems for combined imaging/therapy. Broad Applicability: Targets can be overexpressed in multiple cancer types (e.g., FRα in ovarian, breast, lung).	High Target Affinity & Specificity: Often engineered for very high binding affinity to their target. Well-Established Clinical Use: Extensive clinical data and regulatory approval for several agents. Standardized Protocols: Established dosing, administration, and safety monitoring guidelines. Predictable Biodistribution: Well-characterized pharmacokinetics and clearance pathways [123]

https://doi.org/10.3390/jpm16010036

Table 1. *Cont.*

Aspect	Vitamin-Based Radiopharmaceuticals	Conventional Radiopharmaceuticals
Key Limitations & Challenges	Receptor Heterogeneity: Expression can vary between and within tumors, leading to potential false negatives. Competition with Endogenous Vitamins: High plasma levels of natural vitamins can block binding sites. Off-Target Uptake: Specific organs (e.g., kidneys for folates, liver/kidneys for B12) can show significant accumulation, posing a toxicity risk. Limited Clinical Translation: Most agents are still in preclinical or early clinical stages. Optimization of Pharmacokinetics: Requires careful engineering (e.g., linkers, albumin binders) to improve tumor-to-background ratios.	Immunogenic Potential: Peptide and antibody-based agents can provoke immune responses. Higher Production Costs: Peptide synthesis and monoclonal antibody production are expensive. Toxicities Related to Targets: Off-target binding to healthy tissues expressing the target (e.g., salivary glands for PSMA, kidneys for SSTR). Tumor Resistance Mechanisms: Tumors can downregulate target expression under therapeutic pressure [125].
Clinical Status	Primarily preclinical and early-phase clinical trials. A few agents (e.g., EC20/^{99m}Tc-etarfolatide) have reached clinical studies but are not yet standard of care [126].	Clinically established and approved. Multiple agents are standard care (e.g., Lutathera®, Pluvicto®) for specific indications [127,128].
Ideal Use Case	Precision theranostics for tumors with confirmed overexpression of specific vitamin receptors, especially where conventional targets are absent or as part of combination nano therapy [129].	First-line theranostic approach for cancers with well-defined, highly expressed molecular targets like PSMA (prostate) or SSTR (neuroendocrine) [130].
Potential for Synergy	High potential for integration with nanoparticle drug delivery systems and as radiosensitizing/radioprotective adjuvants due to their biological roles.	Often used in combination with other systemic therapies (e.g., hormone therapy, chemotherapy) and increasingly with immunotherapy.

Table 2. Different radionuclides and targeted agents in preclinical studies with vitamins to treat various forms of cancer.

Cancer Types	Radionuclide	Targeted Agent	Results	Statistical Significance	Vitamin	Reference
Gastric cancer	^{211}At	Anti-TF mAb	Dose-dependent antitumor effects with SA protection	Significant protective effect of SA ($p < 0.05$)	Sodium Ascorbate (SA)	[43]
Gastric cancer	^{68}Ga	DOTA-RGD	High affinity and stability with tumor uptake	Tumor targeting significant ($p < 0.001$)	Folate	[45]
Gastric cancer	^{99m}Tc	HYNIC-NHHN-FA (folate conjugate)	Low tumor uptake, primarily absorbed in stomach and intestines	Tumor targeting significant ($p < 0.05$)	Folate	[50]
Gastric cancer	^{99m}Tc	HYNIC-PEG2-FA	Moderate tumor uptake; reduced uptake with excess folate	Receptor-specific targeting confirmed ($p < 0.05$)	Folate	[51]

https://doi.org/10.3390/jpm16010036

Table 2. *Cont.*

Cancer Types	Radionuclide	Targeted Agent	Results	Statistical Significance	Vitamin	Reference
Gastric cancer	^{99m}Tc	ECG-EDA-folate	Radiolabeling efficiency: >96%; decreased uptake with excess folate	specific targeting and significant reduction in tumor uptake with excess folate ($p < 0.05$)	Folic Acid	[52]
Gastric cancer	^{68}Ga	^{68}Ga-NOTA-folic acid conjugate	Radiolabeling efficiency: >95%; specific uptake by KB cells; biodistribution correlated with kidney retention.	demonstrated strong correlation between tracer and kidney retention. ($p < 0.05$)	Folic Acid	[49]
Gastric cancer	^{177}Lu	cm09 (albumin-binding folate conjugate)	Radiochemical efficiency, >98% Stability, >99% and Serum Protein Biding ~91%	extended blood circulation time enhanced tumor uptake. ($p < 0.05$)	Folic Acid	[44]
Gastric cancer	^{18}F	α- and γ-conjugated fluorinated folate derivatives	Radiochemical purity: >95%; reduced kidney uptake by 50% with γ-regioisomers.	Binding affinity IC50: 1.4–2.2 nM; biodistribution impacted by regioisomers ($p \leq 0.01$)	Folic Acid	[53]
Gastric cancer	^{18}F	3-aza-2-[^{18}F]-fluorofolic acid	High contrast imaging with minimal off-target accumulation.	demonstrated favorable properties for imaging FR-positive tumors.	Folic Acid	[54]
Gastric cancer	^{18}F	[^{18}F]-folic acid derivative	Surpassed previous ^{18}F-labeled radiofolates; highest affinity for FR-positive tumors. radiochemical purity, >95%	Considered the most promising ^{18}F-radioligand for FR-positive tumors.	Folic Acid	[55]
Gastric cancer	^{18}F	[^{18}F]F-fluorodeoxyglucose-folate	Enhanced hydrophilicity; demonstrated high specificity and affinity for folate receptors in cancers and inflammation.	demonstrated potential for clinical translation.	Folic Acid	[57]
Breast cancer	^{177}Lu	DOTA-folate	Tumor inhibition beyond 70 days (NF9006 cells)	Significant tumor growth reduction ($p < 0.01$)	Folate	[60]
Breast cancer	^{89}Zr	^{89}Zirconium-labeled cobalamin (^{89}Zr-Cbl)	6–10-fold higher uptake compared to excess CN-Cbl—High accumulation in kidneys and liver after 48 h.	demonstrated feasibility of tracer for tumor visualization. ($p \leq 0.01$)	Vitamin B12, (Cobalamin)	[65]

https://doi.org/10.3390/jpm16010036

Table 2. *Cont.*

Cancer Types	Radionuclide	Targeted Agent	Results	Statistical Significance	Vitamin	Reference
Breast cancer	^{99m}Tc	^{99m}Tc(CO)3-PTX-FR-NLC,	higher uptake in folate receptor-positive organs, radiolabeling efficiency more than 90%	Tumor accumulation significant ($p < 0.05$)	Folate	[66]
Breast cancer	^{177}Lu	^{177}Lu-DOTA-Folate-Bombesin	High tumor uptake in breast cancer models	Significant tumor inhibition ($p < 0.05$)	Folate	[61]
Breast cancer	^{99m}Tc	^{99m}Tc-Bombesin-Folate	Improved breast tumor imaging and high radiochemical purity (96 ± 2.1%)	Higher tumor-to-muscle ratio ($p < 0.05$)	Folate	[62]
Breast cancer	^{177}Lu	^{177}Lu-Dendrimer-Folate-Bombesin-Gold Nanoparticles	Effective theranostic radiopharmaceutical and radiochemical purity (>95%)	Enhanced imaging and therapy ($p < 0.05$)	Folate	[63]
Breast cancer	^{177}Lu	^{177}Lu-Folate Conjugate with Iron Oxide Nanoparticles	Tumor uptake visualized via SPECT/CT	Enhanced contrast and targeting	Folate	[64]
Breast cancer	^{99m}Tc	Radiolabeled Folate-Conjugated Liposomes	Increased tumor-specific imaging	High affinity for folate receptors ($p < 0.05$)	Folate	[68]
Breast cancer	^{153}Sm	^{153}Sm-Folate-PEI-Chitosan Nanoparticles	High radiochemical purity, (>90%)	Significant tumor localization	Folate	[69]
Breast cancer	^{99m}Tc	^{99m}Tc-HYNFA	Improved imaging contrast and labeling yield: 97–98%; radiochemical purity: 96–98%	Statistically significant uptake ($p < 0.05$)	Folate	[70]
Colorectal cancer	^{64}Cu	B12-en-Bn-NOTA	Tumor uptake: 2.20–4.84% ID/g at 6 h	Tumor uptake significantly reduced with excess B12 ($p < 0.05$)	Vitamin B12	[74]
Colorectal cancer	^{111}In	MORAb-003	Significant tumor uptake (32 ± 5% ID/g at 4 days)	Validated in small group of patients	Folate	[77]
Colorectal cancer	^{89}Zr	^{89}Zr-Labeled Folic Acid-Conjugated Silica	High receptor-specific binding	Strong PET signals	Folic acid	[79]

https://doi.org/10.3390/jpm16010036

Table 2. *Cont.*

Cancer Types	Radionuclide	Targeted Agent	Results	Statistical Significance	Vitamin	Reference
Colorectal cancer	^{64}Cu	^{64}Cu-Folate-Shell Cross-Linked Nanoparticles	Targeted tumor uptake	Effective biodistribution ($p = 0.0001$)	Folate	[75]
Colorectal cancer	^{68}Ga	^{68}Ga-HBED-CC-EDBE-Folate	High radiochemical purity (98%)	Selective tumor accumulation	Folate	[80]
Colorectal cancer	^{99m}Tc	^{99m}Tc-PAMA-Cobalamin	High tumor specificity in clinical study	Improved tumor imaging	Vitamin B12	[82]
Brain cancer	^{18}F	[^{18}F]FOL	Superior tumor-to-brain uptake ratio (TBR) compared to FDG And radiochemical purity was 97.5% ± 1.6	TBR statistically higher for [^{18}F]FOL ($p < 0.05$)	Folate	[88]
Brain cancer	^{18}F	[^{18}F]AlF-NOTA-Folate	Good tumor uptake with reduced kidney accumulation	High specificity and rapid clearance	Folate	[89]
Brain cancer	^{99m}Tc	Vitamin C-coated selenium nanoparticles (SeNPs)	Radiolabeling yield: 96 ± 2%—Stability maintained for over 6 h	demonstrated suitable target-to-non-target ratios in solid tumors.	Vitamin C	[91]
Brain cancer	^{99m}Tc	Radiolabeled Folate Micellar Carriers	High efficiency for brain tumors	Enhanced SPECT imaging ($p < 0.001$)	Folate	[92]
Brain cancer	^{66}Ga, ^{68}Ga	^{66}Ga/^{68}Ga-Folate Conjugates	Tumor uptake validated via PET	High specificity	Folate	[94]
Brain cancer	^{64}Cu	PET/NIR-II Fluorescence Folate Probe	Dual-modality imaging	Enhanced tumor detection ($p < 0.0001$)	Folate	[90]
Brain cancer	^{99m}Tc	^{99m}Tc-Radiolabeled Benzothiazole-Folate	Very high Radiochemicla purity, >99%	Significant uptake observed	Folate	[93]
Brain cancer	^{68}Ga	^{68}Ga-Pteroyl-Lys Conjugates	Selective folate receptor binding and favorable radiolabeling yield (>90%), higher tumor-to-non target ratio	Improved PET contrast, ($p < 0.05$)	Folate	[95]

https://doi.org/10.3390/jpm16010036

Table 2. *Cont.*

Cancer Types	Radionuclide	Targeted Agent	Results	Statistical Significance	Vitamin	Reference
Prostate cancer	^{57}Co, ^{111}In	Radiolabeled vitamin B12 derivatives	Reduced systemic distribution with improved tumor-to-blood ratio.	emphasized improvements in targeted accumulation. ($p < 0.001$)	Vitamin B12	[105]
Prostate cancer	^{99m}Tc	^{99m}Tc-Folate-PEG-Doxorubicin	Antitumor efficiency, radiolabeling yield greater than 90%	Enhanced tumor accumulation ($p < 0.05$)	Folate	[97]
Prostate cancer	^{18}F	^{18}F-Click Radiolabeled Folate	High tumor targeting And radiochemical purity, >95%.	PET-imaging validated	Folate	[102]
Prostate cancer	^{99m}Tc	^{99m}Tc-EC20	High radiochemical yield (>95%)	Superior tumor-to-background contrast	Folate	[99]
Prostate cancer	^{99m}Tc	^{99m}Tc-Labeled Vitamin C	Maximum Radiolabeling yield, $93 \pm 5.0\%$	Favorable pharmacokinetics ($p < 0.05$)	Vitamin C	[103]
Prostate cancer	^{99m}Tc	^{99m}Tc-Dimeric Folic Acid	Strong FR-targeting, (IC50 = 19.06 nM)	High tumor specificity ($p < 0.05$)	Folate	[100]
Prostate cancer	^{99m}Tc	^{99m}Tc-Folate-Isonitrile Complexes	High radiochemical purity, >95%	Improved receptor binding And significant biodistribution ($p < 0.05$, $p < 0.01$)	Folate	[101]
Prostate cancer	^{99m}Tc	^{99m}Tc-Vitamin B12 Derivative	Abolished TC binding for selective uptake and radiochemical purity of PAMA-4-B12 was >95%,	Significant tumor targeting	Vitamin B12	[104]
Ovarian cancer	^{125}I, ^{131}I	[^{125}I]-2 and [$^{125/131}I$]-4 folate conjugates	High stability, FR-specific binding, strong tumor accumulation	Pre-injection with pemetrexed improved imaging ($p < 0.05$)	Folate	[110]
Ovarian cancer	^{18}F	[^{18}F]-2-folate	High radiochemical yield (>80%), purity (>97%), significant tumor uptake	Micro-PET imaging confirmed results ($p < 0.05$)	Folate	[112]
Ovarian cancer	^{18}F	[^{18}F]-FDG-folate and [^{18}F]-8	High yield (>80%), purity (>98%), receptor specificity confirmed	Blocking experiments validated specificity ($p < 0.05$)	Folate	[113]
Ovarian cancer	^{124}I	[^{124}I]-SIB- and [^{124}I]-SIP-folate	High radiochemical yield (>90% and >60%), purity (>98%), strong tumor targeting	Effective tumor uptake in vivo ($p < 0.05$)	Folate	[111]

https://doi.org/10.3390/jpm16010036

Table 2. *Cont.*

Cancer Types	Radionuclide	Targeted Agent	Results	Statistical Significance	Vitamin	Reference
Ovarian cancer	^{47}Sc, ^{177}Lu, ^{90}Y	^{47}Sc-DOTA-folate, ^{177}Lu-folate, ^{90}Y-folate	Tumor growth inhibition (39–43 days vs. 26 days in controls), no severe side effects	^{90}Y-folate showed the highest potency ($p < 0.05$)	Folate	[114]
Ovarian cancer	^{177}Lu	^{177}Lu-FA-DOTA-PEG-PLGA nanoparticles	High labeling efficiency (97–98%), minimal kidney accumulation, tumor localization confirmed	Significant tumor inhibition, no major toxicity ($p < 0.05$)	Folic acid	[115]
Ovarian cancer	^{188}Re	^{188}Re-folate-CDDP/HAS MNP	Apoptosis rates reached 57.16% and significant inhibition tumor growth	Triple combination therapy showed strongest tumor suppression ($p < 0.05$)	Folate	[117]
Ovarian cancer	^{99m}Tc	^{99m}Tc-NP-PEGFA (Folate-functionalized cisplatin nanoparticles)	High cellular uptake	Enhanced blood circulation and tumor accumulation ($p < 0.05$)	Folate	[118]

In contrast, vitamin B12-based agents generally exhibited more moderate but still significant tumor uptake. The PET tracer [^{64}Cu] Cu−B12−en−Bn−NOTA showed uptake in the range of 2.20–4.84% ID/g. A key challenge for B12 derivatives has been high renal accumulation, as seen with.

When comparing radionuclides, diagnostic pairs provided critical insights. For example, studies using the theranostic pair ^{68}Ga (for PET) and ^{177}Lu (for therapy) for the same folate vector often showed correlative high uptake, validating the theranostic principle. The tumor uptake ratios between these isotopes were generally consistent within the same targeting platform, supporting the use of ^{68}Ga imaging for predicting ^{177}Lu therapy efficacy.

A cross-cancer comparison further elucidates the versatility of these agents. The highest tumor uptake values were frequently reported in KB (nasopharyngeal) and ovarian cancer models, which are known for their high folate receptor (FR) expression. For example, folate conjugates in FR-positive KB tumors consistently yielded uptake values above 5% ID/g, with many studies reporting >10% ID/g [44,95]. This contrasts with some gastric and brain cancer models, where initial folate tracers showed lower or more variable uptake (e.g., ~1.7% ID/g in brain [89]), potentially due to differences in FR density, vascularization, or the blood–brain barrier.

Statistical trends from the compiled data (with significance often reported as $p < 0.05$ or higher) confirm that receptor specificity is a major driver of uptake. Blocking experiments with excess cold folate or B12 consistently resulted in a statistically significant reduction (often >50–95%) in tumor accumulation, underscoring the receptor-mediated mechanism.

Conclusion of Meta-Analysis: This quantitative synthesis underscores that folate-based radiopharmaceuticals, particularly those optimized with pharmacokinetic modifiers like PEG or albumin-binding motifs, achieve the highest tumor uptake ratios among vitamin-based agents. While vitamin B12 derivatives show promise, their clinical translation may require further engineering to improve tumor-to-kidney ratios. The consistent performance of the $^{68}Ga/^{177}Lu$-folate pair across studies solidifies its role as a leading candidate for theranostic applications in FR-positive cancers. Future research should focus on standardizing uptake reporting and conducting direct, comparative studies of different vitamin ligands within the same model system to definitively rank their efficacy.

10. Comparison Between Vitamin-Based and Conventional Radiopharmaceuticals

The development of radiopharmaceuticals has evolved from conventional agents targeting specific pathways to innovative vitamin-based systems that exploit the metabolic dependencies of cancer cells. Table 1 below summarizes the key differences, advantages, and challenges between these two approaches.

11. Discussion

This review synthesizes a substantial body of preclinical (from in vitro to in vivo) evidence demonstrating the significant promise of vitamin-based radiopharmaceuticals and nanosystems within the evolving paradigm of precision oncology and theranostics. The rationale behind this approach lies in the elegant exploitation of endogenous biological pathways; vitamins such as folate (B9) and cobalamin (B12) serve as ideal targeting ligands due to their high biocompatibility, low immunogenic potential, and the frequent overexpression of their corresponding receptors on a wide spectrum of tumor cells. The experimental pathway, from the in vitro conjugation and radiolabeling of vitamins to their validation in animal models, consistently demonstrates that these constructs, including prominent examples like [^{68}Ga]Ga-DOTA-folate and [^{177}Lu]Lu-DOTA-folate, exhibit exceptional tumor specificity. This enables not only high-contrast molecular imaging via PET and SPECT but also targeted radionuclide therapy, thereby localizing cytotoxic effects to malignant tissue while largely sparing healthy surroundings. Furthermore, integration of these vitamins into advanced nanosystems further augments their potential by improving pharmacokinetics, prolonging circulation, and enhancing tumor accumulation through both passive targeting and active receptor-mediated uptake.

A critical comparative analysis of the data reveals distinct profiles for different vitamin-based strategies. Folate-based systems currently represent the most advanced and extensively studied class, often achieving remarkably high tumor uptake values, sometimes exceeding 17% ID/g, though they are frequently challenged by significant renal accumulation, an issue that has been creatively mitigated through the use of albumin-binding entities and PEG linkers. In contrast, vitamin B12 derivatives typically exhibit more moderate tumor uptake and face a different primary hurdle: off-target accumulation in the liver and kidneys due to binding with endogenous transport proteins, a challenge that newer derivatives are being engineered to bypass. When compared to conventional, clinically established radiopharmaceuticals such as [^{177}Lu]Lu-PSMA-617, vitamin-based agents offer distinct advantages in terms of low cost and inherent biocompatibility. However, the conventional agents currently hold a superior position in terms of proven clinical efficacy and standardized use for specific indications. This positions vitamin-based theranostics not as a replacement, but as a complementary arsenal, particularly valuable for targeting tumors that lack conventional biomarkers but overexpress vitamin receptors.

Looking forward, a critical evaluation of the field highlights several promising yet underexplored avenues. The research focus has been disproportionately placed on folate and B12, leaving the substantial potential of other vitamins, such as the radioprotective Vitamin E or the receptor-targeting Vitamin A, largely untapped. Furthermore, the true power of these agents may lie in their synergistic potential with other treatment modalities. Preclinical studies, such as those combining [^{177}Lu]Lu-DOTA-folate with immunotherapy,

https://doi.org/10.3390/jpm16010036

demonstrate a powerful capacity to modulate the tumor microenvironment and enhance overall antitumor efficacy, paving the way for novel combination regimens. Some strategies, such as nanoparticles, antibody–drug conjugates, and glutathione-sensing systems, demonstrate complementary roles in theranostics, with each offering distinct advantages in diagnosis, treatment, or both. Several radiolabeled antibodies, including those with [^{99m}Tc] and [^{177}Lu], have successfully localized tumors and exerted potent cytotoxic effects. In particular, [^{99m}Tc] is successfully used for diagnostic purposes in tumor localization in SPECT; similarly, although [^{177}Lu] has been applied as a therapeutic radionuclide, demonstrating potent cytotoxic effects on tumors, it can also be monitored during regression through SPECT imaging, allowing for precise detection and monitoring which shows how these two radionuclides are often used in parallel in in vitro experiments. The FDA has approved several well-established radiopharmaceutical agents for use in oncology, including [^{177}Lu]lu-PSMA-617, [^{177}Lu]lu-DOTATATE, [^{131}I]I-iobenguane (MIBG), 223Ra-dichloride, [^{90}Y]Y-ibritumomab tiuxetan, and [^{153}Sm]Sm-EDTMP [131].

This integrated perspective demonstrates the utility of endogenous biomolecules, such as vitamins, for advanced therapeutic applications. Owing to their good biocompatibility, low immunogenic profile, and well-defined metabolic roles, vitamins serve as exemplary molecular scaffolds for the development of targeted radiopharmaceuticals. The experimental pathway, culminating in these applications, is delineated in Figure 5. This schematic summarizes the workflow from in vitro assessment of vitamin conjugates through to pre-clinical validation and potential clinical translation, specifying the key analytical methodologies employed at each stage of the investigative process.

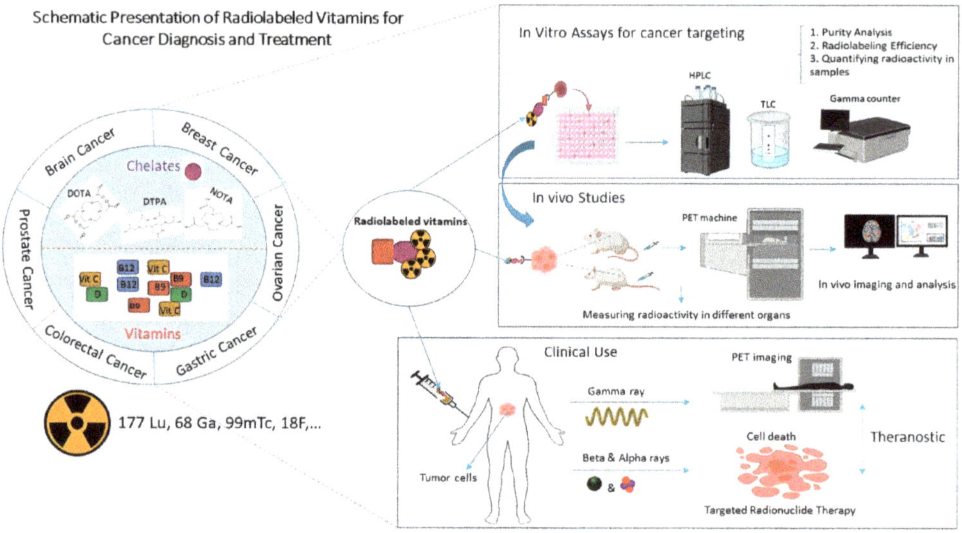

Figure 5. An illustration of the experimental workflow, from in vitro experiments involving vitamins to clinical applications. This schematic presents a theranostic approach to radiolabeled vitamins in various cancers. Radiopharmaceuticals bind to cancer cells selectively, enabling accurate PET/SPECT imaging and targeted radionuclide therapy. In vitro, assays ensure radiolabeling efficiency, while in vivo studies analyze tumor specificity. In clinical studies, gamma emissions aid imaging, whereas beta and alpha particles induce the cancer cells' apoptosis, enhancing personalized cancer treatment approaches.

Despite this promising trajectory, the clinical translation of these innovative systems is contingent upon a clear-eyed acknowledgment of current limitations. A primary constraint

https://doi.org/10.3390/jpm16010036

is the overwhelming reliance on preclinical data; in vitro and small-animal models cannot fully capture the complexity of human tumors and their microenvironments, therefore a robust clinical evaluation is required. The field is also hampered by a lack of standardization in study designs and reporting, making direct comparisons between different agents challenging. Many studies, while demonstrating excellent tumor targeting, lack comprehensive long-term biodistribution and toxicity profiles, especially concerning chronic radiation effects on critical organs like the kidneys. Finally, significant translational barriers persist, including the challenges of scaling up the synthesis of complex nanoconstructs under GMP conditions, navigating regulatory pathways for combination products, and the high costs associated with clinical trials for radiotherapeutics.

Additionally, consistent with precision oncology principles, therapeutic resistance may arise from heterogeneous FR expression, altered receptor recycling, microenvironment-induced modulation, or compensatory folate transport pathways, all of which can reduce the efficacy of FR-targeted imaging or therapy. Integrating these biological, pharmacokinetic, and dosimetric considerations provides a more critical and clinically realistic framework for advancing FR-targeted theranostics. Selecting an appropriate starting dose is important to ensure patient safety, to enable efficiency in reaching the therapeutically relevant dose range [132], and to use data from animal model species and human equivalent models to establish safe starting dosages for first-in-human clinical trials [133]. For instance, the outcome of the therapeutic dose administered is shown in these studies [134,135]. Most studies have employed folate modification to target folate receptor alpha (FRα), which is considered the most therapeutically relevant folate receptor isoform in solid tumors. Also, FRα is preferentially overexpressed in chromosomal instability (CIN)-type gastric cancer, that represented in the majority of the GC studies we mentioned. Although heterogeneity exists between FRα and folate receptor beta (FRβ), most studies have demonstrated that folate-modified agents preferably accumulate in tumors via FRα-mediated endocytosis. Nevertheless, FRα expression may decrease adaptively in response to repeated ligand exposure or therapeutic pressure, potentially reducing tracer accumulation and therapeutic efficacy. Recognizing this receptor plasticity is crucial for optimizing folate-based theranostics and for the development of effective targeting strategies.

Recent advances in nanotechnology have demonstrated considerable potential for developing greener and more cost-effective large-scale technologies, including environmentally sustainable biological processes such as green synthesis. These [136,137] innovations enhance the precision of therapeutic interventions and enable the creation of multifunctional delivery platforms that integrate diagnostic imaging with therapeutic modalities, offering substantial promise for the development of more effective treatment strategies. Thus, future research should focus on the development of advanced molecular designs, exploring innovative biomarkers, and the integration of these therapies with existing modalities, such as immunotherapy, to achieve synergistic outcomes. Realizing the potential of theranostic radionuclides for personalized oncology will be crucial. Further, radioimmunotherapy [138], which combines radiotherapy with immunotherapy, is one of the most advanced treatments, even for the most aggressive forms of cancer, including those resistant to conventional therapies. The support of new Artificial Intelligence tools encompasses an entire treatment process that can be optimized through machine learning [139,140], particularly deep learning algorithms [141]. These technologies can improve dosimetry and treatment response assessment (from in vitro to in vivo), thereby enhancing overall efficiency and personalization in the medical oncology field [142,143], especially in molecular imaging and TRT. The experimental evidence discussed in the manuscript is summarized in Table 2.

https://doi.org/10.3390/jpm16010036

12. Conclusions

Providing exceptional selectivity for both imaging and therapeutic applications, radionuclides play a crucial role in precision medicine. Depending on the radionuclide used, these agents enable targeted imaging and destruction of tumor cells while minimizing damage to surrounding healthy tissues. In this context, vitamin-based radiopharmaceuticals and nanosystems have emerged as an innovative class of agents in oncology and theranostics. Their unique molecular design combines the selective targeting ability of vitamins with the functional versatility of nanomaterials, allowing for improved diagnostic sensitivity and enhanced therapeutic efficacy. Ongoing advancements in radionuclide attachment methods, radiolabeling efficiency, and molecular design continue to strengthen their potential as dual diagnostic and therapeutic platforms, while also aiming to reduce systemic toxicity and improve biocompatibility.

Comparatively, vitamin-functionalized nanosystems offer several advantages over conventional radiopharmaceuticals. Incorporating vitamin ligands, such as folate, facilitates receptor-specific targeting, enhanced cellular uptake, and prolonged circulation. Due to its strong affinity for folate receptors, which are overexpressed in a wide range of malignancies, folate has been studied most extensively among these compounds. Comparing folate-conjugated nanosystems with non-targeted radiolabeled systems, folate-conjugated nanosystems demonstrate superior tumor localization and reduced non-specific biodistribution. However, while folate-based targeting has achieved significant progress in preclinical settings, its clinical translation faces challenges related to heterogeneity in receptor expression and potential interference from endogenous folate. Other vitamins, including vitamins A, C, D, and E, although less investigated, show promise for their radioprotective and antioxidant properties. Vitamin E [144], in particular, has demonstrated the ability to mitigate oxidative stress and radiation-induced tissue injury, suggesting its potential utility as an adjuvant for improving radionuclide therapeutic efficacy.

A critical evaluation of existing studies reveals that, despite substantial progress, significant challenges remain in the optimization and translation of vitamin-based radiopharmaceuticals. One major limitation lies in the stability of radionuclide conjugations with nanocarriers, as unstable linkages can lead to premature release, suboptimal targeting, and unintended systemic exposure. Moreover, radiolabeling efficiency continues to play a key role in both diagnostic accuracy and therapeutic effectiveness. The majority of the available data are derived from in vitro experiments or small-animal models, providing limited insight into pharmacokinetics, dosimetry, long-term safety, and immunogenicity for humans. Furthermore, vitamins play a dual role in radioprotection and radiosensitization. While antioxidant vitamins such as C and E may protect healthy tissues from oxidative damage, if they are not precisely targeted or controlled, they may also attenuate the cytotoxic effects of radionuclide therapy. Therefore, the development of smart nanosystems capable of spatiotemporal regulation of vitamin release within the tumor microenvironment is essential to maximize therapeutic benefits without compromising tumoricidal efficacy.

Vitamin-based radiopharmaceuticals and nanosystems possess several promising biological and therapeutic properties, but their cost-effectiveness is one of the most important considerations for their widespread adoption and clinical translation. Traditional radiopharmaceuticals often involve complex synthesis procedures, expensive targeting ligands such as monoclonal antibodies, and costly radionuclide production processes, which collectively increase overall treatment expense. In contrast, vitamins offer a more economical and readily available class of targeting molecules due to their natural abundance, low molecular weight, and ease of chemical modification. This intrinsic affordability may substantially reduce production costs, especially when integrated into scalable nanoparticle synthesis methods. Furthermore, vitamin-functionalized nanosystems have the potential

https://doi.org/10.3390/jpm16010036

to enhance therapeutic precision, thereby decreasing the need for repeated imaging or treatment cycles, which in turn lowers healthcare costs associated with extended hospital stays and adverse effects management. However, comprehensive cost–benefit analyses remain limited, and economic evaluations comparing vitamin-based nanosystems with conventional radiopharmaceuticals are necessary. Future studies should incorporate pharmacoeconomic modeling to assess the long-term financial sustainability of these systems in clinical oncology, balancing innovation with affordability to ensure equitable patient access to advanced radiotheranostic therapies.

Consequently, vitamin-based radiopharmaceuticals and nanosystems hold significant potential to revolutionize precision oncology and theranostics. With continued innovation in molecular engineering, radionuclide conjugation chemistry, and targeted delivery strategies, these systems offer the potential to improve therapeutic selectivity, minimize systemic toxicity, and enable personalized treatment approaches. Despite the widespread use of folate-based nanosystems, exploring other vitamin ligands with radiosensitizing and radioprotective properties could lead to the development of next-generation radiotheranostic technology. Ultimately, the integration of vitamin-functionalized nanosystems into radionuclide therapy may provide a novel approach to cancer treatment, bridging the gap between molecular imaging, targeted therapy, and patient-centered precision medicine.

Supplementary Materials: The following supporting information can be downloaded at: https://www.mdpi.com/article/10.3390/jpm16010036/s1, Table S1: PRISMA checklist.

Author Contributions: Conceptualization, V.B.; methodology, G.B., A.C. and V.B.; investigation, G.B., M.A., A.C. and V.B.; resources, G.B., P.A., M.A., G.S., C.L., D.D.R., A.T., A.C. and V.B.; data curation, A.C. and V.B.; writing—original draft preparation, G.B. and V.B.; writing—review and editing, G.B., P.A., M.A., G.S., C.L., A.C. and V.B.; visualization, G.B., P.A., M.A., D.D.R., A.T., A.C. and V.B.; supervision, A.C. and V.B.; project administration, A.C.; funding acquisition, P.A. and A.C. All authors have read and agreed to the published version of the manuscript.

Funding: This work was partially supported by the following grant and project: "RADIATIONS" under the PNRR—Next Generation EU, Mission 4, Component 2—Investment 1.5—Cascading Call—Ecosystem of Innovation "THE—Tuscany Health Ecosystem"—code ECS00000017—CUP B83C22003930001, to Albert Comelli; CN00000033, CUP B73C21001300006 from National Center 5 "National Biodiversity Future Center" to Muhammad Ali and Albert Comelli; "INNOVA"—Advanced Diagnostic, Project promoted by Italian Ministry of Health—PNC-E3-2022-23681266 PNCHTS-DA 1, CUP D73C22OO2090001, to Viviana Benfante and Pierpaolo Alongi.

Institutional Review Board Statement: Not applicable.

Informed Consent Statement: Not applicable.

Data Availability Statement: No new data were created or analyzed in this study.

Conflicts of Interest: The authors declare no conflicts of interest.

Abbreviations

Anti-TF mAb	anti-tissue factor monoclonal antibody
^{211}At	astatine-211
ADCs	antibody–drug conjugates
B9	Folate
BC	breast cancer
CIN	chromosomal instability
Cbl	Cobalamin
CDC	silica nanoparticle drug conjugate
CTLA-4	cytotoxic T-lymphocyte antigen 4

https://doi.org/10.3390/jpm16010036

^{57}Co	cobalt-57
^{64}Cu	copper-64
DDS	drug delivery system
DOTA-Mal	maleimido-mono-amide-DOTA
DOX	Doxorubicin
EBV	Epstein–Barr virus
EGFR	epidermal growth factor receptor
FR	folate receptor
FRA	folate receptor alpha
FA-NPs	folate-decorated nanoparticles
^{18}F	fluorine-18
FA	folic acid
FAP	fibroblast activation protein
^{68}Ga	gallium-68
GC	gastric cancer
Gd	Gliadin
GRPR	gastrin-releasing peptide receptors
GBM	glioblastoma multiforme
GS	genomically stable
GEP	Gastroenteropancreatic
HYNIC	hydrazinonicotinic acid
HPLC	high-performance liquid chromatography
HGSC	high-grade serous carcinoma
^{111}In	indium-111
^{124}I	iodine-124
^{125}I	iodine-125
^{131}I	iodine-131
LET	linear Energy Transfer
^{177}Lu	lutetium-177
mAb	monoclonal antibody
MT1-MMP	membrane type-1 matrix metalloproteinase
MRI	magnetic resonance imaging
MDR	multidrug resistance
MSI	microsatellite instability
mCRPC	metastatic castration-resistant prostate cancer
NLCs	nanostructure lipid carriers
NET	neuroendocrine neoplasms
OC	ovarian cancer
PET	positron emission tomography
PEG	polyethylene glycol
PSMA	prostate-specific membrane antigen
PAMAM	poly(amidoamine)
PTX	Paclitaxel
PRRT	peptide receptor radionuclide therapy
^{188}Re	rhenium-188
SA	sodium ascorbate
^{47}Sc	scandium 47
^{153}Sm	samarium-153
SeNPs	selenium nanoparticles
SNPs	silica nanoparticles
SCKs	shell cross-linked nanoparticles
SMWs	micro-scale silica wires
SPECT	Single-photon emission computed tomography
SSTR	somatostatin receptor

https://doi.org/10.3390/jpm16010036

TRT	targeted radionuclide therapy
^{99m}Tc	technetium-99m
TPP	triphenylphosphonium
TLC	Thin-layer chromatography
TC	transcobalamin
TC-II	transcobalamin II
TBR	tumor-to-brain uptake ratio
UPN	uncoated nanoparticles
VEGFR	Vascular endothelial growth factor
WHO	world health organization
^{90}Y	yttrium-90
^{89}Zr	zirconium-89

References

1. Ayalew, B.D.; Abdullah; Khan, S.M.; Alemayehu, Z.G.; Teferi, M.G.; Aboye, B.T.; Woldeyohannes, E.M.; Sime, B.L.; Tewodros, Y.T.; Hundisa, M.I. Role of Emerging Theranostic Technologies in Precision Oncology: Revolutionizing Cancer Diagnosis and Treatment. *Oncologie* **2025**, *27*, 229–238. [CrossRef]
2. Crișan, G.; Moldovean-Cioroianu, N.S.; Timaru, D.-G.; Andrieș, G.; Căinap, C.; Chiș, V. Radiopharmaceuticals for PET and SPECT Imaging: A Literature Review over the Last Decade. *Int. J. Mol. Sci.* **2022**, *23*, 5023. [CrossRef]
3. Cuocolo, A.; Petretta, M. PET and SPECT Specialty Grand Challenge. When Knowledge Travels at the Speed of Light, Photons Take to the Field. *Front. Nucl. Med.* **2021**, *1*, 671914. [CrossRef]
4. Benfante, V.; Stefano, A.; Ali, M.; Laudicella, R.; Arancio, W.; Cucchiara, A.; Caruso, F.; Cammarata, F.P.; Coronnello, C.; Russo, G.; et al. An Overview of In Vitro Assays of 64Cu-, 68Ga-, 125I-, and 99mTc-Labelled Radiopharmaceuticals Using Radiometric Counters in the Era of Radiotheranostics. *Diagnostics* **2023**, *13*, 1210. [CrossRef] [PubMed]
5. Piras, A.; Corso, R.; Benfante, V.; Ali, M.; Laudicella, R.; Alongi, P.; D'Aviero, A.; Cusumano, D.; Boldrini, L.; Salvaggio, G.; et al. Artificial Intelligence and Statistical Models for the Prediction of Radiotherapy Toxicity in Prostate Cancer: A Systematic Review. *Appl. Sci.* **2024**, *14*, 10947. [CrossRef]
6. Qaim, S.M.; Spahn, I. Development of Novel Radionuclides for Medical Applications. *Label. Compd. Radiopharm.* **2018**, *61*, 126–140. [CrossRef] [PubMed]
7. Lau, J.; Rousseau, E.; Kwon, D.; Lin, K.-S.; Bénard, F.; Chen, X. Insight into the Development of PET Radiopharmaceuticals for Oncology. *Cancers* **2020**, *12*, 1312. [CrossRef]
8. Pavone, A.M.; Benfante, V.; Giaccone, P.; Stefano, A.; Torrisi, F.; Russo, V.; Serafini, D.; Richiusa, S.; Pometti, M.; Scopelliti, F.; et al. Biodistribution Assessment of a Novel 68Ga-Labeled Radiopharmaceutical in a Cancer Overexpressing CCK2R Mouse Model: Conventional and Radiomics Methods for Analysis. *Life* **2024**, *14*, 409. [CrossRef]
9. Holik, H.A.; Ibrahim, F.M.; Elaine, A.A.; Putra, B.D.; Achmad, A.; Kartamihardja, A.H.S. The Chemical Scaffold of Theranostic Radiopharmaceuticals: Radionuclide, Bifunctional Chelator, and Pharmacokinetics Modifying Linker. *Molecules* **2022**, *27*, 3062. [CrossRef]
10. Benfante, V.; Stefano, A.; Comelli, A.; Giaccone, P.; Cammarata, F.P.; Richiusa, S.; Scopelliti, F.; Pometti, M.; Ficarra, M.; Cosentino, S.; et al. A New Preclinical Decision Support System Based on PET Radiomics: A Preliminary Study on the Evaluation of an Innovative 64Cu-Labeled Chelator in Mouse Models. *J. Imaging* **2022**, *8*, 92. [CrossRef]
11. Lepareur, N.; Ramée, B.; Mougin-Degraef, M.; Bourgeois, M. Clinical Advances and Perspectives in Targeted Radionuclide Therapy. *Pharmaceutics* **2023**, *15*, 1733. [CrossRef]
12. Sgouros, G.; Bodei, L.; McDevitt, M.R.; Nedrow, J.R. Radiopharmaceutical Therapy in Cancer: Clinical Advances and Challenges. *Nat. Rev. Drug Discov.* **2020**, *19*, 589–608. [CrossRef]
13. Stokke, C.; Kvassheim, M.; Blakkisrud, J. Radionuclides for Targeted Therapy: Physical Properties. *Molecules* **2022**, *27*, 5429. [CrossRef] [PubMed]
14. Sahin, M.C.; Sanli, S. Vitamin-Based Radiopharmaceuticals for Tumor Imaging. *Med. Oncol.* **2023**, *40*, 165. [CrossRef] [PubMed]
15. Lledó, I.; Ibáñez, B.; Melero, A.; Montoro, A.; Merino-Torres, J.F.; San Onofre, N.; Soriano, J.M. Vitamins and Radioprotective Effect: A Review. *Antioxidants* **2023**, *12*, 611. [CrossRef]
16. Giaccone, P.; Benfante, V.; Stefano, A.; Cammarata, F.P.; Russo, G.; Comelli, A. PET Images Atlas-Based Segmentation Performed in Native and in Template Space: A Radiomics Repeatability Study in Mouse Models. In *Image Analysis and Processing—ICIAP 2022 Workshops*; Mazzeo, P.L., Frontoni, E., Sclaroff, S., Distante, C., Eds.; Lecture Notes in Computer Science; Springer International Publishing: Cham, Switzerland, 2022; Volume 13373, pp. 351–361, ISBN 978-3-031-13320-6.

https://doi.org/10.3390/jpm16010036

17. Moudgalya, S.S.; Cahill, N.D.; Borkholder, D.A. Deep Volumetric Segmentation of Murine Cochlear Compartments from Micro-Computed Tomography Images. In Proceedings of the 2020 42nd Annual International Conference of the IEEE Engineering in Medicine & Biology Society (EMBC), Montreal, QC, Canada, 20–24 July 2020; pp. 1970–1975.
18. Shahrokhi, P.; Farahani, A.M.; Tamaddondar, M. Radiolabeled Vitamins as the Potential Diagnostic Probes for Targeted Tumor Imaging. *Bioorganic Chem.* **2022**, *122*, 105717. [CrossRef]
19. Sallam, M.; Nguyen, N.-T.; Sainsbury, F.; Kimizuka, N.; Muyldermans, S.; Benešová-Schäfer, M. PSMA-Targeted Radiotheranostics in Modern Nuclear Medicine: Then, Now, and What of the Future? *Theranostics* **2024**, *14*, 3043–3079. [CrossRef] [PubMed]
20. Ali, M.; Benfante, V.; Di Raimondo, D.; Salvaggio, G.; Tuttolomondo, A.; Comelli, A. Recent Developments in Nanoparticle Formulations for Resveratrol Encapsulation as an Anticancer Agent. *Pharmaceuticals* **2024**, *17*, 126. [CrossRef]
21. Eslami, M.; Memarsadeghi, O.; Davarpanah, A.; Arti, A.; Nayernia, K.; Behnam, B. Overcoming Chemotherapy Resistance in Metastatic Cancer: A Comprehensive Review. *Biomedicines* **2024**, *12*, 183. [CrossRef]
22. Bayda, S.; Adeel, M.; Tuccinardi, T.; Cordani, M.; Rizzolio, F. The History of Nanoscience and Nanotechnology: From Chemical–Physical Applications to Nanomedicine. *Molecules* **2019**, *25*, 112. [CrossRef]
23. Fortune, A.; Aime, A.; Raymond, D.; Kumar, S. Nanotechnology in Medicine: A Double-Edged Sword for Health Outcomes. *Health Nanotechnol.* **2025**, *1*, 9. [CrossRef]
24. Sudimack, J.; Lee, R.J. Targeted Drug Delivery via the Folate Receptor. *Adv. Drug Deliv. Rev.* **2000**, *41*, 147–162. [CrossRef]
25. Yao, Y.; Zhou, Y.; Liu, L.; Xu, Y.; Chen, Q.; Wang, Y.; Wu, S.; Deng, Y.; Zhang, J.; Shao, A. Nanoparticle-Based Drug Delivery in Cancer Therapy and Its Role in Overcoming Drug Resistance. *Front. Mol. Biosci.* **2020**, *7*, 193. [CrossRef] [PubMed]
26. Binnemars-Postma, K.; Storm, G.; Prakash, J. Nanomedicine Strategies to Target Tumor-Associated Macrophages. *Int. J. Mol. Sci.* **2017**, *18*, 979. [CrossRef]
27. Kalli, K.R.; Oberg, A.L.; Keeney, G.L.; Christianson, T.J.H.; Low, P.S.; Knutson, K.L.; Hartmann, L.C. Folate Receptor Alpha as a Tumor Target in Epithelial Ovarian Cancer. *Gynecol. Oncol.* **2008**, *108*, 619–626. [CrossRef]
28. Fadul, A.; Abdalla, E.; Mohamed, A.; Ali, B.; Elamin, N.; Alsayed, A.; Al-Mashdali, A.; Singh, K.; Mohamed, S. Elevated Vitamin B12 Levels in Myeloproliferative Neoplasm (MPN) Patients: A Potential Diagnostic and Prognostic Marker. *JBM* **2024**, *15*, 549–556. [CrossRef]
29. Husseiny, M.M.A.E.; Nilsson, R. The Role of B12 Deficiency and Methionine Synthase in Methionine-Dependent Cancer Cells. *Cancer Metab.* **2025**, *13*, 34. [CrossRef] [PubMed]
30. Moher, D.; Liberati, A.; Tetzlaff, J.; Altman, D.G.; The PRISMA Group. Preferred Reporting Items for Systematic Reviews and Meta-Analyses: The PRISMA Statement. *PLoS Med.* **2009**, *6*, e1000097. [CrossRef] [PubMed]
31. Sung, H.; Ferlay, J.; Siegel, R.L.; Laversanne, M.; Soerjomataram, I.; Jemal, A.; Bray, F. Global Cancer Statistics 2020: GLOBOCAN Estimates of Incidence and Mortality Worldwide for 36 Cancers in 185 Countries. *CA Cancer J. Clin.* **2021**, *71*, 209–249. [CrossRef]
32. Siegel, R.L.; Miller, K.D.; Jemal, A. Cancer Statistics, 2019. *CA Cancer J. Clin.* **2019**, *69*, 7–34. [CrossRef]
33. Leake, P.-A.; Cardoso, R.; Seevaratnam, R.; Lourenco, L.; Helyer, L.; Mahar, A.; Law, C.; Coburn, N.G. A Systematic Review of the Accuracy and Indications for Diagnostic Laparoscopy Prior to Curative-Intent Resection of Gastric Cancer. *Gastric Cancer* **2012**, *15*, 38–47. [CrossRef]
34. Yang, L. Incidence and Mortality of Gastric Cancer in China. *WJG* **2006**, *12*, 17. [CrossRef]
35. Nagtegaal, I.D.; Odze, R.D.; Klimstra, D.; Paradis, V.; Rugge, M.; Schirmacher, P.; Washington, K.M.; Carneiro, F.; Cree, I.A. the WHO Classification of Tumours Editorial Board. The 2019 WHO Classification of Tumours of the Digestive System. *Histopathology* **2020**, *76*, 182–188. [CrossRef] [PubMed]
36. Tan, M.C.; Graham, D.Y. Screening for Gastric Cancer: Focus on the Ants Instead of the Ant Hill. *Clin. Gastroenterol. Hepatol.* **2021**, *19*, 1990–1991. [CrossRef]
37. Wu, K.; Nie, Y.; Guo, C.; Chen, Y.; Ding, J.; Fan, D. Molecular Basis of Therapeutic Approaches to Gastric Cancer. *J. Gastro. Hepatol.* **2009**, *24*, 37–41. [CrossRef] [PubMed]
38. Yin, M.; Hu, Z.; Tan, D.; Ajani, J.A.; Wei, Q. Molecular Epidemiology of Genetic Susceptibility to Gastric Cancer: Focus on Single Nucleotide Polymorphisms in Gastric Carcinogenesis. *Am. J. Transl. Res.* **2009**, *1*, 44–54. [PubMed]
39. Lochhead, P.; El-Omar, E.M. Gastric Cancer. *Br. Med. Bull.* **2008**, *85*, 87–100. [CrossRef]
40. Sohn, B.H.; Hwang, J.-E.; Jang, H.-J.; Lee, H.-S.; Oh, S.C.; Shim, J.-J.; Lee, K.-W.; Kim, E.H.; Yim, S.Y.; Lee, S.H.; et al. Clinical Significance of Four Molecular Subtypes of Gastric Cancer Identified by The Cancer Genome Atlas Project. *Clin. Cancer Res.* **2017**, *23*, 4441–4449. [CrossRef]
41. Murphy, G.; Pfeiffer, R.; Camargo, M.C.; Rabkin, C.S. Meta-Analysis Shows That Prevalence of Epstein–Barr Virus-Positive Gastric Cancer Differs Based on Sex and Anatomic Location. *Gastroenterology* **2009**, *137*, 824–833. [CrossRef]
42. Basirinia, G.; Ali, M.; Comelli, A.; Sperandeo, A.; Piana, S.; Alongi, P.; Longo, C.; Di Raimondo, D.; Tuttolomondo, A.; Benfante, V. Theranostic Approaches for Gastric Cancer: An Overview of In Vitro and In Vivo Investigations. *Cancers* **2024**, *16*, 3323. [CrossRef]

https://doi.org/10.3390/jpm16010036

43. Takashima, H.; Koga, Y.; Manabe, S.; Ohnuki, K.; Tsumura, R.; Anzai, T.; Iwata, N.; Wang, Y.; Yokokita, T.; Komori, Y.; et al. Radioimmunotherapy with an ^{211}At-labeled Anti–Tissue Factor Antibody Protected by Sodium Ascorbate. *Cancer Sci.* **2021**, *112*, 1975–1986. [CrossRef]
44. Müller, C.; Struthers, H.; Winiger, C.; Zhernosekov, K.; Schibli, R. DOTA Conjugate with an Albumin-Binding Entity Enables the First Folic Acid–Targeted ^{177}Lu-Radionuclide Tumor Therapy in Mice. *J. Nucl. Med.* **2013**, *54*, 124–131. [CrossRef] [PubMed]
45. Si, Z.; Cheng, Y.; Xu, Z.; Shi, D.; Shi, H.; Cheng, D. Exploration of ^{68}Ga-DOTA-MAL as a Versatile Vehicle for Facile Labeling of a Variety of Thiol-Containing Bioactive Molecules. *ACS Omega* **2023**, *8*, 4747–4755. [CrossRef]
46. Fani, M.; Wang, X.; Nicolas, G.; Medina, C.; Raynal, I.; Port, M.; Maecke, H.R. Development of New Folate-Based PET Radiotracers: Preclinical Evaluation of 68Ga-DOTA-Folate Conjugates. *Eur. J. Nucl. Med. Mol. Imaging* **2011**, *38*, 108–119. [CrossRef] [PubMed]
47. Fani, M.; Tamma, M.-L.; Nicolas, G.P.; Lasri, E.; Medina, C.; Raynal, I.; Port, M.; Weber, W.A.; Maecke, H.R. In Vivo Imaging of Folate Receptor Positive Tumor Xenografts Using Novel ^{68}Ga-NODAGA-Folate Conjugates. *Mol. Pharm.* **2012**, *9*, 1136–1145. [CrossRef]
48. Brand, C.; Longo, V.A.; Groaning, M.; Weber, W.A.; Reiner, T. Development of a New Folate-Derived Ga-68-Based PET Imaging Agent. *Mol. Imaging Biol.* **2017**, *19*, 754–761. [CrossRef]
49. Jain, A.; Mathur, A.; Pandey, U.; Bhatt, J.; Mukherjee, A.; Ram, R.; Sarma, H.D.; Dash, A. Synthesis and Evaluation of a 68Ga Labeled Folic Acid Derivative for Targeting Folate Receptors. *Appl. Radiat. Isot.* **2016**, *116*, 77–84. [CrossRef] [PubMed]
50. Lu, J.; Pang, Y.; Xie, F.; Guo, H.; Li, Y.; Yang, Z.; Wang, X. Synthesis and in Vitro/in Vivo Evaluation of ^{99m}Tc-Labeled Folate Conjugates for Folate Receptor Imaging. *Nucl. Med. Biol.* **2011**, *38*, 557–565. [CrossRef]
51. Xie, F.; Zhang, C.; Yu, Q.; Pang, Y.; Chen, Y.; Yang, W.; Xue, J.; Liu, Y.; Lu, J. Novel ^{99m}Tc Radiolabeled Folate Complexes with PEG Linkers for FR-Positive Tumor Imaging: Synthesis and Biological Evaluation. *RSC Adv.* **2014**, *4*, 32197–32206. [CrossRef]
52. Kim, M.H.; Kim, W.H.; Kim, C.G.; Kim, D.-W. Synthesis and Evaluation of 99mTc-Labeled Folate-Tripeptide Conjugate as a Folate Receptor-Targeted Imaging Agent in a Tumor-Bearing Mouse Model. *Nucl. Med. Mol. Imaging* **2015**, *49*, 200–207. [CrossRef]
53. Boss, S.D.; Betzel, T.; Müller, C.; Fischer, C.R.; Haller, S.; Reber, J.; Groehn, V.; Schibli, R.; Ametamey, S.M. Comparative Studies of Three Pairs of α- and γ-Conjugated Folic Acid Derivatives Labeled with Fluorine-18. *Bioconjugate Chem.* **2016**, *27*, 74–86. [CrossRef]
54. Betzel, T.; Müller, C.; Groehn, V.; Müller, A.; Reber, J.; Fischer, C.R.; Krämer, S.D.; Schibli, R.; Ametamey, S.M. Radiosynthesis and Preclinical Evaluation of 3′-Aza-2′-[^{18}F]Fluorofolic Acid: A Novel PET Radiotracer for Folate Receptor Targeting. *Bioconjugate Chem.* **2013**, *24*, 205–214. [CrossRef]
55. Ross, T.L.; Honer, M.; Müller, C.; Groehn, V.; Schibli, R.; Ametamey, S.M. A New ^{18}F-Labeled Folic Acid Derivative with Improved Properties for the PET Imaging of Folate Receptor–Positive Tumors. *J. Nucl. Med.* **2010**, *51*, 1756–1762. [CrossRef]
56. Spartivento, G.; Benfante, V.; Ali, M.; Yezzi, A.; Di Raimondo, D.; Tuttolomondo, A.; Lo Casto, A.; Comelli, A. Revolutionizing Periodontal Care: The Role of Artificial Intelligence in Diagnosis, Treatment, and Prognosis. *Appl. Sci.* **2025**, *15*, 3295. [CrossRef]
57. Fischer, C.R.; Müller, C.; Reber, J.; Müller, A.; Krämer, S.D.; Ametamey, S.M.; Schibli, R. [^{18}F]Fluoro-Deoxy-Glucose Folate: A Novel PET Radiotracer with Improved in Vivo Properties for Folate Receptor Targeting. *Bioconjugate Chem.* **2012**, *23*, 805–813. [CrossRef]
58. Hong, R.; Xu, B. Breast Cancer: An Up-to-date Review and Future Perspectives. *Cancer Commun.* **2022**, *42*, 913–936. [CrossRef] [PubMed]
59. Li, H.; Liu, Z.; Yuan, L.; Fan, K.; Zhang, Y.; Cai, W.; Lan, X. Radionuclide-Based Imaging of Breast Cancer: State of the Art. *Cancers* **2021**, *13*, 5459. [CrossRef]
60. Guzik, P.; Siwowska, K.; Fang, H.-Y.; Cohrs, S.; Bernhardt, P.; Schibli, R.; Müller, C. Promising Potential of [^{177}Lu]Lu-DOTA-Folate to Enhance Tumor Response to Immunotherapy—A Preclinical Study Using a Syngeneic Breast Cancer Model. *Eur. J. Nucl. Med. Mol. Imaging* **2021**, *48*, 984–994. [CrossRef] [PubMed]
61. Aranda-Lara, L.; Ferro-Flores, G.; Azorín-Vega, E.; Ramírez, F.D.M.; Jiménez-Mancilla, N.; Ocampo-García, B.; Santos-Cuevas, C.; Isaac-Olivé, K. Synthesis and Evaluation of Lys^1 (α,γ-Folate)Lys^3 (^{177}Lu-DOTA)-Bombesin(1–14) as a Potential Theranostic Radiopharmaceutical for Breast Cancer. *Appl. Radiat. Isot.* **2016**, *107*, 214–219. [CrossRef] [PubMed]
62. Aranda-Lara, L.; Ferro-Flores, G.; Ramírez, F.D.M.; Ocampo-García, B.; Santos-Cuevas, C.; Díaz-Nieto, L.; Isaac-Olivé, K. Improved Radiopharmaceutical Based on 99mTc-Bombesin–Folate for Breast Tumour Imaging. *Nucl. Med. Commun.* **2016**, *37*, 377–386. [CrossRef]
63. Mendoza-Nava, H.; Ferro-Flores, G.; Ramírez, F.D.M.; Ocampo-García, B.; Santos-Cuevas, C.; Aranda-Lara, L.; Azorín-Vega, E.; Morales-Avila, E.; Isaac-Olivé, K. ^{177}Lu-Dendrimer Conjugated to Folate and Bombesin with Gold Nanoparticles in the Dendritic Cavity: A Potential Theranostic Radiopharmaceutical. *J. Nanomater.* **2016**, *2016*, 1039258. [CrossRef]
64. Gupta, A.; Shin, J.H.; Lee, M.S.; Park, J.Y.; Kim, K.; Kim, J.H.; Suh, M.; Park, C.R.; Kim, Y.J.; Song, M.G.; et al. Voxel-Based Dosimetry of Iron Oxide Nanoparticle-Conjugated ^{177}Lu-Labeled Folic Acid Using SPECT/CT Imaging of Mice. *Mol. Pharm.* **2019**, *16*, 1498–1506. [CrossRef]

https://doi.org/10.3390/jpm16010036

65. Kuda-Wedagedara, A.N.W.; Workinger, J.L.; Nexo, E.; Doyle, R.P.; Viola-Villegas, N. ^{89}Zr-Cobalamin PET Tracer: Synthesis, Cellular Uptake, and Use for Tumor Imaging. *ACS Omega* **2017**, *2*, 6314–6320. [CrossRef] [PubMed]
66. Ucar, E.; Teksoz, S.; Ichedef, C.; Kilcar, A.Y.; Medine, E.I.; Ari, K.; Parlak, Y.; Sayit Bilgin, B.E.; Unak, P. Synthesis, Characterization and Radiolabeling of Folic Acid Modified Nanostructured Lipid Carriers as a Contrast Agent and Drug Delivery System. *Appl. Radiat. Isot.* **2017**, *119*, 72–79. [CrossRef] [PubMed]
67. Temma, T.; Sano, K.; Kuge, Y.; Kamihashi, J.; Takai, N.; Ogawa, Y.; Saji, H. Development of a Radiolabeled Probe for Detecting Membrane Type-1 Matrix Metalloproteinase on Malignant Tumors. *Biol. Pharm. Bull.* **2009**, *32*, 1272–1277. [CrossRef] [PubMed]
68. Silindir-Gunay, M.; Karpuz, M.; Ozturk, N.; Yekta Ozer, A.; Erdogan, S.; Tuncel, M. Radiolabeled, Folate-Conjugated Liposomes as Tumor Imaging Agents: Formulation and in Vitro Evaluation. *J. Drug Deliv. Sci. Technol.* **2019**, *50*, 321–328. [CrossRef]
69. Mollarazi, E.; Jalilian, A.R.; Johari-daha, F.; Atyabi, F. Development of ^{153}Sm-Folate-Polyethyleneimine-Conjugated Chitosan Nanoparticles for Targeted Therapy: ^{153}Sm-Folate-PEI-Conjugated Chitosan Nanoparticles. *J. Label. Compd. Radiopharm.* **2015**, *58*, 327–335. [CrossRef]
70. Guo, Z.; You, L.; Shi, C.; Song, M.; Gao, M.; Xu, D.; Peng, C.; Zhuang, R.; Liu, T.; Su, X.; et al. Development of a New FR-Targeting Agent ^{99m}Tc-HYNFA with Improved Imaging Contrast and Comparison of Multimerization and/or PEGylation Strategies for Radio-Folate Modification. *Mol. Pharm.* **2017**, *14*, 3780–3788. [CrossRef]
71. Baidoun, F.; Elshiwy, K.; Elkeraie, Y.; Merjaneh, Z.; Khoudari, G.; Sarmini, M.T.; Gad, M.; Al-Husseini, M.; Saad, A. Colorectal Cancer Epidemiology: Recent Trends and Impact on Outcomes. *CDT* **2021**, *22*, 998–1009. [CrossRef]
72. Dariya, B.; Aliya, S.; Merchant, N.; Alam, A.; Nagaraju, G.P. Colorectal Cancer Biology, Diagnosis, and Therapeutic Approaches. *Crit. Rev. Oncog.* **2020**, *25*, 71–94. [CrossRef]
73. Gudkov, S.; Shilyagina, N.; Vodeneev, V.; Zvyagin, A. Targeted Radionuclide Therapy of Human Tumors. *Int. J. Mol. Sci.* **2015**, *17*, 33. [CrossRef]
74. Ikotun, O.F.; Marquez, B.V.; Fazen, C.H.; Kahkoska, A.R.; Doyle, R.P.; Lapi, S.E. Investigation of a Vitamin B_{12} Conjugate as a PET Imaging Probe. *ChemMedChem* **2014**, *9*, 1244–1251. [CrossRef]
75. Rossin, R.; Pan, D.; Qi, K.; Turner, J.L.; Sun, X.; Wooley, K.L.; Welch, M.J. 64Cu-Labeled Folate-Conjugated Shell Cross-Linked Nanoparticles for Tumor Imaging and Radiotherapy: Synthesis, Radiolabeling, and Biologic Evaluation. *J. Nucl. Med.* **2005**, *46*, 1210–1218.
76. Cheal, S.M.; Patel, M.; Yang, G.; Veach, D.; Xu, H.; Guo, H.; Zanzonico, P.B.; Axworthy, D.B.; Cheung, N.-K.V.; Ouerfelli, O.; et al. An *N* -Acetylgalactosamino Dendron-Clearing Agent for High-Therapeutic-Index DOTA-Hapten Pretargeted Radioimmunotherapy. *Bioconjugate Chem.* **2020**, *31*, 501–506. [CrossRef]
77. Smith-Jones, P.M.; Pandit-Taskar, N.; Cao, W.; O'Donoghue, J.; Philips, M.D.; Carrasquillo, J.; Konner, J.A.; Old, L.J.; Larson, S.M. Preclinical Radioimmunotargeting of Folate Receptor Alpha Using the Monoclonal Antibody Conjugate DOTA–MORAb-003. *Nucl. Med. Biol.* **2008**, *35*, 343–351. [CrossRef] [PubMed]
78. Kim, G.G.; Lee, J.Y.; Choi, P.S.; Kim, S.W.; Park, J.H. Tumor Targeting Effect of Triphenylphosphonium Cations and Folic Acid Coated with Zr-89-Labeled Silica Nanoparticles. *Molecules* **2020**, *25*, 2922. [CrossRef]
79. Kim, G.G.; Jang, H.M.; Park, S.B.; So, J.-S.; Kim, S.W. Synthesis of Zr-89-Labeled Folic Acid-Conjugated Silica (SiO2) Microwire as a Tumor Diagnostics Carrier for Positron Emission Tomography. *Materials* **2021**, *14*, 3226. [CrossRef]
80. Choi, P.S.; Lee, J.Y.; Park, J.H.; Kim, S.W. Synthesis and Evaluation of $^{68}G_A$-HBED-CC-EDBE-folate for positron-emission tomography Imaging of Overexpressed Folate Receptors on CT26 Tumor Cells. *Label. Comp Radiopharm.* **2018**, *61*, 4–10. [CrossRef] [PubMed]
81. Khatik, R.; Dwivedi, P.; Junnuthula, V.R.; Sharma, K.; Chuttani, K.; Mishra, A.K.; Dwivedi, A.K. Potential in Vitro and in Vivo Colon Specific Anticancer Activity in a HCT-116 Xenograft Nude Mice Model: Targeted Delivery Using Enteric Coated Folate Modified Nanoparticles. *RSC Adv.* **2015**, *5*, 16507–16520. [CrossRef]
82. Sah, B.-R.; Schibli, R.; Waibel, R.; Von Boehmer, L.; Bläuenstein, P.; Nexo, E.; Johayem, A.; Fischer, E.; Müller, E.; Soyka, J.D.; et al. Tumor Imaging in Patients with Advanced Tumors Using a New ^{99m}Tc-Radiolabeled Vitamin B12 Derivative. *J. Nucl. Med.* **2014**, *55*, 43–49. [CrossRef]
83. Benfante, V.; Vetrano, I.G.; Ali, M.; Purpura, P.; Gagliardo, C.; Feraco, P.; Longo, C.; Bartolotta, T.V.; Toia, P.; Calisto, O.; et al. An Update on DOTA-Peptides PET Imaging and Potential Advancements of Radioligand Therapy in Intracranial Meningiomas. *Life* **2025**, *15*, 617. [CrossRef]
84. Agus, D.B.; Gambhir, S.S.; Pardridge, W.M.; Spielholz, C.; Baselga, J.; Vera, J.C.; Golde, D.W. Vitamin C Crosses the Blood-Brain Barrier in the Oxidized Form through the Glucose Transporters. *J. Clin. Investig.* **1997**, *100*, 2842–2848. [CrossRef] [PubMed]
85. Est, C.B.; Murphy, R.M. An in Vitro Model for Vitamin A Transport across the Human Blood–Brain Barrier. *eLife* **2023**, *12*, RP87863. [CrossRef]
86. Ale, Y.; Nainwal, N. Progress and Challenges in the Diagnosis and Treatment of Brain Cancer Using Nanotechnology. *Mol. Pharm.* **2023**, *20*, 4893–4921. [CrossRef]

https://doi.org/10.3390/jpm16010036

87. Bailly, C.; Vidal, A.; Bonnemaire, C.; Kraeber-Bodéré, F.; Chérel, M.; Pallardy, A.; Rousseau, C.; Garcion, E.; Lacoeuille, F.; Hindré, F.; et al. Potential for Nuclear Medicine Therapy for Glioblastoma Treatment. *Front. Pharmacol.* **2019**, *10*, 772. [CrossRef]
88. Miner, M.W.G.; Liljenbäck, H.; Virta, J.; Kärnä, S.; Viitanen, R.; Elo, P.; Gardberg, M.; Teuho, J.; Saipa, P.; Rajander, J.; et al. High Folate Receptor Expression in Gliomas Can Be Detected in Vivo Using Folate-Based Positron Emission Tomography with High Tumor-to-Brain Uptake Ratio Divulging Potential Future Targeting Possibilities. *Front. Immunol.* **2023**, *14*, 1145473. [CrossRef]
89. Liang, H.; Chen, Z.; Mo, C.; Tang, G. Synthesis and Preclinical Evaluation of [^{18}F]AlF-NOTA-Asp$_2$-PEG$_2$-Folate as a Novel Folate-Receptor-Targeted Tracer for PET Imaging. *Label. Comp. Radiopharm.* **2024**, *67*, 334–340. [CrossRef] [PubMed]
90. Shi, X.; Xu, P.; Cao, C.; Cheng, Z.; Tian, J.; Hu, Z. PET/NIR-II Fluorescence Imaging and Image-Guided Surgery of Glioblastoma Using a Folate Receptor α-Targeted Dual-Modal Nanoprobe. *Eur. J. Nucl. Med. Mol. Imaging* **2022**, *49*, 4325–4337. [CrossRef]
91. Korany, M.; Mahmoud, B.; Ayoub, S.M.; Sakr, T.M.; Ahmed, S.A. Synthesis and Radiolabeling of Vitamin C-Stabilized Selenium Nanoparticles as a Promising Approach in Diagnosis of Solid Tumors. *J. Radioanal. Nucl. Chem.* **2020**, *325*, 237–244. [CrossRef]
92. Upadhaya, P.; Hazari, P.P.; Mishra, A.K.; Dutta, B.; Hassan, P.; Patravale, V. Radiolabelled Folate Micellar Carriers as Proposed Diagnostic Aid for CNS Tumors by Nasal Route. *Drug Deliv. Transl. Res.* **2023**, *13*, 2604–2613. [CrossRef] [PubMed]
93. Nosrati, S.; Molavipordanjani, S.; Emami, S.; Abedi, S.M.; Talebpour Amiri, F.; Hosseinimehr, S.J. ^{99m}Tc-Radiolabeled Imidazo [2,1-b]Benzothiazole Derivatives as Potential Radiotracers for Glioblastoma. *J. Radioanal. Nucl. Chem.* **2020**, *323*, 205–211. [CrossRef]
94. Mathias, C.J.; Lewis, M.R.; Reichert, D.E.; Laforest, R.; Sharp, T.L.; Lewis, J.S.; Yang, Z.-F.; Waters, D.J.; Snyder, P.W.; Low, P.S.; et al. Preparation of 66Ga- and 68Ga-Labeled Ga(III)-Deferoxamine-Folate as Potential Folate-Receptor-Targeted PET Radiopharmaceuticals. *Nucl. Med. Biol.* **2003**, *30*, 725–731. [CrossRef]
95. Zhang, X.; Yu, Q.; He, Y.; Zhang, C.; Zhu, H.; Yang, Z.; Lu, J. Synthesis and Biological Evaluation of ^{68}Ga-labeled Pteroyl-Lys Conjugates for Folate Receptor-targeted Tumor Imaging. *Label. Compd. Radiopharm.* **2016**, *59*, 346–353. [CrossRef] [PubMed]
96. Sekhoacha, M.; Riet, K.; Motloung, P.; Gumenku, L.; Adegoke, A.; Mashele, S. Prostate Cancer Review: Genetics, Diagnosis, Treatment Options, and Alternative Approaches. *Molecules* **2022**, *27*, 5730. [CrossRef]
97. Ak, G.; Yurt Lambrecht, F.; Sanlier, S.H. Radiolabeling of Folate Targeted Multifunctional Conjugate with Technetium-99m and Biodistribution Studies in Rats. *J. Drug Target.* **2012**, *20*, 509–514. [CrossRef]
98. Dhas, N.L.; Ige, P.P.; Kudarha, R.R. Design, Optimization and in-Vitro Study of Folic Acid Conjugated-Chitosan Functionalized PLGA Nanoparticle for Delivery of Bicalutamide in Prostate Cancer. *Powder Technol.* **2015**, *283*, 234–245. [CrossRef]
99. Leamon, C.P.; Parker, M.A.; Vlahov, I.R.; Xu, L.-C.; Reddy, J.A.; Vetzel, M.; Douglas, N. Synthesis and Biological Evaluation of EC20: A New Folate-Derived,^{99m} Tc-Based Radiopharmaceutical. *Bioconjugate Chem.* **2002**, *13*, 1200–1210. [CrossRef]
100. Guo, Z.; Gao, M.; Song, M.; Shi, C.; Zhang, P.; Xu, D.; You, L.; Zhuang, R.; Su, X.; Liu, T.; et al. Synthesis and Evaluation of 99mTc-Labeled Dimeric Folic Acid for FR-Targeting. *Molecules* **2016**, *21*, 817. [CrossRef] [PubMed]
101. Feng, J.; Zhang, X.; Ruan, Q.; Jiang, Y.; Zhang, J. Preparation and Evaluation of Novel Folate Isonitrile 99mTc Complexes as Potential Tumor Imaging Agents to Target Folate Receptors. *Molecules* **2021**, *26*, 4552. [CrossRef] [PubMed]
102. Ross, T.L.; Honer, M.; Lam, P.Y.H.; Mindt, T.L.; Groehn, V.; Schibli, R.; Schubiger, P.A.; Ametamey, S.M. Fluorine-18 Click Radiosynthesis and Preclinical Evaluation of a New ^{18}F-Labeled Folic Acid Derivative. *Bioconjugate Chem.* **2008**, *19*, 2462–2470. [CrossRef]
103. Yigit, U.S.; Lambrecht, F.Y.; Unak, P.; Biber, F.Z.; Medine, E.I.; Cetinkaya, B. Preparation of ^{99m}Tc Labeled Vitamin C (Ascorbic Acid) and Biodistribution in Rats. *Chem. Pharm. Bull.* **2006**, *54*, 1–3. [CrossRef]
104. Schibli, R.; Waibel, R.; Schaefer, N.; Burger, I.; Blaeuenstein, P.; Johayem, A.; Fischer, E.; Nexø, E. Pharmacokinetic of a New Tc-99m Labeled Vitamin B12 Derivative with Abolished Binding to TC: A Story of Mice and Man. *J. Nucl. Med.* **2010**, *51*, 485.
105. Waibel, R.; Treichler, H.; Schaefer, N.G.; Van Staveren, D.R.; Mundwiler, S.; Kunze, S.; Küenzi, M.; Alberto, R.; Nüesch, J.; Knuth, A.; et al. New Derivatives of Vitamin B12 Show Preferential Targeting of Tumors. *Cancer Res.* **2008**, *68*, 2904–2911. [CrossRef] [PubMed]
106. Matulonis, U.A.; Sood, A.K.; Fallowfield, L.; Howitt, B.E.; Sehouli, J.; Karlan, B.Y. Ovarian Cancer. *Nat. Rev. Dis. Primers* **2016**, *2*, 16061. [CrossRef]
107. Abedi, S.M.; Mardanshahi, A.; Shahhosseini, R.; Hosseinimehr, S.J. Nuclear Medicine for Imaging of Epithelial Ovarian Cancer. *Future Oncol.* **2016**, *12*, 1165–1177. [CrossRef]
108. Benfante, V.; Salvaggio, G.; Ali, M.; Cutaia, G.; Salvaggio, L.; Salerno, S.; Busè, G.; Tulone, G.; Pavan, N.; Di Raimondo, D.; et al. Grading and Staging of Bladder Tumors Using Radiomics Analysis in Magnetic Resonance Imaging. In *Image Analysis and Processing—ICIAP 2023 Workshops*; Foresti, G.L., Fusiello, A., Hancock, E., Eds.; Lecture Notes in Computer Science; Springer Nature: Cham, Switzerland, 2024; Volume 14366, pp. 93–103, ISBN 978-3-031-51025-0.
109. Boca, B.; Caraiani, C.; Telecan, T.; Pintican, R.; Lebovici, A.; Andras, I.; Crisan, N.; Pavel, A.; Diosan, L.; Balint, Z.; et al. MRI-Based Radiomics in Bladder Cancer: A Systematic Review and Radiomics Quality Score Assessment. *Diagnostics* **2023**, *13*, 2300. [CrossRef]

https://doi.org/10.3390/jpm16010036

110. Reber, J.; Struthers, H.; Betzel, T.; Hohn, A.; Schibli, R.; Müller, C. Radioiodinated Folic Acid Conjugates: Evaluation of a Valuable Concept To Improve Tumor-to-Background Contrast. *Mol. Pharm.* **2012**, *9*, 1213–1221. [CrossRef] [PubMed]
111. AlJammaz, I.; Al-Otaibi, B.; Al-Rumayan, F.; Al-Yanbawi, S.; Amer, S.; Okarvi, S.M. Development and Preclinical Evaluation of New ^{124}I-Folate Conjugates for PET Imaging of Folate Receptor-Positive Tumors. *Nucl. Med. Biol.* **2014**, *41*, 457–463. [CrossRef]
112. Jammaz, I.A.; Al-Otaibi, B.; Amer, S.; Okarvi, S.M. Rapid Synthesis and in Vitro and in Vivo Evaluation of Folic Acid Derivatives Labeled with Fluorine-18 for PET Imaging of Folate Receptor-Positive Tumors. *Nucl. Med. Biol.* **2011**, *38*, 1019–1028. [CrossRef]
113. Al Jammaz, I.; Al-Otaibi, B.; Amer, S.; Al-Hokbany, N.; Okarvi, S. Novel Synthesis and Preclinical Evaluation of Folic Acid Derivatives Labeled with 18F-[FDG] for PET Imaging of Folate Receptor-Positive Tumors. *Nucl. Med. Biol.* **2012**, *39*, 864–870. [CrossRef]
114. Siwowska, K.; Guzik, P.; Domnanich, K.A.; Monné Rodríguez, J.M.; Bernhardt, P.; Ponsard, B.; Hasler, R.; Borgna, F.; Schibli, R.; Köster, U.; et al. Therapeutic Potential of 47Sc in Comparison to 177Lu and 90Y: Preclinical Investigations. *Pharmaceutics* **2019**, *11*, 424. [CrossRef] [PubMed]
115. Guo, Z.; Du, Y.; Zhao, J.; Sha, S.; Wang, J. ^{177}Lu-FA-DOTA-PEG-PLGA Nanoparticles Show Antitumor Efficiency in Targeting Ovarian Cancer. *Clin. Exp. Obstet. Gynecol.* **2024**, *51*, 118. [CrossRef]
116. Wu, F.; Chen, P.-M.; Gardinier, T.C.; Turker, M.Z.; Venkatesan, A.M.; Patel, V.; Khor, T.; Bradbury, M.S.; Wiesner, U.B.; Adams, G.P.; et al. Ultrasmall Folate Receptor Alpha Targeted Enzymatically Cleavable Silica Nanoparticle Drug Conjugates Augment Penetration and Therapeutic Efficacy in Models of Cancer. *ACS Nano* **2022**, *16*, 20021–20033. [CrossRef]
117. Tang, Q.; Chen, D. Study of the Therapeutic Effect of 188Re Labeled Folate Targeting Albumin Nanoparticle Coupled with Cis-Diamminedichloroplatinum Cisplatin on Human Ovarian Cancer. *Bio-Med. Mater. Eng.* **2014**, *24*, 711–722. [CrossRef]
118. Oumzil, K.; Khiati, S.; Camplo, M.; Koquely, M.; Chuttani, K.; Chaturvedi, S.; Mishra, A.K.; Barthélémy, P. Nucleolipids as Building Blocks for the Synthesis of ^{99m}Tc-Labeled Nanoparticles Functionalized with Folic Acid. *New J. Chem.* **2014**, *38*, 5240–5246. [CrossRef]
119. Fallah, J.; Agrawal, S.; Gittleman, H.; Fiero, M.H.; Subramaniam, S.; John, C.; Chen, W.; Ricks, T.K.; Niu, G.; Fotenos, A.; et al. FDA Approval Summary: Lutetium Lu 177 Vipivotide Tetraxetan for Patients with Metastatic Castration-Resistant Prostate Cancer. *Clin. Cancer Res.* **2023**, *29*, 1651–1657. [CrossRef]
120. Urso, L.; Nieri, A.; Uccelli, L.; Castello, A.; Artioli, P.; Cittanti, C.; Marzola, M.C.; Florimonte, L.; Castellani, M.; Bissoli, S.; et al. Lutathera® Orphans: State of the Art and Future Application of Radioligand Therapy with ^{177}Lu-DOTATATE. *Pharmaceutics* **2023**, *15*, 1110. [CrossRef]
121. Kluge, K.; Lotz, V.; Einspieler, H.; Haberl, D.; Spielvogel, C.; Amereller, D.; Kramer, G.; Grubmüller, B.; Shariat, S.; Haug, A.; et al. Imaging and Outcome Correlates of ctDNA Methylation Markers in Prostate Cancer: A Comparative, Cross-Sectional [^{68}Ga]Ga-PSMA-11 PET/CT Study. *Clin. Epigenetics* **2025**, *17*, 36. [CrossRef]
122. Hofman, M.S.; Violet, J.; Hicks, R.J.; Ferdinandus, J.; Thang, S.P.; Akhurst, T.; Iravani, A.; Kong, G.; Ravi Kumar, A.; Murphy, D.G.; et al. [^{177}Lu]-PSMA-617 Radionuclide Treatment in Patients with Metastatic Castration-Resistant Prostate Cancer (LuPSMA Trial): A Single-Centre, Single-Arm, Phase 2 Study. *Lancet Oncol.* **2018**, *19*, 825–833. [CrossRef] [PubMed]
123. Bodei, L.; Cremonesi, M.; Grana, C.M.; Fazio, N.; Iodice, S.; Baio, S.M.; Bartolomei, M.; Lombardo, D.; Ferrari, M.E.; Sansovini, M.; et al. Peptide Receptor Radionuclide Therapy with 177Lu-DOTATATE: The IEO Phase I-II Study. *Eur. J. Nucl. Med. Mol. Imaging* **2011**, *38*, 2125–2135. [CrossRef]
124. Bleeker, G.; Schoot, R.A.; Caron, H.N.; De Kraker, J.; Hoefnagel, C.A.; Van Eck, B.L.; Tytgat, G.A. Toxicity of Upfront 131I-Metaiodobenzylguanidine (131I-MIBG) Therapy in Newly Diagnosed Neuroblastoma Patients: A Retrospective Analysis. *Eur. J. Nucl. Med. Mol. Imaging* **2013**, *40*, 1711–1717. [CrossRef]
125. Liu, M.; Svirskis, D.; Proft, T.; Loh, J.; Yin, N.; Li, H.; Li, D.; Zhou, Y.; Chen, S.; Song, L.; et al. Progress in Peptide and Protein Therapeutics: Challenges and Strategies. *Acta Pharm. Sin. B* **2025**, *15*, 6342–6381. [CrossRef]
126. Yamada, Y.; Nakatani, H.; Yanaihara, H.; Omote, M. Phase I Clinical Trial of ^{99m}Tc-Etarfolatide, an Imaging Agent for Folate Receptor in Healthy Japanese Adults. *Ann. Nucl. Med.* **2015**, *29*, 792–798. [CrossRef] [PubMed]
127. Tran, H.H.; Yamaguchi, A.; Manning, H.C. Radiotheranostic Landscape: A Review of Clinical and Preclinical Development. *Eur. J. Nucl. Med. Mol. Imaging* **2025**, *52*, 2685–2709. [CrossRef] [PubMed]
128. Ninatti, G.; Lee, S.T.; Scott, A.M. Radioligand Therapy in Cancer Management: A Global Perspective. *Cancers* **2025**, *17*, 3412. [CrossRef]
129. Xu, M.; Yang, L.; Lin, Y.; Lu, Y.; Bi, X.; Jiang, T.; Deng, W.; Zhang, L.; Yi, W.; Xie, Y.; et al. Emerging Nanobiotechnology for Precise Theranostics of Hepatocellular Carcinoma. *J. Nanobiotechnol.* **2022**, *20*, 427. [CrossRef]
130. Watabe, T.; Hirata, K.; Iima, M.; Yanagawa, M.; Saida, T.; Sakata, A.; Ide, S.; Honda, M.; Kurokawa, R.; Nishioka, K.; et al. Recent Advances in Theranostics and Oncology PET: Emerging Radionuclides and Targets. *Ann. Nucl. Med.* **2025**, *39*, 909–921. [CrossRef]
131. Bodei, L.; Herrmann, K.; Schöder, H.; Scott, A.M.; Lewis, J.S. Radiotheranostics in Oncology: Current Challenges and Emerging Opportunities. *Nat. Rev. Clin. Oncol.* **2022**, *19*, 534–550. [CrossRef]

https://doi.org/10.3390/jpm16010036

132. Elmeliegy, M.; Udata, C.; Liao, K.; Yin, D. Considerations on the Calculation of the Human Equivalent Dose from Toxicology Studies for Biologic Anticancer Agents. *Clin. Pharmacokinet.* **2021**, *60*, 563–567. [CrossRef] [PubMed]
133. Blanchard, O.L.; Smoliga, J.M. Translating Dosages from Animal Models to Human Clinical Trials—Revisiting Body Surface Area Scaling. *FASEB J.* **2015**, *29*, 1629–1634. [CrossRef]
134. Govindan, S.V.; Cardillo, T.M.; Rossi, E.A.; Trisal, P.; McBride, W.J.; Sharkey, R.M.; Goldenberg, D.M. Improving the Therapeutic Index in Cancer Therapy by Using Antibody–Drug Conjugates Designed with a Moderately Cytotoxic Drug. *Mol. Pharm.* **2015**, *12*, 1836–1847. [CrossRef]
135. Tosca, E.M.; Borella, E.; Piana, C.; Bouchene, S.; Merlino, G.; Fiascarelli, A.; Mazzei, P.; Magni, P. Model-based Prediction of Effective Target Exposure for MEN1611 in Combination with Trastuzumab in HER2 -positive Advanced or Metastatic Breast Cancer Patients. *CPT Pharmacom. Syst. Pharma.* **2023**, *12*, 1626–1639. [CrossRef] [PubMed]
136. Bharadwaj, K.K.; Rabha, B.; Pati, S.; Sarkar, T.; Choudhury, B.K.; Barman, A.; Bhattacharjya, D.; Srivastava, A.; Baishya, D.; Edinur, H.A.; et al. Green Synthesis of Gold Nanoparticles Using Plant Extracts as Beneficial Prospect for Cancer Theranostics. *Molecules* **2021**, *26*, 6389. [CrossRef]
137. Ali, M.; Benfante, V.; Stefano, A.; Yezzi, A.; Di Raimondo, D.; Tuttolomondo, A.; Comelli, A. Anti-Arthritic and Anti-Cancer Activities of Polyphenols: A Review of the Most Recent In Vitro Assays. *Life* **2023**, *13*, 361. [CrossRef] [PubMed]
138. Azadinejad, H.; Farhadi Rad, M.; Shariftabrizi, A.; Rahmim, A.; Abdollahi, H. Optimizing Cancer Treatment: Exploring the Role of AI in Radioimmunotherapy. *Diagnostics* **2025**, *15*, 397. [CrossRef]
139. Ali, M.; Benfante, V.; Cutaia, G.; Salvaggio, L.; Rubino, S.; Portoghese, M.; Ferraro, M.; Corso, R.; Piraino, G.; Ingrassia, T.; et al. Prostate Cancer Detection: Performance of Radiomics Analysis in Multiparametric MRI. In *Image Analysis and Processing—ICIAP 2023 Workshops*; Foresti, G.L., Fusiello, A., Hancock, E., Eds.; Lecture Notes in Computer Science; Springer Nature: Cham, Switzerland, 2024; Volume 14366, pp. 83–92, ISBN 978-3-031-51025-0.
140. Ali, M.; Benfante, V.; Basirinia, G.; Alongi, P.; Sperandeo, A.; Quattrocchi, A.; Giannone, A.G.; Cabibi, D.; Yezzi, A.; Di Raimondo, D.; et al. Applications of Artificial Intelligence, Deep Learning, and Machine Learning to Support the Analysis of Microscopic Images of Cells and Tissues. *J. Imaging* **2025**, *11*, 59. [CrossRef]
141. Lo Casto, A.; Spartivento, G.; Benfante, V.; Di Raimondo, R.; Ali, M.; Di Raimondo, D.; Tuttolomondo, A.; Stefano, A.; Yezzi, A.; Comelli, A. Artificial Intelligence for Classifying the Relationship between Impacted Third Molar and Mandibular Canal on Panoramic Radiographs. *Life* **2023**, *13*, 1441. [CrossRef]
142. Cairone, L.; Benfante, V.; Bignardi, S.; Marinozzi, F.; Yezzi, A.; Tuttolomondo, A.; Salvaggio, G.; Bini, F.; Comelli, A. Robustness of Radiomics Features to Varying Segmentation Algorithms in Magnetic Resonance Images. In *Image Analysis and Processing—ICIAP 2022 Workshops*; Mazzeo, P.L., Frontoni, E., Sclaroff, S., Distante, C., Eds.; Lecture Notes in Computer Science; Springer International Publishing: Cham, Switzerland, 2022; Volume 13373, pp. 462–472, ISBN 978-3-031-13320-6.
143. Li, H.; Lee, C.H.; Chia, D.; Lin, Z.; Huang, W.; Tan, C.H. Machine Learning in Prostate MRI for Prostate Cancer: Current Status and Future Opportunities. *Diagnostics* **2022**, *12*, 289. [CrossRef]
144. Norman, H.A.; Butrum, R.R.; Feldman, E.; Heber, D.; Nixon, D.; Picciano, M.F.; Rivlin, R.; Simopoulos, A.; Wargovich, M.J.; Weisburger, E.K.; et al. The Role of Dietary Supplements during Cancer Therapy. *J. Nutr.* **2003**, *133*, 3794S–3799S. [CrossRef] [PubMed]

Journal of
Personalized Medicine

MDPI

Review

Personalized Immunotherapy for T Cell Lymphomas: From Immune Escape to Precision Therapeutics

Joshua M. L. Casan [1,2,3,*,†], Xiao Jing Ong [1,3,†], Carrie van der Weyden [1,2], Costas K. Yannakou [4,5], Joe Zhu [1,3,‡], Criselle D'Souza [1,3,‡], Paul Neeson [1,3,‡] and H. Miles Prince [1,2,4,5,‡]

1 The Sir Peter MacCallum Department of Oncology, Faculty of Medicine, Dentistry and Health Science, University of Melbourne, Melbourne, VIC 3010, Australia; xiaojing.ong@petermac.org (X.J.O.); carrie.vanderweyden@petermac.org (C.v.d.W.); joe.zhu@petermac.org (J.Z.); criselle.dsouza@petermac.org (C.D.); paul.neeson@petermac.org (P.N.); miles.prince@petermac.org (H.M.P.)
2 Department of Clinical Hematology, Peter MacCallum Cancer Centre, Melbourne, VIC 3000, Australia
3 Cancer Immunology Program, Peter MacCallum Cancer Centre, Melbourne, VIC 3000, Australia
4 Epworth HealthCare, Melbourne, VIC 3121, Australia
5 Department of Clinical Pathology, Faculty of Medicine, Dentistry and Health Science, University of Melbourne, Melbourne, VIC 3010, Australia
* Correspondence: joshua.casan@petermac.org
† These authors contributed equally to this work.
‡ These authors also contributed equally to this work.

Abstract: Despite recent progress in lymphoma immunotherapy, outcomes for patients with peripheral T cell lymphomas (PTCLs) remain poor. The challenge of PTCLs reflects the profound biological heterogeneity and relative rarity of this disease group and its resistance to conventional chemotherapy, as well as the formidable challenge of generating definitive clinical evidence. However, deepening insight into the immunogenomic and microenvironmental basis of PTCL has revealed diverse mechanisms of immune escape, spanning defects in antigen presentation, apoptotic signaling, adhesion, and extensive tumor microenvironmental remodeling. These vulnerabilities provide a sound rationale for novel immunotherapeutic strategies—checkpoint inhibitors, CAR-T and NK cell platforms, bispecific antibodies, oncolytic viruses, and immunomodulatory agents. Early studies show encouraging but inconsistent activity, and the variability in response highlights the urgent need for biomarker-driven stratification to deliver personalized approaches and clinically meaningful efficacy. This review synthesizes the current literature on the immune dysregulation of PTCLs, as well as advances in PTCL immunotherapy, outlining the biological rationale underpinning these approaches. We discuss approaches to molecular, transcriptomic, and microenvironmental profiling with circulating biomarkers that could enable adaptive trial designs and personalized treatment strategies. Together, these developments chart a path away from empiricism and toward precision therapy in PTCLs.

Keywords: T cell lymphoma; peripheral T-cell lymphomas (PTCL); immunotherapy; tumor microenvironment (TME); immune checkpoint inhibitors; CAR-T cell therapy; biomarkers

1. Introduction

Peripheral T cell lymphomas (PTCLs) are a biologically and clinically heterogeneous group of malignancies that remain among the most challenging lymphomas to treat. PTCLs collectively account for approximately 10–15% of non-Hodgkin lymphomas worldwide but remain rare in Western populations, where they comprise less than 5% of cases [1]. Their incidence and subtype distribution show marked geographic variation, reflecting distinct pathogenetic and environmental influences [1]. Within this broad category, there are more than 30 distinct subtypes, with highly variable clinicopathological presentation and outcomes [2]. Their rarity and diversity have historically meant treatment strategies are extrapolated from B cell lymphoma, despite fundamental biological differences. Consequently, conventional chemotherapy regimens, while still used frontline, often yield only transient responses, and outcomes for relapsed or refractory disease remain abysmal [2,3]. Increasing evidence from molecular and immunogenomic profiling has elucidated the profound immune dysregulation underpinning PTCL biology, including defects in antigen presentation, deregulated apoptotic pathways, altered adhesion signaling, and remodeling of the tumor microenvironment. These discoveries confirm what clinical practice has repeatedly suggested: that PTCL pathobiology involves many distinct immune escape mechanisms that demand tailored therapeutic approaches.

The rapid evolution of novel immunotherapeutics has generated unprecedented opportunities to exploit such vulnerabilities. Checkpoint inhibitors, engineered cellular therapies, such as Chimeric Antigen Receptor (CAR)-T and CAR-NK cells, bispecific antibodies, oncolytic viruses, and immunomodulatory drugs are promising treatments that continue to evolve and transform outcomes for cancer patients. However, the variable efficacy of these agents across different cancers highlights the limitations of "one-size-fits-all" therapy and the urgency of developing biomarker-driven patient selection frameworks. Current personalized approaches are still in their infancy, often limited to subgroup analyses or exploratory biomarker studies, but they represent the first steps towards implementing true precision medicine in cancer generally and PTCL specifically. By integrating genomic, immunophenotypic, and microenvironmental data, it may be possible to stratify patients more effectively, match them to the therapies most likely to succeed, and avoid futile or harmful interventions. This review explores the current state of PTCL immunotherapy, the biological rationale underpinning these strategies, and the future directions that may ultimately deliver durable and personalized disease control. The focus of this article is on PTCLs, though relevant data from cutaneous T cell lymphoma (CTCL) will be discussed where relevant and important realms of overlap will be acknowledged.

2. Immunobiology of Peripheral T Cell Lymphomas (PTCLs)

T cell lymphomas (TCLs) represent a heterogeneous group of malignancies, arising from either innate lymphoid cells, such as natural killer (NK) and gamma-delta ($\gamma\delta$) T cells, or from CD8+ and, more commonly, CD4+ T-helper cells of the adaptive immune compartment. Multiple tumor-intrinsic mechanisms have been shown to contribute to T cell lymphomagenesis, including the acquisition of genomic alterations in the JAK-STAT signaling pathways, T cell receptor (TCR), T cell activation-related genes (CD28, CD40, PI3K-AKT, AP-1), and, in some subtypes, the RHOA pathway and epigenetic modifier genes. Multiple reviews have described these intrinsic defects in detail [4,5].

The interaction between TCL cells and their tumor microenvironment (TME) contributes another layer of complexity in this lymphomagenesis process. The immune system plays a crucial role in tumor immune surveillance, eliminating transformed cells under normal circumstances [6]. However, TCL cells can evolve and acquire tumor-intrinsic changes, such as downregulation of antigen presentation and adhesion molecules, upregulation of "don't eat me" signals, and dysregulated apoptotic signals, that allow them to escape immune destruction. In parallel, the TME can be remodeled into a pro-tumorigenic, immune-suppressive niche through the recruitment of immunosuppressive cells, the secretion of inhibitory cytokines, the upregulation of immune checkpoint, and vascular remodeling, thereby further supporting tumor growth and survival [7,8]. This section will provide an in-depth insight into these processes within the context of TCL (Figure 1).

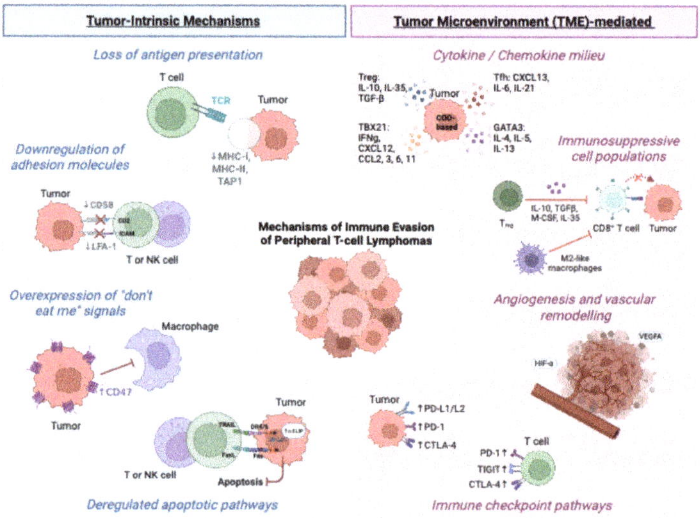

Figure 1. Schematic representation of tumor-intrinsic and tumor-extrinsic immune evasion pathways in peripheral T cell lymphomas. Malignant T cells evade immune surveillance through impaired antigen presentation (HLA/TAP loss), adhesion molecule downregulation (CD58/LFA-1), upregulation of anti-phagocytic signals (CD47), and resistance to apoptosis (Fas/TRAIL pathways). In parallel, the tumor microenvironment is reshaped into an immunosuppressive niche, mediated by regulatory T cells, M2-like macrophages, inhibitory cytokines, and angiogenesis. Together, these mechanisms foster immune escape and therapeutic resistance.

Understanding the escape from tumor immune surveillance is not only critical for elucidating disease biology but also for identifying patient-specific vulnerabilities that can be exploited by personalized immunotherapeutic strategies aimed at reprogramming the tumor–immune interface. Emerging modalities such as checkpoint inhibitors, CAR-T cells, and TME-modulating agents provide opportunities to translate these insights into biomarker-driven strategies for PTCLs, a group of lymphomas that still lack effective standard treatments.

2.1. Tumor-Intrinsic Immune Surveillance Escape Mechanisms

2.1.1. Loss of Antigen Presentation

CD8+ T cell recognition of malignant cells requires the expression of tumor antigens on Major Histocompatibility Complex Class 1 (MHC-1) molecules [9]. PTCL tumor cells can evade immune surveillance by perturbing antigen presentation pathways, which reduce their immunogenic stimulus. High-throughput sequencing studies in peripheral T cell lymphoma, not otherwise specified (PTCL-NOS), have identified frequent loss-of-function mutations in pathways involved in immune surveillance, which include the components of MHC-1 (*HLA-A* and *HLA-B*) and the MHC Class II trans-activator *CIITA* [10,11]. Similar alterations have also been reported in extranodal NK/T cell lymphomas (ENKTL), where mutations in *HLA-A*, *β2M*, and *TAP1* correlate with more advanced disease stage [12], while approximately 50% of cases of adult T cell leukemia/lymphoma (ATLL) also harbor HLA Class 1 and/or *β2M* mutations [13,14].

Defects in the TAP1 gene, a component of the antigen processing machinery, and the HLA Class I genes (HLA-A, HLA-B, and HLA-C) enable tumor cells to evade immune destruction by CD8+ T cells due to impaired presentation of tumor antigens. Loss of MHC-II through the CIITA gene impairs the presentation of tumor-derived antigens to

CD4+ T-helper cells, affecting dendritic cell priming and potentially impacting DC function cross-presentation. Together, these findings highlight antigen presentation defects as a recurring mechanism of impaired immune recognition in PTCL, enabling malignant clones to escape CD8+ T cell-mediated cytotoxicity, promoting disease progression.

2.1.2. Downregulation of Adhesion Molecules

Although the downregulation of MHC class I molecules allows cancer cells to evade cytotoxic T cell-mediated killing, it may paradoxically render them more vulnerable to NK cell-mediated cytotoxicity, since the loss of MHC-I abrogates inhibitory signaling through Killer Immunoglobulin-like Receptors (KIRs) [15]. Accordingly, tumor cells have also evolved other mechanisms, such as the downregulation of adhesion molecules (CD58 and LFA-1) to escape killing by cytotoxic immune cells. Following engagement of the T cell receptor to MHC molecules, CD58 (LFA-3) and LFA-1 play key roles in the formation of immunological synapses, stabilizing and enhancing cell-to-cell adhesion [16,17]. Loss of CD58 in tumor cells has been shown to compromise CAR-T cell activity, driving tumor-intrinsic resistance to T cell killing [16]. Across T/NK cell lymphoma subtypes, CD58 expression is frequently lost, affecting >50% of cases in most PTCL categories, with the highest prevalence in ENKTL (83.3%), followed by PTCL-NOS (63.6%) and anaplastic large cell lymphoma (ALCL) (58%), underscoring its potential role in immune escape [10,18]. Similarly, genomic alteration of *CD58* has also been reported in ATLL, specifically in the acute form [13,19].

Beyond T cell interactions, CD58 is indispensable for NK cell-mediated cytotoxicity, and loss of CD58 in melanoma and B-lymphoblastic leukemia lines confers resistance to NK cell attack [16]. Putting this in the context of T cell lymphoma, the loss of CD58 expression may cause therapeutic resistance to monoclonal antibody therapies (mogamulizumab), which heavily rely on NK cell antibody-directed cell cytotoxicity (ADCC), underscoring its potential role in immune escape [18].

In addition, reduced expression of LFA-1, an integrin required for stable immune synapse formation, has been observed in ATLL cell lines, further contributing to tumor immune evasion [20]. These findings highlight adhesion molecule dysregulation as a recurrent mechanism of resistance in PTCL and support its evaluation as a biomarker to guide personalized T/NK cell-directed immunotherapies, including CAR-T and CAR-NK strategies.

2.1.3. Overexpression of "Don't Eat Me" Signals

Overexpression of CD47 was first identified in acute myeloid leukemia (AML), where its upregulation is linked to adverse outcomes [21]. Subsequently, CD47 overexpression has been documented across various cancers, including both hematologic and solid tumors [22,23]. CD47 contributes to tumor immune escape by binding to signal regulatory protein alpha (SIRPα) on myeloid cells, delivering a "don't eat me" signal that prevents tumor cell phagocytosis by macrophages [24]. Consistent with this, single-cell transcriptomic profiling of nodal T follicular helper lymphoma angioimmunoblastic type (nTFHL-AI) demonstrated significantly higher expression of CD47 in malignant T-follicular helper (Tfh) T cells and B cells from relapsed/refractory (*r/r*) samples compared with newly diagnosed samples [25]. Relapsed/refractory samples exhibit a reduction in phagocytosis by myeloid cells, suggesting that CD47 overexpression confers a survival advantage during immune selection [25]. CD47 overexpression occurs in other PTCL subtypes, including PTCL-NOS and ALCL, although expression levels vary across tumor samples [26,27]. CD47's established role in tumor immune evasion may represent a targetable vulnerability in personalized therapeutic approaches and has prompted the development of an anti-CD47 monoclonal antibody, which blocks the CD47-SIRPα interaction to promote phagocytosis of tumor cells. Multiple preclinical studies have now provided a rationale for testing this agent in TCL [23,27–30]. Interestingly, phase I studies of anti-CD47 (TTI-621) in 12 PTCL and 29 CTCL patients achieved an overall response rate (ORR) of 18% (2/11) and 21% (6/29), respectively (NCT02663518) [31], with 4 of 5 Sezary Syndrome (SS) patients having a prominent decrease in malignant clones 8 days after infusion [30]. This agent has also been demonstrated to potentiate responses to anti-PD-L1 checkpoint inhibitors in preclinical studies [32], which may provide further rationale for combination treatment [23,27–30]. Despite significant enthusiasm for CD47 targeting pathways given the therapeutic rationale and early clinical data, further trials to date across the spectrum of non-PTCL hematologic malignancies have not wholly delivered on this promise due to perceived lack of efficacy and/or potential toxicities, including significant anemia [33]. Future pathways for development in a competitive environment are not assured.

2.1.4. Deregulated Apoptotic Pathways

In addition to extrinsic escape mechanisms, TCL cells utilize intrinsic survival strategies, most notably deregulated apoptotic pathways, which confer a selective survival advantage. Mutations of the *Fas* gene are frequently identified in ENKTL (50–60% of cases in two independent studies), resulting in resistance to Fas–FasL-mediated apoptosis and implicating this aberrancy in disease pathogenesis [34,35].

TNF-related apoptosis-inducing ligand (TRAIL)-mediated apoptosis represents another apoptotic pathway, initiated through binding of TRAIL to the death receptors DR4 and DR5. Notably, despite receptor expression on primary ATLL cells and cell lines, most are resistant to TRAIL-mediated apoptosis, indicative of a further means of apoptosis evasion [36]. TRAIL resistance in ATLL is mediated through the increased expression of anti-apoptotic proteins, including Bcl-xL, via activation of NF-κB by the Human T lymphotropic virus 1 (HTLV-1) Tax protein [36].

Further resistance results from overexpression of cellular FLICE inhibitory protein (c-FLIP), which also protects TCLs from apoptosis and contributes to tumor progression [37].

Deregulated apoptosis pathways may undermine the efficacy of immunotherapies, as T and NK cell-mediated cytotoxicity relies not only on perforin/granzyme but also on Fas-FasL and TRAIL-DR4/5 interactions to eliminate tumor cells [38]. Defects in these pathways may provide an additional layer of immune evasion and could potentially lead to resistance to T and NK cell-based therapies. Again, a more comprehensive understanding of these mechanisms could yield targeted therapeutic approaches that overcome this tumor survival advantage.

2.2. Tumor Microenvironment (TME)-Mediated Immunosuppression

The tumor microenvironment (TME) is a complex network of interactions between tumor cells and local cellular and non-cellular related factors. This includes non-malignant cells, such as immune cells, stromal cells, and fibroblasts, as well as surrounding blood vessels, the extracellular matrix (ECM), and other growth factors or cytokines [7].

2.2.1. Cytokine and Chemokine Milieu of PTCLs

In PTCLs, the composition of the TME varies substantially between subtypes and is likely influenced by the lymphoma cell-of-origin (T-helper (Th)1, Th2, Th17, Tfh or Treg) [26,39,40]. The cell-of-origin defines the cytokine and chemokine profile, which governs immune cell recruitment and drives progressive remodeling of the TME. As an example, PTCL-NOS can be classified into two categories, namely PTCL-TBX21 and PTCL-GATA3 [40]. PTCL-TBX21 is characterized by a T-helper 1 (Th1)-dominant signature, with upregulation of Th1-related genes such as *IFNg*, *CXCL12*, *CCL2*, *CCL3*, *CCL6*, and *CCL11*. In contrast, GATA3-enriched cases exhibit overexpression of T-helper 2 (Th2) cytokines, including IL-4, IL-5, and IL-13 [40]. Additionally, the recently updated WHO designation of nodal T follicular helper lymphomas (nTFHLs) as a diagnostic entity, incorporating the previous diagnoses of angioimmunoblastic T cell lymphoma, follicular T cell lymphoma, and PTCL with T follicular helper phenotype [41], underscores the common feature within this group of a clonal proliferation of T-follicular helper (Tfh) cells, marked by overexpression of CXCL13 [42], IL-6, and IL-21 [43,44]. Furthermore, adult T cell leukemia/lymphoma (ATLL) is known to express FOXP3, a marker of regulatory T cells (Tregs) [45]. Tregs are known to secrete IL-10, IL-35, and TGF-β, which dampen the immune responses and potentially contribute to systemic immunosuppression [46].

Understanding the difference in the cytokine milieu may help elucidate the differences in TME signatures across different PTCL subtypes. This is shown where PTCL-TBX21 is associated with an enrichment in pro-inflammatory cells, likely due to the upregulated Th1 genes, evidenced by the enrichment of histiocytes in 89% of cases, with the remaining 11% consisting of a mixed immune cell infiltrate of lymphocytes, eosinophils, plasma cells, and histiocytes. This contrasts with PTCL-GATA3, which is characterized by low or absent immune cell infiltration [47,48]. The resulting cytokine skew suppresses TH1-mediated anti-tumor immunity, promoting an immune-excluded microenvironment which provides a molecular explanation for the paucity of inflammatory infiltrate observed in PTCL-GATA3. This may provide insights into the significantly better prognosis of PTCL-TBX21 cases, highlighting the need to convert the immune-excluded TME of PTCL-GATA3 into a more inflammatory one.

In nTFHL, recurrent cooperating lesions in *TET2*, *DNMT3A*, *IDH2*, and *RHOA*, together with aberrant PI3K-pathway activation, establish and sustain the TFH transcriptional program [49]. In n-TFHL angioimmunoblastic-type (nTFHL-AI), recent studies have revealed that the malignant Tfh population accounts for only 7–32% of the total cells [50,51]. Although they constitute only a minority of cells within the TME, the overexpression of Tfh cytokines [37,38] promotes the recruitment and expansion of B cells, plasma cells, and follicular dendritic cells (FDCs) [43,44]. Inducible T cell costimulator ligand (ICOSL), which is abundantly expressed on follicular FDCs, activated monocytes, and myeloid dendritic cells (mDCs), engages ICOS on malignant Tfh cells to drive proliferation and survival. This interaction activates downstream signaling cascades, including the PI3K–AKT and NF-κB pathways, which enhance metabolic fitness, cytokine secretion, and resistance to apoptosis. Beyond supporting malignant clone expansion, ICOS–ICOSL signaling reinforces the aberrant Tfh transcriptional program and promotes reciprocal crosstalk with surrounding immune and stromal cells, sustaining a permissive tumor microenvironment [50]. These data underscore the importance of cytokine-mediated TME remodeling in establishing a pro-tumorigenic niche.

Similarly, in ENKTL, single-cell transcriptomics have revealed that the tumor cells foster an immunosuppressive TME through enhanced expression of chemokines CCL3, CCL4, and CCL5, recruiting immune cells such as macrophages via their corresponding receptors CCR1 and CCR5 [52]. Additionally, ENKTL tumor cells can express DPP4, which cleaves CXCL2, CXCL9, and CXCL10, chemokines that recruit T cells and NK cells into the tumor microenvironment, depleting the number of anti-tumor effector cells [52].

2.2.2. Immunosuppressive Cell Populations

Through chemokine/cytokine signaling, TCLs can recruit and expand multiple immunosuppressive cell types into the TME. In ENKTL, macrophages recruited into the TME can be skewed toward an immunosuppressive phenotype (M2-like) and interact with tumor-infiltrating T cells through the expression of immune checkpoints, such as CD80/CD86-CTLA4, PD-L1/PD-L2-PD-1, and Galectin-9-TIM3 [52,53]. Beyond TAMs, nTFHL-AI samples also show expansion of non-malignant CD4$^+$FoxP3$^+$ regulatory T cells (Tregs) compared with healthy lymph node controls. Tregs are known to secrete IL-10, IL-35, and TGF-β, which dampen the immune response and may contribute to tumor immune evasion [43,46,50,51].

Improving our understanding of the dynamic interplay among immune cell subsets is important for devising therapeutic approaches that can recalibrate the tumor microenvironment, shifting it from a state of immune suppression to one that facilitates durable antitumor immunity.

2.2.3. Angiogenesis and Vascular Remodeling

TCL cells also adapt the TME through vascular remodeling, particularly by upregulating pro-angiogenic factors such as vascular endothelial growth factor (VEGF). In nTFHL-AI, increased VEGF expression in both lymphoma cells and endothelial cells causes remodeling of lymphoid structure, which develops an extensive network of high endothelial venules (HEVs) and FDCs adjacent to malignant Tfh cells [43,54,55]. In another PTCL subtype—anaplastic lymphoma kinase (ALK)-positive anaplastic large cell lymphoma (ALCL)—rearrangement of the ALK gene has also been shown to dysregulate the expression of Hypoxia-Inducible Factor (HIF-α) and subsequently VEGFA. In tumor xenografts, ALK knockdown was shown to reduce VEGFA expression, decrease tumor vessels in tumor xenografts, and control tumor growth [56]. Again, this pathogenic interaction highlights the therapeutic potential of disrupting the pro-tumorigenic microenvironment. Notably, this concept is supported by a case in which an nTFHL-AI patient achieved complete remission after treatment with the anti-VEGF antibody bevacizumab [57].

2.2.4. Immune Checkpoint Pathways

The TME of TCLs is often characterized by profound T cell dysfunction and immune exhaustion. For example, in nTFHL-AI, recurrent loss of function in TET2 is found in >60% of cases, often preceding co-occurring RHOA G17V and IDH2 R172 mutations [50]. In mouse models, TET2 deficiency and RHOA mutations promote TFH polarization via ICOS/PI3K-MAPK signaling, leading to lymphoma development [58], while IDH2 further augments this process through TET inhibition [59]. These events promote chronic antigenic stimulation combined with progressive immune exhaustion, evidenced where CD8$^+$ T cells frequently display heightened expression of immune checkpoint receptors, including PD-1, TIGIT, and CTLA-4. In the relapsed/refractory setting, the absolute number of CD8$^+$ T cells declines relative to treatment-naïve disease; however, the residual population demonstrates further enrichment of these inhibitory receptors, suggesting progressive functional exhaustion in advanced disease [25,51]. In ENKTL, malignant cells also display marked upregulation of immune checkpoint molecules. Functional studies demonstrate that co-culture with normal T cells drives an exhaustion phenotype, characterized by increased checkpoint receptor expression and impaired IFN-γ production [52,53]. Similarly, ATLL tumor cells often upregulate immune checkpoint molecules, including PD-1, PD-L1, and CTLA-4, inhibiting T cell function and promoting immune evasion [13]. Notably, in ATLL, PD-L1 expression on tumor cells correlates with inferior outcomes [60,61], whereas PD-L1 expression on non-malignant microenvironmental cells is associated with significantly improved overall survival [60]. This dichotomy underpins the complexity of the tumor–immune interface: tumor-derived PD-L1 promotes immune evasion, while PD-L1 expression in microenvironmental cells may instead signify active anti-tumor immunity. These observations provide important context for the potential application of immune checkpoint inhibitors in ATLL, where prognosis remains poor.

In summary, accumulated evidence demonstrates that TCLs employ a diverse array of immune evasion strategies, including impaired antigen presentation, disruption of adhesion molecules, defective apoptotic signaling, and recruitment of immunosuppressive myeloid populations. These mechanisms not only shape the tumor microenvironment but also create subtype-specific vulnerabilities that may ultimately prove exploitable in a personalized manner. By integrating molecular and immunologic profiling, it is increasingly possible to stratify patients according to the dominant pathways of immune escape in their disease. This framework provides the biological rationale for the therapeutic strategies discussed in the following sections, including checkpoint inhibition, engineered cellular therapies, bispecific antibodies, and approaches that reprogram the tumor–immune interface.

3. Immunotherapy and Immune-Modulating Agents in TCL

3.1. Checkpoint Inhibitors in T Cell Lymphoma

Countervailing cancer immune evasion via blockade of immune checkpoint axes has revolutionized the management of many malignancies, including lymphomas, particularly Hodgkin lymphoma (HL). However, the use of these immune checkpoint inhibitors (ICIs), which leverage and augment T cell cytotoxic responses as a core mechanism of action, present a particular paradox when deployed against malignant T cells. In T cell lymphoma, PD-1 is not just an immune evasion pathway but also a cell-intrinsic constraint on malignant T cell proliferation, acting as a tumor suppressor in cell-based and murine models [62]. Mechanistically, PD-1 engagement restrains aberrant TCR-driven PI3K–AKT signaling and downstream MYC activation. Accordingly, PD-1 axis inhibition risks potentiating T cell lymphoma progression, a phenomenon termed the PD-1 paradox [62]. The PD-1 paradox was manifested in early trials of PD-1 inhibitors in ATLL, where multiple patients developed disease hyperprogression upon treatment, prompting study termination [63,64]. However, subsequent trials have not reproduced this disastrous complication (including in patients with ATLL) [65], and ICIs have demonstrable activity in some PTCL and CTCL patients, either as monotherapy or as part of combination regimens. These observations highlight the duality of PD-1's role in T cell lymphomas and emphasize the importance of molecular and microenvironmental stratification to safely utilize checkpoint blockade in PTCL. Occasional "elite responders" achieve spectacular and durable responses. Consistent with the heterogeneity of TCL pathobiology, response rates vary considerably between disease contexts and studies, underscoring the urgent need to incorporate biomarker response predictors in patient selection.

3.1.1. PD-1/PD-L1 Blockade in PTCL

ICI efficacy in PTCL varies significantly with disease subtype and context. Initial phase I and II studies of PD-1 inhibitor (pembrolizumab or nivolumab) monotherapy in relapsed/refractory PTCL reported widely varying ORRs, ranging from 17.6% in the AVAIL-T study to 40% in the study published by Lesokhin et al., reflecting participant heterogeneity and small cohort size (Table 1) [66–68]. Responses were only transient, and median progression-free survival (PFS) was <4 months for the patients with PTCLs in these trials.

The largest prospective trial of an ICI in PTCLs was reported by Shi et al. In it, the PD-1 inhibitor geptanolimab was deployed through a single-arm, phase II, multicenter study on relapsed/refractory PTCLs; of the 89 patients with reported data, the ORR was 40.4%, with a complete response rate (CRR) of 14.4% [69]. However, response rates varied significantly between PTCL subtypes, with the best response documented in patients with ENKTL (63.2%, 12/19), compared to ALK+ALCL (53.8%, 7/13), ALK-negative ALCL

(42.9%, 3/7), and PTCL-NOS (17.9%, 5/28) [69]. Additionally, several non-randomized studies have investigated the use of ICIs as maintenance therapy following autologous stem cell transplantation (auSCT), demonstrating the safety of this strategy, but with evidence of long-term efficacy still awaited [70,71]. See Table 1 for additional details on clinical evidence for ICIs in PTCLs.

Of importance, patients with relapsed/refractory ENKTL defy the broader PTCL trend, consistently demonstrating high rates of response to PD-1 axis ICIs across multiple studies [69,72–78] (Table 1). ORRs in these studies frequently exceed 50%, including CR rates of up to 31.3%. However, response duration is highly variable, with median PFS not reached in several studies, whereas others reported modest PFS rates averaging several months. In ENKTL, superior response to ICI is thought to be mediated by the near-universal association of the disease with Epstein–Barr Virus (EBV). EBV plays a fundamental role in the pathogenesis of ENKTL, and EBV-encoded proteins expressed during viral latency can cause aberrant expression of NF-κB, PI3K/AKT, JAK/STAT, and other signaling pathways [79]. Perturbed JAK/STAT signaling can upregulate PD-L1 expression on tumor cells generating an immunosuppressive tumor microenvironment [80]. Additional evidence suggests that EBV-derived miRNAs can also promote PD-L1 expression [81]. These phenomena render these tumors dependent on immune evasion and thus more vulnerable to checkpoint inhibition.

Furthermore, ICI therapy may augment the presentation viral antigens, enhancing immune stimulation and anti-tumor immune responses [82]. These findings prompt consideration of whether EBV status is a potential biomarker of ICI response in PTCLs; however, this conjecture remains incompletely addressed by existing data. Given the challenge of recruiting sizable cohorts of PTCL patients, studies have not generally reported responses stratified by EBV status. In non-Hodgkin lymphoma (NHL) more broadly, Kim et al. reported that EBV positivity was associated with improved ICI responses, though the responder cohort was enriched with ENKTL patients ($n = 6/7$ responders), limiting generalizability [75].

Beyond EBV positivity, other biomarkers of ICI response have been explored, but a robust predictive method remains elusive.

3.1.2. Immune Checkpoint Expression

PD1, *PD-L1*, and *PD-L2* expression has been repeatedly investigated, as have levels of soluble PD-L1. However, assessment methods and scoring techniques vary considerably, as does the utility of these metrics across different lymphoma subtypes. Unfortunately, no cogent tool based on PD-L1/PD-L2 tumor or TME expression has proven of sufficient clinical benefit, and documented responses to PD-L1-negative tumors indicate the lack of discriminative power for these pathological factors [83]. Some studies do indeed report superior outcomes in cases with higher PD-L1 expression; however, attribution is difficult as responders are enriched for ENKTL cohorts [69]. Overall, as a biomarker of ICI response, PD1/PD-L1/PD-L2 expression assessment suffers from a lack of standardization in assessment, biological complexity, variability across disease subtypes, and inconsistent clinical correlation, and it cannot be considered a reliable indicator of ICI response in PTCLs.

3.1.3. Tumor Mutational Burden

Tumor mutational burden (TMB), defined as the total number of somatic mutations per coding unit of the genome (typically as mutations per megabase (mut/Mb)), has emerged as a biomarker of ICI response in multiple solid organ cancer contexts [84–86]. This is thought to reflect a proportional relationship between TMB and the degree of tumor neoantigen expression and, therefore, immunogenicity [87]. However, TMB has yielded inconsistent results in hematological malignancies, where the mutational burden is highly variable between disease entities (but trends lower than that seen in archetypical ICI responsive solid cancers like melanoma) [88–91]. Although some studies have demonstrated a potential relationship between TMB and ICI response in some lymphoma subtypes, data are neither robust nor consistent [92]. Unsurprisingly, such data are far less developed in the PTCL context specifically, but panel-based sequencing (with its attendant limitations) suggests a lower TMB in TCLs compared to B cell lymphomas [91].

3.1.4. Microsatellite Instability (MSI) and Deficient Mismatch Repair (dMMR)

Microsatellites are repetitive genomic motifs of 1–6 nucleotides distributed across the genome and contribute to chromatin organization, DNA stability, and gene expression regulation. However, their repetitive nature predisposes microsatellites to replication errors during DNA synthesis. Ordinarily, such errors are corrected by the DNA mismatch repair (MMR) system. When this repair system is dysfunctional—termed deficient mismatch repair (dMMR)—microsatellite sequences accumulate insertion–deletion mutations, resulting in microsatellite instability (MSI) [93]. MSI-high and dMMR phenotypes are associated with greater mutational loads, leading to an elevated neoantigen burden, which can enhance tumor immunogenicity and drive strong responses to immune checkpoint inhibition in some cancers [94,95]. However, dMMR and MSI rarely occur in lymphoma, and in contrast to solid organ cancers, these factors cannot be used to predict response to ICIs for hematological cancer [96–98]. Again, the paucity of any data in PTCLs precludes meaningful discussion, though MSI has been shown in a subset of monomorphic epitheliotropic intestinal T cell lymphoma (MEITL) and ATLL cases and could be explored further [99,100].

3.1.5. Chr 9p Structural Variants

Chromosome 9p24.1 includes the loci of *CD274* (encoding the PD-L1 checkpoint) and *PDCD1LG2* (encoding PD-L2), and structural variants (SVs) affecting this region have proven amongst the most reproducible indicators of ICI response in lymphoma. In classical Hodgkin lymphoma, copy number gains, focal amplifications, and translocations at 9p24.1 are strongly associated with overexpression of PD-L1/PD-L2 and can be coupled with JAK2-driven STAT signaling, further enhancing PD-L1 transcription. These variants induce PD-1 axis dependency and underpin the efficacy of PD-1 inhibitors in this disease, with objective response rates exceeding 65–85% across multiple trials [101–104].

In non-Hodgkin lymphomas, 9p24.1 SVs are less common but remain clinically relevant. In primary mediastinal B cell lymphoma (PMBCL), 9p24.1 structural changes are also associated with high PD-L1 expression and impressive ICI responses [105,106]. In PTCLs, the frequency of 9p24.1 alterations is incompletely defined, but published genomic datasets suggest they occur at lower prevalence than in Hodgkin lymphoma or PMBCL [107]. Rates vary significantly between TCL subtypes, however, with high rates in EBV-driven disease generally reflected in the ENKTL cohort, where 9p24.1 SVs were found in 23% of cases, as well as in 15% of cases of EBV-positive PTCL-NOS [107]. Data can be inconsistent, however, as Ng and colleagues showed only low rates of 9p24.1 SV in EBV-driven T/NK cell lymphomas despite documented overexpression of PD-L1, suggesting alternative mechanisms leading to checkpoint upregulation [108]. SVs involving *CD274* are also documented in mycosis fungoides with large cell transformation, with small numbers of patients demonstrating high rates of disease response, though these responses appeared to be ephemeral [109]. In ATLL, a variety 9p24.1 SVs have been documented in approximately 10–25% of patients, but correlation with ICI response is unknown [110,111]. Though a promising biomarker of ICI response in HL, ENKTL, and PMBCL, the independent predictive power of chromosome 9p SVs for ICI response in TCL remains unproven, though some data suggest this possibility.

3.1.6. PD-1/PD-L1 Blockade Combination Regimens in PTCL

Numerous efforts have been made to augment responses to ICIs in TCL by deploying them in combination with other targeted therapeutics or with conventional cytotoxic therapies (Table 1).

The addition of the histone deacetylase inhibitor (HDACi) romidepsin to pembrolizumab has been investigated in relapsed/refractory PTCL, with the most recent data reporting high response rates, particularly in the nTFHL subtypes (ORR 85.7%, CRR 57.1%) [112]. With a median duration of follow-up of 40 months, median PFS for nTFHL patients was not reached, but it was only 1.23 months in the PTCL NOS cohort [112]. Other pembrolizumab combination trials include partnering with pralatrexate (NCT03598998) and the multi-arm Embolden study with pembrolizumab added to decitabine, decitabine and pralatrexate, or pralatrexate (NCT03240211). Embolden reported initial data in 2022, demonstrating responses in heavily pre-treated patients (2/3 patients receiving the triplet regimen responded), but further data are awaited to draw meaningful conclusions on safety and efficacy [113]. In relapsed/refractory ENKTL, a further multi-agent regimen (PCET) is under investigation, utilizing the HDACi chidamide, etoposide, and thalidomide combined with the PD-1 target monoclonal antibody toripalimab. Early data are extremely limited ($n = 3$), but all patients responded (2 CRs, 1 PR). [114]

Additional combinations under active study in TCL include pembrolizumab with brentuximab vedotin (NCT05313243); camrelizumab (PD-1 inhibitor) with pegasparaginase and apatinib (VEGFR2 inhibitor) in ENKTL (NCT04366128); nivolumab with chemotherapy for relapsed ALCL (NCT07013565); duvelisib and nivolumab in mycosis fungoides (MF) and Sezary Syndrome (SS) (NCT04652960); sintilimab (PD-L1 inhibitor) with gemcitabine and oxaliplatin (NCT04127227); and durvalumab with different combinations of pralatrexate, romidepsin, and oral azacitidine (NCT03161223).

Despite a compelling biological rationale, clinical responses to PD-1 and PD-L1 blockade in PTCLs have been inconsistent overall, and most promising results have been largely confined to ENKTL and TFH-derived subtypes. Most PTCL-NOS and ALK-negative ALCLs derive little benefit, and PD-1-associated hyperprogression has been observed in ATLL and occasionally in other subtypes. Even within CTCL, response rates are variable, reflecting the influence of tumor-intrinsic genotype, cytokine milieu, and immune context [115]. Current predictive biomarkers have shown limited reliability, underscoring that checkpoint efficacy in PTCL cannot yet be confidently forecast. Collectively, these findings indicate that checkpoint inhibition alone is insufficient for most PTCL and highlight the need for deeper biomarker discovery and rational combination strategies. Emergent work examining the interplay of molecular profiling and PD-L1 expression, for example, suggests a potential way to focus research efforts [116]. Integration of immune-gene profiling, spatial transcriptomics, and multi-omic signatures will be critical to define the subsets most likely to benefit and to convert these biologic insights into effective, personalized immunotherapeutic regimens.

Table 1. Studies evaluating checkpoint inhibitor therapy in peripheral T cell lymphoma, organized by monotherapy versus combination regimens and by disease subtype.

Trial and Phase	Line of Therapy	No of Patients (TCL Cohort)	Regimen	ORR	CR	Median PFS	OS	Notes	Reference
Checkpoint inhibitor monotherapy studies—mixed PTCL									
AVAIL-T **NCT03046953**	Median 3 prior lines Range 1–7	Total: 34 AITL: 11 PTCL NOS: 17 ENKTL: 4 ALCL: 1 Transformed MF: 1	Avelumab monotherapy	17.6%	0%	2.9 months	8.9 months	N/A	[65]
Phase I **NCT01592370**		5	Nivolumab monotherapy	40%	0%	14 weeks		N/A	[67]
Phase II **NCT03075553**	Median 2 prior line Range 1–6	12 AITL: 6 PTCL NOS: 3 ALCL ALK-: 1 EATL: 1 HSTCL: 1	Nivolumab monotherapy	33%	16.7%	2.7 months	6.7 months	Median DOR: 3.6 months Hyperprogression in 4 patients (3 AITL and 1 HSTCL)	[114]
GXPLORE-002 **Phase II** **NCT03502629**	Median 2 prior line	102 (89 in full analysis set) PTCL NOS: 41 ENKTL: 23 ALCL ALK-: 12 ALCL ALK+: 7 EATL: 3 MF: 3 Others: 12	Geptanolimab monotherapy	40.4%	14.6%	2.7 months	14.6 months	DOR: 11.4 months ORR by disease subtype ENKTL: 63.2% ALCL ALK-: 53.8% ALCL ALK+: 42.9% PTCL NOS: 17.9% PD-L1 ≥50% enriched (ORR 53.3% vs. 25%)	[68]
Phase II **NCT02535247**	Median 2 prior lines Range 1–9	18 (13 evaluable) PTCL NOS: 7 TFH: 4 Transformed MF: 3	Pembrolizumab monotherapy	33%	27%	3.2 months	10.6 months	Halted early after futility analysis	[66]
Pembrolizumab maintenance post ASCT **Phase II** **NCT02362997**	N/A	21 PTCL NOS: 11 AITL: 4 ENKTL: 3 ALCL ALK-: 2 MEITL: 1	Pembrolizumab monotherapy Post ASCT maintenance study	N/A	N/A	18-month PFS: 83.6%	18-month OS: 94.4%	N/A	[70]
Duvelisib maintenance post ASCT **Phase II** **NCT04331119**	N/A	12 (5 PTCL) ALCL: 3 PTCL NOS: 1 AITL: 3	Duvelisib monotherapy Post ASCT maintenance study	N/A	N/A	Note reported	Not reported	N/A	[69]
Checkpoint inhibitor monotherapy studies—ENKTL									

Table 1. *Cont.*

Trial and Phase	Line of Therapy	No of Patients (TCL Cohort)	Regimen	ORR	CR	Median PFS	OS	Notes	Reference
ORIENT-4 **Phase II** **NCT03228836**	Median 3 prior lines	28	Sintilimab monotherapy	75%	21.4%	Not reported	NR 2yr OS: 78.6%	Median DOR: 4.1 months Pseudoprogression in 17.9%	[75]
Avelumab **Phase II** **NCT 03439501**	Median ≥2 prior lines	21	Avelumab monotherapy	38%	24%	2.7 months	NR	Response by PDL1 expression: High PD-L1: 73% Low PD-L1: 0%	[77]
GEMSTONE-201 **Phase II** **NCT03595657**	Median 1 prior lines	80	Sugemalimab monotherapy	44.9%	35.9%	Not reported	NR 18-month OS: 57.9%	Median DOR: NR	[115]
Pembrolizumab **(Retrospective case series)**	Median 2 prior lines Range 1–5	7	Pembrolizumab monotherapy	100%	71.4%	Not reported	Not reported	Non-trial study	[71]
Pembrolizumab (Retrospective case series)	Median 4 prior lines Range 3–10	7	Pembrolizumab monotherapy	57%	28.6%	4.8 months	5 months	Non-trial study DOR: 4.1 months	[74]
Pembrolizumab (Retrospective case series)		14	Pembrolizumab monotherapy	44%	35.7%	Not reported??	N/A	N/A	[74]
Checkpoint inhibitor combination studies—Mixed PTCL									
Pembrolizumab + Romidepsin **Phase I/II** **NCT03278782**	Median 2.5 prior lines	20 (14 evaluable for efficacy) PTCL NOS: 7 TFH: 15 AITL: 2 Transformed MF: 3 ALCL: 3 ENKTL: 2	Pembrolizumab + Romidepsin	50%	35.7%	Not reported	Not reported	Hyperprogression occurred in 2 patients	[116]
Camrelizumab + Apatinib **Phase II** **NCT03701022**	Median 3 prior lines Range 1–6	ENKTL: 7 PTCL NOS: 6 AITL: 5 ALCL ALK-: 2	Camrelizumab + Apatinib	30%	10%	5.6 months	16.7 months	DOR: not reached Patients with PD-L1 expression ≥ 50% vs. <50% ORR (66.7% vs. 40%). The two patients with the highest PD-L1 expression showed PFS of 18.2 and 22.3 months, respectively.	[117]
PCET (Retrospective case series)	Median 2 prior lines Range 1–6	ENKTL: 3	PCET: toripalimab + chidamide + etoposide + thalidomide	100%	66.7%	Not reported	Not reported	Non-trial study	[113]

Abbreviations: AITL, angioimmunoblastic T cell lymphoma; ALCL, anaplastic large cell lymphoma; ALK, anaplastic lymphoma kinase; ALK-, ALK-negative; ALK+, ALK-positive; ASCT, autologous stem cell transplantation; CR, complete response; DOR, duration of response; EATL, enteropathy-associated T cell lymphoma; ENKTL, extranodal natural killer/T cell lymphoma; HSTCL, hepatosplenic gamma delta T cell lymphoma; MEITL, monomorphic epitheliotropic intestinal T cell lymphoma; MF, mycosis fungoides; N/A, not applicable; NR, not reached; ORR, overall response rate; OS, overall survival; PCET, PD-1 antibody + chidamide + etoposide + thalidomide; PD, progressive disease; PD-L1, programmed death-ligand 1; PFS, progression-free survival; PTCL, peripheral T cell lymphoma; PTCL NOS, peripheral T cell lymphoma not otherwise specified; TCL, T cell lymphoma; TFH, T-follicular helper.

3.2. Engineered Cellular Therapies (CAR-T, CAR-NK)

Over the past decade, adoptive cell transfer (ACT) therapy has demonstrated significant efficacy in treating various cancers, particularly in B cell malignancies. Anti-tumor lymphocytes used in ACT therapy include naturally occurring tumor-infiltrating lymphocytes (TILs) or lymphocytes that have been genetically engineered to express an anti-tumor T cell receptor (TCR) or chimeric antigen receptor (CAR). CAR-T cell therapy has emerged as the leading advance, distinguished by its unprecedented efficacy in relapsed/refractory B cell malignancies [117–119]. Recognition of tumor antigens by CARs is achieved through an antigen-binding domain commonly derived from the variable regions of antibodies [120]. Therefore, antigen recognition by CAR bypasses the need for peptide presentation on MHC molecules, where its downregulation in PTCL samples is one of the mechanisms by which tumors evade host immunity, as described above. Given this, there is considerable interest in adopting CAR-T cell therapy for the treatment of T cell lymphomas. However, there are several challenges due to the sharing of antigens between malignant cells and normal T cells, which can lead to the depletion of healthy T cells, causing profound immunosuppression (T cell aplasia), CAR-T cell fratricide (self-killing of CAR-T cells), and contamination of CAR T cell products during manufacturing. In the following section, we will review CAR-T and CAR-NK targets (Figure 2) currently under clinical investigation for PTCLs (Table 2) and summarize their therapeutic potential. To date, no CAR-/TCR-T therapies have been approved for this disease group.

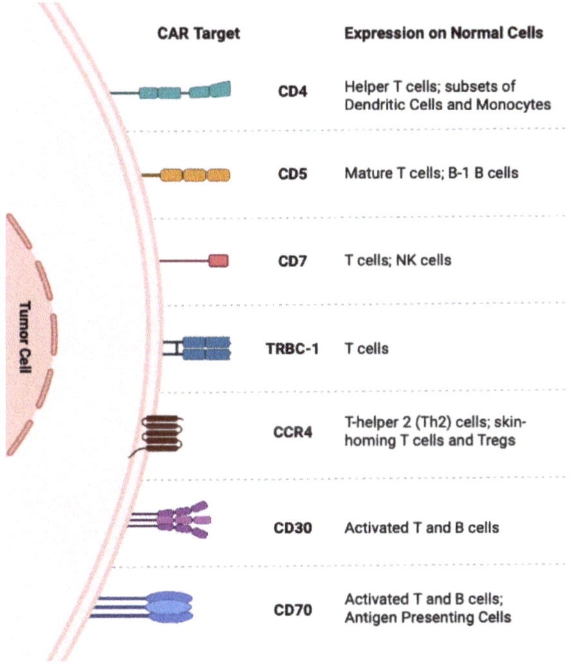

Figure 2. Surface antigens currently under clinical or preclinical investigation as CAR-T targets in peripheral T cell lymphomas. Pan-T cell antigens (CD4, CD5, CD7) present challenges due to T cell aplasia and fratricide, prompting safety-switch strategies and gene-editing approaches. More selective targets (TRBC1/2) exploit clonal restriction of the malignant TCR to spare healthy T cell compartments. Additional targets with more restricted or disease-specific expression, such as CD30, CCR4, and CD70, may improve therapeutic windows. These approaches highlight both the opportunities and unique challenges of CAR-T therapy in T cell lymphoma.

3.2.1. CD4

CD4 is a membrane glycoprotein expressed on T cells that serves as a co-receptor for the T cell receptor (TCR). In healthy individuals, approximately 40–50% of T lymphocytes are CD4+ T cells [121,122]. Upon antigenic stimulation, these cells differentiate into diverse T-helper subsets that coordinate and regulate adaptive immune responses [122]. In PTCL, the malignant clone is most often $CD4^{+}$, representing approximately two-thirds of cases, whereas $CD8^{+}$ PTCLs account for only 15–25%, with the remainder typically double-negative and, more rarely, double-positive [123]. Owing to this, Pinz et al. developed CAR-T cells targeting CD4 and demonstrated significant anti-tumor efficacy both in vitro against the Karpas 299 ALCL line and in mouse xenograft models [124]. Despite the remarkable efficacy in preclinical studies, concerns arise surrounding the safety of depleting healthy CD4+ T cells in patients, as CD4+ T cells play a crucial role in providing help to multiple immune effectors, including antibody production by B cells, licensing of dendritic cells to enhance CD8+ T cell functions, and other direct effector functions through cytokine secretion. Unlike the depletion of B cells, which can be tolerated or compensated through intravenous immunoglobulin infusion, the depletion of CD4+ T cells leads to profound immunosuppression, rendering patients vulnerable to opportunistic infections, a situation akin to HIV-associated depletion of CD4+ T cells. To circumvent this, the group has engineered a CD52 alemtuzumab safety switch to deplete the infused CD4 CAR-T cells and reverse the CD4+ T cell aplasia, shortening the window of immunosuppression [125]. Currently, there are multiple ongoing phase I trials of CD4 CAR-T cells in T cell lymphoma (NCT04162340, NCT04712864, NCT03829540). Preliminary data from the first three patients in the NCT04162340 clinical trial showed that two patients treated with CD4 CAR-T cells engineered to secrete an IL-15/IL-15Rα complex achieved durable complete remissions for 15 months and 8 months, respectively, and the third patient achieved a durable partial response (PR) [126]. Importantly, none of the three patients experienced severe opportunistic infections, neurotoxicity, or grade 3 and above cytokine release syndrome (CRS), indicating that the CD4 CAR-T cells were well tolerated in these patients. Better insights into the safety and tolerability of CD4 CAR-T cells are anticipated with the enrolment of more patients and the publication of these phase I studies.

3.2.2. CD5

In 2015, CD5-targeting CAR-T cells were developed by Mamonkin et al. to target T cell acute lymphoblastic leukemia (T-ALL) and T cell lymphomas [127]. CD5 is a surface glycoprotein expressed on all mature T cells and a subset of B cells, serving as a negative regulator of cellular activation [128]. Reflecting their post-thymic origin, malignant clones in PTCL frequently express CD5, with studies reporting positivity in ~63% of cases, though there is notable variation in expression patterns between subtypes [129]. Nodal Tfh lymphoma, PTCL-NOS, and ATLL have the highest proportion of patients with CD5-expressing tumors (>75%), whereas low expression is observed in ENKTL, breast-implant-associated (BIA) ALCL, and hepatosplenic TCL (HSTCL) [129]. Despite CAR-T cell fratricide caused by CD5 expression on mature T cells, Mamonkin et al. successfully generated CD5 CAR-T cells, as the surviving CAR-T cells downregulated surface CD5 expression [127]. Importantly, this loss of CD5 did not compromise the cells' effector function, which demonstrated preserved cytotoxicity in vitro and in vivo against preclinical models of T-ALL and T cell lymphoma. Supporting this, CD5-knockout CAR-T cells have been shown to exhibit augmented CAR-T cell function, consistent with CD5's role as a negative regulator of T cell activation [130].

While CAR-T fratricide can be mitigated by gene editing or expanding CD5-downregulated T cells, off-tumor targeting of normal T cells remains a concern. The risk of prolonged T cell aplasia has also prompted the development of safety switches in CD5 CAR-T cells. Inclusion of CD52 or truncated Epidermal Growth Factor Receptor (tEGFR) safety switches allows for antibody-mediated depletion (anti-CD52 and anti-EGFR, respectively) of these CAR-T cells in the event of unacceptable toxicity [131,132].

A recently published phase I clinical trial of autologous CD5 CAR-T cells (NCT03081910) targeting relapsed/refractory T cell lymphomas has shown a tolerable safety profile, with no patient experiencing CRS of grade 3 or higher [133]. However, three out of nine patients experienced prolonged cytopenias that persisted beyond 28 days. Although prior case reports described remarkable responses of CD5 CAR-T cells in ALK$^+$ ALCL [134] and T cell lymphoblastic lymphoma (T-LBL) [135], outcomes in this clinical trial were modest. Among nine treated patients, four had progressive disease (PD), one achieved stable disease (SD) but subsequently died following salvage therapy, one achieved a partial response (PR), and three achieved complete responses (CRs). At the end of follow-up, only two patients remained alive: one with nTFHL-AI who attained CR and subsequently underwent allogeneic hematopoietic stem cell transplantation (allo-HSCT) and another who relapsed after an initial CR. Six patients died of lymphoma progression and one from allo-HSCT complications. This limited efficacy may reflect the heavily pre-treated nature of the cohort (median of five prior therapies, up to eighteen in one patient), which likely compromised T cell fitness for autologous CAR-T manufacturing. Notably, clinical responses were confined to patients treated with CAR-T products generated using a shortened manufacturing protocol. This suggests that a minimally differentiated CAR-T product may be crucial for expansion and persistence. Additional challenges with autologous CD5 CAR-T manufacturing for T cell lymphoma include malignant cell contamination, as observed in a study from Hill et al., in which a CAR-T product had to be abandoned before infusion, as well as the potential for a long interval from apheresis to CAR-T cell infusion, with two patients dying from disease progression in this study while awaiting receipt of CAR-T cells [133].

Allogeneic CD5 CAR-T cells offer potential benefits by reducing the time to CAR-T infusion, ensuring T cell fitness, and preventing malignant clone contamination. Encouragingly, a phase II trial of allogeneic CD5 CAR-T cells in *r/r* T-ALL (NCT05032599) demonstrated a 100% response rate in 16 patients, suggestive also of their potential utility in the treatment of CD5-positive PTCL [136].

3.2.3. CD7

CD7 is a pan-T cell antigen expressed by most peripheral T cells [137], NK cells, and in more than 95% of T-lymphoblastic leukemia/lymphoma (T-ALL and T-LBL) [138]. Its expression in PTCL tumors varies considerably between subtypes, with 25% to 79% of cases being positive or partly positive [139]. In contrast to CD5-targeted CAR-T cells, which undergo only transient fratricide followed by complete loss of CD5 expression on the CAR-T population, CD7-targeted CAR-T cells are vulnerable to substantial fratricide following CAR transduction due to the high physiologic expression of CD7 on normal T cells [140]. Consequently, several strategies have been developed to yield fratricide-resistant CD7 CAR-T cells, including knocking out CD7 via genome editing [140], intracellular protein expression blockade (PEBL) [138], and pharmacologic inhibition of CAR signaling [141]. These approaches enabled the successful generation of CD7-targeting CAR-T cells, which possess significant anti-tumor activity both in vitro and in vivo. Interestingly, Lu et al. were able to develop a "naturally selected" CD7-targeting CAR-T cell therapy without additional manipulation of the T cell genome or culture conditions [142]. These naturally selected CAR-T cells undergo self-destruction (fratricide), and those that survive this process become the final CAR-T product. This study demonstrated that despite lower folds of expansion in these naturally selected CD7-targeting CAR-T (NS7CAR) cells, manufacturing was still able to be scaled successfully for clinical application. The researchers hypothesized that the surviving NS7CAR T cells had escaped fratricide due to antigenic masking or intracellular sequestration of CD7 by the CAR. Promisingly, in this phase I study of NS7CAR-T cells in T-ALL and T-LBL patients (NCT04572308), 19 out of 20 patients achieved minimal residual disease-negative (MRD-negative) CR in the bone marrow [142].

Thereafter, a further trial evaluated NS7CAR T cell therapy in CD7-positive *r/r* PTCL (NCT04928105) [143]. Preliminary data from the first five patients treated showed a remarkable response, where three patients achieved CR and one had a PR. CD7 CAR-T cells also demonstrated a manageable safety profile in these patients, with no patient experiencing grade $\geq$ 3 CRS or neurotoxicity. However, prolonged depletion of healthy T and NK cells following infusion of CD7 CAR-T cells remains a concern. While not observed in the PTCL trial, a follow-up study in T-ALL reported infections in 6 of the 12 patients who did not undergo allogeneic SCT consolidation, including 4 infection-related deaths [144]. These findings underscore the need for larger patient cohorts and extended follow-up to fully elucidate the safety and efficacy of CD7 CAR-T cells in PTCL. An additional limitation is CD7 downregulation, a frequent phenomenon in PTCLs [145]; hence, patient stratification is critical to ensure that the benefits of CD7 CAR-T cell therapy outweigh the risks. Ongoing clinical trials (NCT05290155, NCT05059912, NCT06925464, NCT04004637, NCT05979792, NCT04480788, NCT04264078, NCT05377827) will provide valuable insights into the efficacy and safety of this treatment.

3.2.4. TRBC-1

The T cell receptor (TCR) is a transmembrane complex consisting of two distinct protein chains. In humans, approximately 95% of T cells express an $\alpha\beta$ TCR, formed by alpha (α) and beta (β) chains, and the remaining 5% of T cells express a $\gamma\delta$ TCR, composed of a gamma (γ) and a delta (δ) chain. Within $\alpha\beta$ T cells, the β chain is unique to each T cell clone and is structured into variable (V), diversity (D), joining (J), and constant (C) regions. The constant (C) region of the beta (β) chain is encoded by two mutually exclusive genes, TRBC1 and TRBC2. Hence, T cells expanding from the same clone express the same TCRβ constant gene, either TRBC1 or TRBC2. Because PTCL arises from mature T cells, clonal lymphoma cells typically exhibit monoclonality at the TRBC locus (when derived from $\alpha\beta$ T cells), with homogeneous expression of either TRBC1 or TRBC2 [146–148]. Leveraging this clonality, Maciocia et al. developed TRBC1-targeting CAR-T cell therapy TRBC1+ tumors [146], aiming to ensure that healthy T cells expressing TRBC2 remained unaffected. Preliminary in vitro studies affirmed this hypothesis, and the investigators demonstrated TRBC1-targeting CAR-T cell therapy depleted only TRBC1-expressing tumors and normal T cells, sparing TRBC2-expressing T cells. Notably, in the phase I/II trial of TRBC1-CAR T cell therapy (NCT03590574) [149], the CAR-T therapy was well tolerated, with no severe adverse events, as evidenced by the absence of immune cell-associated neurotoxicity syndrome (ICANS) or dose-limiting toxicity. Only one patient experienced grade 3 CRS, which resolved within three days. Out of the nine evaluable patients, four achieved a complete response (CR) and two had a partial response (PR). Unfortunately, only two of the four that achieved a complete response had an ongoing remission at 15 and 18 months, whereas all other patients eventually developed progressive disease. Given the inability to readily detect the CAR-T cells in the peripheral blood, the lack of durable remission is likely attributable to limited expansion and persistence of the CAR-T cells. Concerningly, a recent study suggested that normal T cells may eliminate anti-TRBC1 CAR-T cells, potentially contributing to their limited persistence [150]. Additional contributors to poor CAR-T persistence may include fratricidal killing by non-malignant T cells, a bias toward effector-like differentiation, and the compromised fitness of autologous T cells rendered dysfunctional and exhausted by prior therapies [151]. Nevertheless, TRBC1-targeting CAR-T cell therapy holds promise as a novel treatment for PTCL patients, and sustained remission may be achieved by improving CAR-T cell manufacturing (e.g., using allogeneic CAR-T cells or generating Tstem-like CAR-T cells). Given TRBC1 targeting excludes a substantial number of patients to be eligible, the development of TRBC2-targeting CAR-T cell therapy is also currently underway for TRBC2-positive PTCL tumors [152]. Such approaches will spare a considerable fraction of the healthy residual T cell population, mitigating the risks of T cell compartmental ablation seen with pan T antigen targeting strategies.

3.2.5. CD30

CD30 is a membrane glycoprotein from the tumor necrosis factor (TNF) receptor family and is frequently overexpressed in classical Hodgkin lymphoma (HL) and ALCL [153,154], with expression observed in 93–100% of cases in both ALK-positive and ALK-negative ALCL tumors [139,155]. Multiple studies have also characterized its expression in other PTCL subtypes, including PTCL-NOS (16–58%), nTFHL-AI (21.42–63%), ATLL (39–55.5%), enteropathy-associated T cell lymphoma (EATL, 50–100%), ENKTL (46–70%). In contrast, MEITL and HSTCL show no detectable CD30 expression on tumors [139,155,156]. Given its restricted expression of only a small subset of activated T and B cells in healthy adults [154], CD30 has been regarded as a safe and attractive tumor target compared to other pan-T cell markers, leading to the successful development of brentuximab vedotin, a CD30 antibody–drug conjugate, which is discussed in more detail later in this review [157–160]. However, outside of durable responses in patients with ALCL, responses to brentuximab can be brief in other PTCL subtypes, mirroring the 22% 5-year PFS reported in HL. On the other hand, CAR-T cells may provide more durable disease control due to their persistence and formation of memory subsets [161]. Consistent with this, a patient with EATL who received CD30 CAR-T cell therapy made from allogeneic-donor stem cells achieved a complete response and remained in remission for 24 months [162].

In a phase I dose escalation study of CD30 CAR-T cells by Ramos et al. (NCT01316146), one of two enrolled ALCL patients achieved CR, and no CAR-T infusion-related toxicities were observed [163]. By contrast, Wang et al. reported treatment-related fatalities [164], including a Hodgkin lymphoma patient with high tumor burden who died of pleural hemorrhage with massive CD30 CAR-T infiltration and an ALCL patient who died of infection, possibly linked to targeting of normal $CD30^{+}$ T cells. Nevertheless, two of three ALCL patients in that trial achieved durable CRs lasting over one year [164].

CD30 CAR-T cells have also been evaluated as consolidation following autologous HSCT with BEAM conditioning in a mixed patient population with either Hodgkin lymphoma (HL) or PTCL [98] (NCT02663297). While this approach yielded encouraging outcomes in the HL cohort (2-year PFS 73%), five of six patients with PTCL (four with ALCL, one with nTFHL-AI, and one with PTCL-NOS) died during follow-up, four from disease progression and one from unrelated lung cancer, highlighting the limited efficacy for TCL in this setting. Seeking to improve this, Grover et al. (NCT03602157) are evaluating whether co-expressing CCR4 on CD30 CAR-T cells can enhance tumor homing [165]. Ultimately, larger PTCL-specific studies are required to define the therapeutic potential of CD30 CAR-T cells and to clarify the biological basis for the differing responses observed between HL and PTCL.

3.2.6. CD70

CD70, the ligand for the costimulatory receptor CD27 within the Tumor Necrosis Factor (TNF) receptor–ligand superfamily, is normally expressed on antigen-presenting cells and activated T cells [166,167]. However, dysregulated expression can drive aberrant CD27-CD70 signaling, which has been implicated in various solid tumors and hematological cancers, including T cell lymphomas [168]. CD70 is aberrantly overexpressed across several T cell lymphoma subtypes, notably in cutaneous T cell lymphoma (CTCL), including MF and primary cutaneous ALCL, and in certain PTCL subtypes, such as PTCL-NOS, systemic ALK-negative ALCL, nTFHL-AI, and acute-type ATLL [169–171]. Functionally, CD70 has also been implicated in promoting tumor growth and facilitating immune escape [168]. CD70's direct pathophysiological role coupled with its overexpression in T cell lymphomas make it a promising candidate for targeting.

Several CD70-directed therapeutics have been developed, including the antibody–drug conjugate SGN-CD70a [171], the monoclonal antibody cusatuzumab [172], and, more recently, allogeneic CD70-targeting CAR-T cells (CTX130), which have recent published data from a phase I study (NCT04502446) [173]. In this first-in-human phase I trial of allogeneic CD70-targeting CAR-T cells for relapsed/refractory T cell lymphoma, 18 of 39 patients achieved an objective response, including 10 with PTCLs (4 CRs and 6 PRs). These results highlight encouraging activity in a population with few effective options. Safety signals included a case of dose-limiting toxicity in a PTCL-NOS patient who developed hemophagocytic lymphohistiocytosis and grade 4 cytokine release syndrome (CRS). Overall, CRS was the most common serious adverse event, occurring in 28% of patients. Notably, no graft-versus-host disease (GvHD) was observed, supporting the feasibility of healthy donor-derived CAR-T platforms. A separate phase I/II trial (NCT06492304) is currently evaluating another further modified allogeneic CD70-directed CAR-T product, CTX131, in relapsed/refractory hematologic malignancies [173].

Besides the use of allogeneic T cells, another promising approach is CD70-targeted CAR-NK cells derived from induced pluripotent stem cells (iPSCs), which may mitigate the risk of GvHD due to their lack of TCR expression and serve as an off-the-shelf therapeutic for patients. CD70 CAR-NK cells developed by Wang et al. have been gene-edited to knock out CD70 expression, thereby avoiding fratricide, and engineered to express a high-affinity, non-cleavable CD16 and an IL-15 receptor α/IL-15 fusion protein (IL15RF), which improves antibody-dependent cellular cytotoxicity and persistence [174]. These CD70 CAR-NK cells were able to eradicate T cell lymphoma cells both in vitro and in mouse xenograft models using the MT4 ATLL cell line and represent a promising novel approach [174]. A phase I dose escalation study of these CD70 CAR-NK cells for the treatment of relapsed/refractory TCL and AML is currently active (NCT06696846).

3.2.7. CCR4

CCR4 is a chemokine receptor involved in T cell migration into the skin and is highly expressed on neoplastic T cells of CTCL (~62%) [175], ATLL (~90%) [176], and certain PTCL subtypes, including ALK-negative ALCL (~66.7%), PTCL-NOS (38%), and nTFHL-AI (34.8%) [177,178]. Higher CCR4 expression has also been correlated with disease severity [179,180]. CCR4 is a validated therapeutic target in TCL: mogamulizumab, a humanized, defucosylated anti-CCR4 monoclonal antibody (KW-0761) has received FDA approval for the treatment of *r/r* CTCL [181–184]. Despite initial activity with mogamulizumab, response durability is often limited [181,182,184,185]. Seeking to build on the achievements of mogamulizumab, CCR4-targeting CAR-T cells have been developed by Perera et al. [186] and Watanabe et al. [187]. In preclinical TCL models, Perera et al. demonstrated that CCR4-targeting CAR-T cells caused significant tumor lysis against multiple TCL cell lines, with superior efficacy observed in adult T cell leukemia (ATLL) and ALK-negative ALCL lines, concordant with CCR4 expression profiles in those diseases [186]. Significant tumor control was also achieved in ATLL murine xenografts treated with CCR4 CAR-T cells.

A further advantage of targeting CCR4 is the depletion of immunosuppressive Th2 cells and Tregs, enabling reactivation of endogenous anti-tumor responses that can act synergistically to improve outcomes [185,188]. This was demonstrated by Watanabe et al. [187], who showed that their CCR4 CAR-T product is enriched in Th1 cells due to fratricide of Th2 and Treg cells, possibly yielding improved anti-tumor efficacy and engraftment compared to CD19 CAR-T cells. However, Treg depletion may risk potentiating autoimmune adverse effects, which may prove a specific risk with CCR4-targeting CAR-T cells. The ongoing phase I trial of CCR4 CAR T cells for PTCL and CTCL (NCT07055477) should provide further insights into the safety profile of this agent.

3.2.8. Other Targets in Preclinical Development

The development of CAR-T cell therapy for TCLs is rapidly evolving, with many other targets currently in preclinical development. These include CD3 [189], CD26 [190], B7-H3 [191], and CCR8 [192], CD37 [193], and CD56 [194].

Engineered cellular therapies directed against a range of PTCL targets have demonstrated proof-of-concept anti-tumor activity. However, particular challenges remain including fratricide, antigen overlap, and toxicity. Various innovations such as TRBC-restricted, CD30- or CCR4-targeted constructs and allogeneic gene-edited products are promising means of overcoming these issues. However, balancing potency, safety, and persistence while ensuring viable immune reconstitution represents the greater challenge of these agents in T cell malignancies compared to B cell lymphoma. The following section considers how novel multi-specific and antibody-based strategies might complement or substitute cell therapy in this space.

3.3. Bispecific Antibodies in T Cell Lymphoma

T cell-engaging bispecific antibodies have proven to be an invaluable development in cancer immunotherapy, offering an off-the-shelf strategy to redirect endogenous T or NK cells against tumors. They are an established modality in the B cell lymphoma armamentarium [195]. However, these agents are more challenging to deploy in a TCL context. As with CAR-T cells, targeting common T cell antigens that are simultaneously present on healthy T cells risks induction of T cell aplasia. Furthermore, therapies that induce effector T cell interaction with a T cell target can result in unintended T cell fratricide, as discussed in relation to CAR-T cell design [196]. Nonetheless, there is a growing portfolio of agents under development with promising early clinical data.

Leveraging the proven efficacy of the antibody–drug conjugate brentuximab vedotin, CD30 has emerged as an antigen of interest for bispecific antibody development. Circumventing the risk of fratricide, AFM13 is a first-in-class tetravalent bispecific antibody that binds CD30 and CD16a. CD16a is expressed on natural killer (NK) cells and macrophages, and AFM13 has been termed an innate cell engager (ICE) as a result. In preclinical studies, AFM13 achieved potent NK cell activation, enhancing cytokine production and killing $CD30^{+}$ lymphoma targets in vitro. When combined with cytokine-preactivated peripheral blood or cord blood NK cells, AFM13 induced CAR-like activity with strong anti-tumor effects and improved survival outcomes in $CD30^{+}$ lymphoma xenograft models [197].

An initial phase I study on AFM13 in heavily pre-treated patients with Hodgkin lymphoma demonstrated an ORR of 11.5%, though the disease control rate (defined as the sum of ORR and stable disease rate) was 61.5% [198]. Thereafter, a small phase Ib/II trial in patients with TCL with cutaneous involvement (CTCL or ALCL with cutaneous involvement) achieved an ORR of 40% (n = 14) [199]. Notably, responses to AFM13 monotherapy in HL were modest, and more substantial activity has been observed in combination with checkpoint inhibitors, where combination with pembrolizumab in *r/r* HL showed evidence of synergy with an ORR of 83%. Safety of the combination appeared comparable to either agent alone, and such a strategy could be adopted for PTCLs [200].

More recently, a phase II open-label study (REDIRECT) was performed in relapsed/refractory CD30+ PTCL. Of 108 patients treated on REDIRECT, the ORR was 32.4% (CR:10.2%), with a higher response rate seen in nTFHL-AI (53.3%). The median duration of response was 2.3 months, and the treatment proved tolerable, with no cases of cytokine release syndrome [201].

Given the mechanism of action, a new phase I study of AFM13 in combination with cord-blood-derived, cytokine-preactivated allogeneic NK cells has shown impressive efficacy in relapsed/refractory CD30+ lymphoma [202]. In this approach, NK cells are isolated from cryopreserved cord blood units, briefly preactivated with cytokines such as IL-12, IL-15, and IL-18 and expanded ex vivo using feeder cells before being precomplexed with AFM13 just prior to infusion. This generates an NK cell product that is highly enriched for $CD56^{+}/CD16^{+}$ effector cells. Patients received 2–4 cycles of lymphodepleting chemotherapy followed by infusion of the AFM13–NK product, along with weekly AFM13 dosing. Among 42 patients treated (37 with Hodgkin lymphoma and 5 with T cell lymphoma), the overall response rate was 92.9% and the complete response rate was 66.7%. At a median follow-up of 20 months, the 2-year event-free survival (EFS) and OS rates were 26.2% and 76.2%, respectively. Durable responses were evident, with 11 patients who had achieved CR maintaining this response for 14–40 months. No CRS or graft-versus-host disease occurred [202]. In this study, the trial population was dominantly composed of patients with Hodgkin lymphoma; of the patients with TCL, one died of unrelated causes and the other four all progressed. One patient achieved CR (duration ~ 12 months) and two achieved PR, with no response in the remaining two participants. Nonetheless, the TCL population had received a median of seven prior lines of therapy, representing a highly refractory cohort; it is therefore difficult to draw meaningful conclusions about the efficacy of this combination in the TCL context. A key advantage of this strategy is that cord blood-derived NK products do not require HLA matching and can be manufactured in advance, representing an "off-the-shelf" cellular immunotherapy, contrasting with the complex, bespoke production required for autologous CAR-T cells.

Responses to CD30/CD3 bispecific antibodies in Hodgkin lymphoma appear modest in the absence of checkpoint blockade, and consistent with this limited single-agent activity, Genmab has recently discontinued development of GEN3017 in relapsed/refractory CD30-positive lymphomas as part of a strategic pipeline reprioritization [203]. Hence, the future of these agents as monotherapies is uncertain.

Beyond CD30, several other bispecific antibodies are under development for TCL. Efforts to overcome the risk of T cell fratricide with TRBC1/2-targeting therapies continue but remain in the preclinical space [204].

GNC-038 is a first-in-class octavalent CD19/CD3/4-1BB/PD-L1 tetra-specific antibody, GNC-038. It functions as a T cell engager that can target both CD19 and PDL1. Accordingly, there are potential applications in both B cell and T cell malignancies, and this agent may counteract T cell-mediated inhibition based on its PD-L1-targeting capability. GNC-038 is being investigated in both acute lymphoblastic leukemia and lymphoma [205]. A further trial is underway specifically in NK/T cell lymphoma (NCT05627856).

ONO-4685 is a novel PD-1/CD3 bispecific antibody which has demonstrated preclinical activity against PD-1-expressing T cell malignancies, with dose-dependent granzyme-B-mediated killing in cell lines and in humanized mouse xenograft models [206]. A phase I trial in relapsed/refractory peripheral and cutaneous T cell lymphomas is now underway (NCT05079282). A key challenge in applying CD3-engaging bispecifics to PTCLs is the risk of engaging the malignant T cells themselves. In addition to triggering fratricide, this engagement could cause paradoxical tumor activation and major toxicities; the safety of this approach remains uncertain and must be carefully considered.

An intriguing variation on both conventional bispecific and genetically modified cellular therapies is the antibody-armed T cell (AATC). Unlike CAR-T cells, which require genetic modification and permanent receptor expression, autologous T cells can be "armed" ex vivo with a therapeutic bispecific antibody [207]. The arming is transient and produces effector cells that can immediately redirect cytotoxicity toward target tumor cells without genome editing or complex manufacturing. NCT05544968 is a first-in-human, phase I/II study of CD30 biAb-AATC, armed with a CD30/CD3 bispecific antibody. It is designed to treat relapsed/refractory $CD30^+$ hematologic malignancies in pediatric and young-adult patients, with safety, feasibility, and early efficacy endpoints; the trial is scheduled to commence in late 2025.

3.4. Oncolytic Viruses

Oncolytic virus therapy is an emerging approach for cancer treatment. In 2015, the FDA approved T-Vec (talimogene laherparepvec), a second-generation oncolytic virus, for the treatment of melanoma [208]. The concept of oncolytic viruses originated from observations of tumor regression in patients following naturally acquired systemic viral infections. Oncolytic viruses, whether naturally occurring or genetically engineered, exert their anti-tumor effect by selectively replicating in cancer cells, stimulating host anti-tumor responses to cause immunogenic cell death [208,209].

The oncolytic effect of viral infection was highlighted in T cell lymphoma patients during the SARS-CoV-2 (COVID-19) pandemic. Three case reports have reported tumor regression after infection with the SARS-CoV-2 virus. One patient with MF achieved complete remission, while another with SS and a third with NK/T cell lymphoma experienced transient responses [210–212]. The virus likely exerted immunomodulatory properties through the induction of cytokine "storm", which led to the reinvigoration of anti-tumor immunity in these patients.

Early clinical exploration of oncolytic virus therapy in T cell lymphoma dates to 2005, when Heinzerling et al. [213] evaluated the oncolytic effect of measles virus in five patients with CTCL. These patients received two cycles of therapy, with each cycle consisting of two intra-tumoral injections of live measles virus, followed by a subcutaneous injection of IFN-alfa 72 h and 24 h before each viral dose. Five of the six treated lesions (one patient received treatment for two lesions) showed tumor regression, with one of the treated lesions completely disappearing, highlighting the potential of this modality [213]. Consistent results were observed in the phase I study (NCT03017820) of a single dose of vesicular stomatitis virus (VSV) expressing interferon-β (IFN-β) with the sodium iodide symporter (NIS), where five out of seven patients with relapsed/refractory TCL demonstrated regression in one or more tumors, and three achieving a clinical response (two with PR and one with CR) [214]. Importantly, no dose-limiting toxicities were observed, CRS was limited to grade 1/2 [214].

More recently, preclinical studies of a rat protoparvovirus, H-1 (H-1PV), demonstrated that the virus can infect and stimulate oncolytic activity in CTCL cell lines (HH, HuT78, and MyLa) and CTCL tumor spheroids while sparing healthy T cells and PBMCs [215]. Although most data regarding oncolytic viruses in TCL is derived from the CTCL context, these early findings suggest potential applicability in patients with PTCL. Three clinical trials of oncolytic viruses involving PTCL patients are currently active (NCT06508463, NCT05387226, NCT03017820).

There is significant potential for combining oncolytic viruses with orthogonal immunotherapeutic modalities. Numerous studies have demonstrated their capacity to reinvigorate antitumor immunity by remodeling the tumor microenvironment (TME) from an immune-suppressed "cold" state to an inflamed "hot" state [209]. This immunologic shift may enhance responsiveness to immune checkpoint inhibitors, CAR-T cell therapy, and bispecific T cell engagers. Combining oncolytic viruses with ICI immunotherapy has been evaluated in advanced melanoma, where adding an oncolytic virus to ipilimumab (anti-CTLA-4) improved response rates compared with ipilimumab alone (39% vs. 18%) [216]. Such combinations have not been investigated in patients with TCL but represent an intriguing area for future investigation.

3.5. Immunomodulatory Imide Drugs (IMiDs)

Immunomodulatory imide drugs (IMiDs) are structural analogues of thalidomide with potent anti-cancer and immunomodulatory properties [217]. The class includes thalidomide, lenalidomide, and pomalidomide. These drugs not only exhibit direct cytotoxicity against tumor cells but can also modulate the TME via their anti-angiogenic effects, T cell co-stimulation, and enhancing antibody-dependent cellular cytotoxicity (ADCC) of NK cells [217,218].

The use of lenalidomide as monotherapy in PTCL has been explored in multiple phase II trials across various disease subtypes, where it has shown a tolerable safety profile and comparable efficacy, with ORRs of 22–30%, respectively [219–221]. Response rates differ by disease subtype, with nTFHL-AI (ORR 31%) [219] and ATLL patients (ORR 42%) [222], responding better to lenalidomide as monotherapy. These results align with case reports in nTFHL-AI with refractory disease, where single-agent thalidomide has successfully induced a treatment response, with one patient achieving complete remission [223,224]. In these studies, the investigators demonstrated that thalidomide therapeutically modulates the tumor microenvironment in nTFHL-AI, reducing EBV-driven proliferation of monoclonal B cells, which likely contribute to the pro-tumorigenic TME [223].

Whilst IMiDs as a single agent were able to induce clinical response, PTCL patients do eventually relapse, with a progression-free survival of approximately 4 months [220,222]. Subsequent studies have investigated the utility of combining IMiDs with multi-agent chemotherapy regimens. In PTCL, the addition of thalidomide to standard CHOP (cyclophosphamide, adriamycin, vincristine, and prednisone) improved CR rates (mixed frontline and relapsed patient cohort) from 36.4% in the control (chemotherapy alone) group to 50% in the combination group [225]. Encouragingly, a phase II trial of an all-oral regimen of chidamide plus prednisone, cyclophosphamide, and thalidomide (CPCT) for *r/r* PTCL patients achieved an ORR of 71.1% (32/45) and a 28.9% CR rate, with a PFS of 8.5 months [226]. The clinical utility of IMiDS in first-line treatment has also been demonstrated in a trial comparing standard CHOP therapy versus GDPT (gemcitabine, cisplatin, prednisone, thalidomide) in newly diagnosed PTCL patients, where the ORR and CR rates of the GDPT group were significantly superior to the CHOP group (ORR 66.3% vs. 50% $p = 0.042$, CR 42.9% vs. 27.6% $p = 0.049$) [227].

Due to their immune-modulating properties, IMiDs have been investigated in combination with immunotherapies. In CTCL, a phase II trial of the combination of anti-PD-L1 and lenalidomide showed a significantly better ORR compared to durvalumab alone (58% vs. 36%) [228]. While this combination has not been investigated in PTCLs, a few studies have shown possible synergistic effects that may offer benefits to PTCL patients as well. In a small series of three *r/r* ENKTL patients, an anti-PD1 antibody combined with chidamide, etoposide, and thalidomide led to two CRs and one PR, suggesting a possible synergistic effect of IMiDs with immunotherapies [114]. However, enhanced efficacy may be accompanied by increased toxicity, as in the phase III trial of IMiD-anti-PD1 combination treatment in multiple myeloma, where a higher frequency of serious adverse events and treatment-related deaths resulted in termination of these studies [229,230]. Nevertheless, IMiDs have been shown to synergize with monoclonal antibody treatment in a B cell lymphoma context [231]. This is likely due to their ability to enhance NK-mediated ADCC and consequently could be investigated in combination with monoclonal antibodies or ADCs such as mogamulizumab (anti-CCR4) and brentuximab vedotin (anti-CD30) in *r/r* PTCL patients. In a phase I dose escalation study, the combination of lenalidomide with brentuximab vedotin showed promising responses, with two out of six patients achieving CRs and three patients achieving PRs (NCT03302728) [232]. Additionally, a phase II trial examining the same combination (NCT03409432) showed an ORR of 27.8% for CTCL (2 of 18 CRs) and 50% for PTCL (3 of 8 CRs) [233]. As previously mentioned, multiple clinical trials are investigating lenalidomide in combination with anti-PD1 (NCT04231370, NCT05182957, NCT01919619), anti-PD1 and chemotherapy (NCT04040491, NCT04038411), and anti-PDL1 (NCT03011814, NCT03054532). Besides enhancing NK cell activity, IMiDs are also known to provide co-stimulation to T cells, polarize the TME into Th1, and promote T cell survival [217], underscoring the rationale for combination with T cell-based cancer immunotherapies like CAR-T cell therapy and bispecific antibodies. Currently, the combination of IMiDs with CAR-T cell therapy or bispecifics is being trialed in multiple myeloma [218], and if successful, it could prompt consideration of combination therapy in TCL patients as well.

3.6. Other Agents

3.6.1. Denileukin Diftitox

Denileukin diftitox is a recombinant fusion protein in which human interleukin-2 is conjoined to diphtheria toxin fragments A/B, delivering the toxin into cells that express the high-affinity IL-2 receptor (CD25). Once bound to CD25, the complex is internalized and the diphtheria toxin broadly arrests protein synthesis, leading to cell death. As discussed with CCR4-targeting therapies, denileukin diftitox also depletes $CD25^+$ regulatory T cells, offering a dual rationale though modulation of the TME and augmentation of tumor immune responses.

A pivotal phase III trial in relapsed/refractory $CD25^+$ CTCL demonstrated an ORR of 44% (CR 34%), with a median response duration of 6.9 months. Median progression-free survival was significantly longer (over 2 years) in the denileukin arms versus ~124 days in placebo. Toxicities included infusion reactions, elevated liver enzymes, hypoalbuminemia, and the characteristic capillary leak syndrome [234]. The original formulation was withdrawn in 2014 for manufacturing reasons, but an improved-purity version (CXDL) has since been developed.

The registrational phase III of denileukin diftitox CXDL in relapsed/refractory CTCL reported an ORR of 36.2% (CR 8.7%) and median DOR of 8.9 months, leading to FDA approval in 2024 [235]. Smaller phase II studies in PTCL have also shown single-agent activity, with ORR around 40–50% (particularly in $CD25^+$ cases), and early efforts have combined the drug with CHOP in frontline PTCL, establishing feasibility.

The CONCEPT trial evaluated the addition of denileukin diftitox to CHOP in previously untreated PTCL. In this phase II study ($n = 49$), the overall response rate was 65%, with complete responses in 45% of patients. At a median follow-up of 25.6 months, the median DOR was approximately 30 months, median PFS was 12 months, and median OS had not been reached, with an estimated OS rate of 63% at last analysis [236]. These data suggest that a subset of patients achieved durable remissions; however, no longer-term (>5 year) follow-up of this cohort has been reported.

Denileukin diftitox is a clinically validated option in CTCL, with potential applications in PTCL, though careful monitoring for capillary leak and hepatic toxicity is required, and longer-term outcome data would be valuable.

3.6.2. Brentuximab Vedotin

The antibody–drug conjugate brentuximab vedotin (BV) combines a CD30 monoclonal antibody with the antimitotic agent monomethyl auristatin E. Phase I/II studies suggested clinical utility in TCL, with the most pronounced benefits observed in patients with CTCL and systemic ALCL (sALCL) in these early trials [237–239]. In the phase II trial of BV patients with sALCL, the ORR was 86%, with a CR rate of 57% and a median duration of response of 12.6 months [238]. Long-term follow-up at five years confirmed that this treatment was able to deliver durable disease control to a substantial number of patients, with median overall survival (OS) not reached. In the 38 patients who achieved a CR, neither median OS nor PFS were reached. Sixteen patients of this group had not required additional therapy apart from a consolidative auSCT, with eight patients being auSCT recipients and another eight patients not receiving auSCT or any further anti-cancer treatment after conclusion of study participation [240].

By way of contrast, the phase II data for brentuximab vedotin in patients with relapsed/refractory PTCL reported by Horwitz et al. demonstrated substantially reduced efficacy in histologic subtypes other than sALCL. ORR was 41%, and CR was observed in 8 of 35 participants (22%); however, median PFS was a short 6.7 months in patients with nTFHL-AI and only 1.6 months in patients with PTCL-NOS [241].

Combination strategies have also been explored in PTCL, most notably the phase III ECHELON 2 trial, which compared BV in combination with the cytotoxic backbone of cyclophosphamide, doxorubicin, and prednisolone (BV-CHP) against the standard-of-care CHOP (cyclophosphamide, doxorubicine, vincristine, and prednisolone) in patients with newly diagnosed CD30-positive PTCL. In this study of 452 patients, of whom 70% had sALCL, 3-year OS was 77% versus 69% (HR 0.66, $p = 0.02$), with median PFS of 48.2 months versus 20.8 months (HR 0.71, $p = 0.01$) [158]. At 5 years of follow-up, these results were sustained, with estimated 5-year PFS of 51% for BV-CHP compared to 43% for CHOP. Estimated 5-year OS was 70% and 61%, respectively [242].

While CTCL is not the predominant focus of this review, it is worth noting the results of the phase III ALCANZA study in patients with CD30-positive relapsed or refractory CTCL, in whom BV was compared to physician's choice of either oral methotrexate or bexarotene. A total of 128 patients were included. Outcome data favored BV treatment, with an objective response lasting 4 or more months (ORR4) being 54.7% in the BV group versus 12.5% in the physician's choice group ($p < 0.001$), and ORR of 65.6% versus 20.3% ($p < 0.001$). The CR rate was 17.2% versus 1.6% ($p = 0.002$). Median PFS was 16.7 months for BV-treated patients versus 3.5 months for the physician's choice cohort (HR 0.38, $p = 0.001$), with a median follow-up of 36.8 months [157]. The final analysis of the data at a median follow-up of 45.9 months continued to demonstrate clinical benefit from BV treatment in this group of patients [243].

3.6.3. Lacutamab

Lacutamab, also known as IPH4102, is a fully humanized monoclonal antibody targeting KIR3DL2, an inhibitory immune receptor usually expressed on small numbers of CD8-positive T cells and NK cells in health which is upregulated and highly expressed in selected subtypes of CTCL [244–248]. Assessment of the mode of action of lacutamab in preclinical work in CTCL suggested a highly tumor-specific effect causing antibody-dependent cell death and phagocytosis, with reduced tumor growth and prolonged survival in animal models [244,249]. Phase I–II trials confirmed clinical benefit with good tolerance in patients with SS and MF, with long-term results from the phase II study in SS recently reported showing ORR of 42.9% and median duration of response of 25.6 months (range, 11—not evaluable) [250–252].

Later research confirmed that KIR3DL2 is also upregulated in certain PTCL subtypes when assessed in vivo by either flow cytometric methods or immunohistochemistry, with highest rates of expression observed in PTCL-NOS and AITL [253]. Preclinical work in PTCL suggested a combinational effect on cell death in PTCL in tumor models when lacutamab was used with cytotoxic agents, either CHOP or pralatrexate [254].

Based on encouraging results for lacutamab in CTCL and bolstered by the preclinical data in PTCL, a phase Ib trial (NCT05321147) was developed to explore the efficacy and safety of lacutamab monotherapy in relapsed/refractory PTCL [255]. However, interim results from this study suggested a lack of sufficient efficacy, which in early 2024 led to discontinuation of the PTCL monotherapy development pathway, with a refocus predominantly on lacutamab monotherapy in CTCL and combination strategies in PTCL [256]. The phase II randomized non-comparative clinical trial of lacutamab in combination with gemcitabine and oxaliplatin (GemOx) versus GemOx alone (KILT study; NCT04984837) is ongoing in patients with *r/r* PTCL [257].

3.6.4. Mogamulizumab

Mogamulizumab, a CCR4 monoclonal antibody, has demonstrable clinical benefit in CTCL, particularly in advanced disease with a leukemic component. The phase III MAVORIC study compared mogamulizumab in comparison to the HDACi–vorinostat in patients with *r/r* MF and SS, stratified according to stage. Median PFS was 7.7 months for mogamulizumab versus 3.1 months for vorinostat (HR 0.53, 95% CI 0.41–0.69, $p < 0.0001$), with similar rates of adverse events between both groups. For patients with SS, HR was 0.32 (95% CI, 0.21–0.49) [182]. Improved ORR and time to next treatment (TTNT) appeared to correlate to the degree of blood involvement, with ORR among patients with a high burden of Sezary cells being 37.4% for mogamulizumab-treated patients versus 3.2% for vorinostat-treated patients ($p < 0.0001$) [258].

An optimal therapeutic niche for mogamulizumab in patients with PTCL is still being delineated. Phase II data from selected studies suggested an ORR between 11.4 and 34%, although the latter study included both PTCL and CTCL patients [185,259]. Post marketing surveillance data from Ishitsuka et al., Japan, reported an ORR of 34.5% in their PTCL cohort, with highest responses in patients with nTFHL-AI (50%) [260]. Durable responses are not guaranteed, as noted elsewhere in this review.

It is important to note, however, that there seems to be a specific clinical benefit to the use of mogamulizumab in patients with ATLL, particularly in the setting of relapsed/refractory disease. Data is predominantly drawn from small case series and selected phase II studies at present, but the agent appears active and well tolerated either given as monotherapy or in combination, and larger-scale trials are key [261–265].

3.6.5. MEDI-570

As elucidated earlier in this review, the high expression of the inducible T cell costimulator (ICOS) on Tfh, coupled with an evolving understanding of the role ICOS in lymphomagenesis, led to the development of clinical trials of MEDI-570, a human afucosylated, IgG kappa monoclonal anibody targeting ICOS. Initial trials in the autoimmune disorder systemic lupus erythematosus (NCT01127321) were terminated due to emergent side effects deemed unacceptable in the setting of a chronic inflammatory disease [266]; however, the observation of a significant reduction in memory CD4-positive ICOS-positive cells in the study population refocused interest in the utility of this agent in nTFHL. The phase I dose escalation study (NCT02520791) explored intravenous administration of MEDI-570 once every three weeks in a cohort of patients with relapsed/refractory PTCL. Twenty-three patients were included, including eighteen in the dose escalation phase, with patients having received a median of three prior lines of treatment. Of these, 17 had nTFHL (nTFHL-AI in 16 patients, follicular TFHL in 1). No DLTs were observed. Treatment-emergent adverse events (TEAEs) included predominantly grade 1–2 side effects, including infusion-related reactions (IRRs) (48% of the patients), fatigue (35% of the patients), and nausea (30% of the patients), while grade 3–4 TEAEs were predominantly reduced CD4 counts (57% of the patients), lymphopenia, and anemia, as well as a grade 3 IRR in one patient leading to augmented mandatory premedication for subsequent subjects. ORR was 30% (7/23 patients), with 2 patients achieving a CR and 5 achieving PR. All responding patients had nTFHL-AI, with ORR in patients with this subtype being 44%. Median PFS for nTFHL-AI patients was 2.9 months (95% CI: 1.9–6.7 months), while median OS was 17.1 months [267]. Further study is needed to identify the optimal therapeutic niche for this agent, noting also the potential for rational combinations.

Collectively, these emerging immunotherapeutic modalities demonstrate the growing capacity to target both tumor-intrinsic and microenvironmental mechanisms of immune escape in PTCL. Checkpoint inhibitors, engineered cellular therapies, bispecific antibodies, antibody–drug conjugates, and immunomodulatory agents act through complementary mechanisms that together broaden the therapeutic landscape. Figure 3 summarizes these strategies and the diverse immunologic axes they engage to restore effective anti-tumor immunity. Though exciting, future research must seek to define which patient subgroups will benefit most from which therapy and identify rational approaches to therapy combination, sequencing, and monitoring.

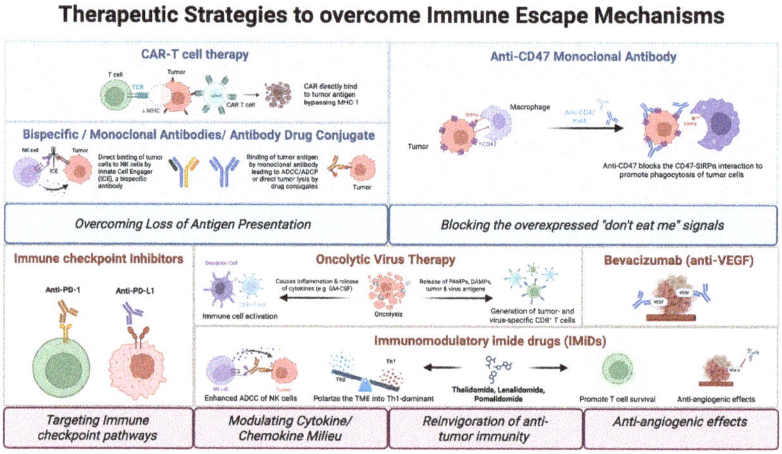

Figure 3. Therapeutic strategies to overcome immune escape mechanisms in peripheral T cell lymphomas. Approaches include CAR-T and CAR-NK cell therapies, bispecific and antibody–drug conjugates that overcome loss of antigen presentation; anti-CD47 antibodies that block "don't-eat-me" signals; checkpoint inhibitors and oncolytic viruses that modulate tumor–immune interactions; and immunomodulatory agents that reshape the cytokine milieu and promote T cell activation. Together, these strategies exemplify the convergence of cellular, molecular, and immunologic modalities toward personalized immunotherapy in PTCL.

Table 2. Studies evaluating cellular therapies, oncolytic viruses, and immunomodulatory agents in peripheral T cell lymphoma, organized by therapeutic approach and target.

Regimen	Phase	Trial	Prior Lines of Therapy	No of Patients (TCL Cohort)	ORR	CR	Median PFS	OS	Reference
CAR-T Cell Therapies									
CD4-specific CAR-T	Phase I	NCT04162340	N/A	(Preliminary data) Total: 3 SS: 1 Transformed MF: 1 AITL: 1	100% (2 CR, 1 PR)	66% (2 out of 3)	N/A	N/A	[130]
	Phase I	NCT04712864	Active, Not Recruiting						
	Phase I	NCT03829540	Recruiting						
CD5-specific CAR-T	Phase I	NCT03081910 (MAGENTA)	Median: 5 lines (Range 2–18)	Total: 9 MF/SS: 1 CTCL: 1 AITL: 2 PTCL: 4 ATLL: 1	44% (2 CRs, 1 PR, 1 mixed radiographic response)	22% (2 out of 9)	N/A	N/A	[137]
	Phase I	NCT04767308	(Range 2–6)	(Preliminary data) Total: 3 AITL: 2 SPTCL: 1	100% (1 CR, 2 PR)	33% (1 out of 3)	N/A	N/A	[136]
	Phase I	NCT04594135	Unknown status						Preclinical and preliminary clinical data of 1 patient [135]
	Phase I	NCT06633341	Recruiting						
	Phase I	NCT07022964	Recruiting						
CD7-specific CAR-T	Phase I	NCT04928105	Median: 6 (Range: 2–12)	(Preliminary data) Total: 5 PTCL-NOS: 2 MEITL: 1 HSTCL: 1 NKTCL: 1	80% (3 CR, 1 PR)	60% (3 out of 5)	N/A	N/A	[148]
	Phase I	NCT05377827	N/A	(Preliminary data) Total: 5 PTCL:1 T-PLL:2 Gamma-delta TCL: 2	80% (2 CR, 2 PR, 1 SD)	40% (2 out of 5)	N/A	N/A	[268]
	Phase I	NCT04004637	Unknown status						Preliminary data on T-ALL/T-LBL [269]
	Phase I	NCT05290155	Completed, results not published						
	Phase II	NCT05059912	Unknown status						

Table 2. *Cont.*

Regimen	Phase	Trial	Prior Lines of Therapy	No of Patients (TCL Cohort)	ORR	CR	Median PFS	OS	Reference
CD7-specific CAR-T	Phase I/II	NCT06925464	Recruiting						
	Phase I	NCT05979792	Not yet recruiting						
	Phase I	NCT04480788	Unknown status						
	Phase I	NCT04264078	Unknown status						
	Phase I	NCT04934774	Unknown status						
	Phase I	NCT04823091	Recruiting						
	Phase I	NCT05995028	Recruiting						
	N/A	NCT07008872	Not yet recruiting						
	N/A	NCT05620680	Recruiting						
TRBC1-specific CAR-T	Phase I/II	NCT03590574 (AUTO4)	Median: 2 (Range 1–5)	Total: 10 AITL: 4 PTCL-NOS: 5 ALCL: 1	66.6% (6 of 9)	44.4% (4 of 9)	Median 4.7 months	Median OS was not reached	[270]
	Phase I	NCT04828174	Trial suspended						
CD30-specific CAR-T	Phase I	NCT01316146	N/A	Total: 9 Hodgkin's lymphoma: 7 ALCL: 2	33.3% (3 of 9)	33.3% (3 of 9)	N/A	N/A	[169]
	Phase I	ChiCTR-OPN-16009069	N/A	Total: 9 Hodgkin's lymphoma: 6 ALCL: 3	77.7% (7 CR)	77.7%	Median 13 months		[170]
	Phase I	NCT04526834	Active, not recruiting						
	Phase I	NCT07048353	Not yet recruiting						
	Phase I	NCT05208853	Unknown status						
	Phase I	NCT02917083 (RELY-30)	Recruiting						
	Phase I	NCT04653649	Unknown status						
	Phase II	NCT04083495	Recruiting						
	Phase I	NCT06494371	Recruiting						
Allogeneic CD30 CAR-EBVST cells	Phase I	NCT04288726	Recruiting						
Allogeneic CD30 CAR-EBVST cells with constitutive IL7R (C7R)	Phase I	NCT06176690	Not yet recruiting						
CCR4-expressing CD30-specific CAR-T cells	Phase I	NCT03602157	Recruiting						

Table 2. *Cont.*

Regimen	Phase	Trial	Prior Lines of Therapy	No of Patients (TCL Cohort)	ORR	CR	Median PFS	OS	Reference
CD30-specific CAR-T as consolidation after BEAM and autologous HSCT	Phase I	NCT02663297	83% of patients have one line of salvage therapy before autologous HSCT, 17% required second line of therapy	Total: 21 Hodgkin's lymphoma: 11 ALCL: 4 AITL: 1 PTCL-NOS: 1 Grey zone lymphoma: 1	At median follow-up of 48.2 months, 5 patients with T cell lymphoma have died	N/A	Median 32.3 months	Not reached	[171]
Allogeneic CD70-specific CAR-T cells	Phase I	NCT04502446 (COBALT-LYM)	Median: 2.5 for PTCL, 5 for CTCL	Total: 39 PTCL: 22 (9 ATLL, 8 PTCL-NOS, 4 AITL, 1 ALCL) CTCL: 17	46.2% (18 of 39)	19.4% (6 of 39)	N/A	N/A	[179]
	Phase I/II	NCT06492304	Recruiting						
CCR4-specific CAR-T cells	Phase I	NCT07055477	Recruiting						
CD37-specific CAR-T cells	Phase I	NCT04136275	Median 6 (range 3–8)	Total: 5 Double-hit HGBCL: 2 CTCL:1 Hodgkin's lymphoma: 1 NKTCL: 1	80% (3 CR)	60% (3 of 5)	N/A	N/A	[193]
CD56-specific CAR-T	Phase II	NCT05941156	Recruiting						
CAR-NK Cell Therapies									
CD5-specific CAR-NK	Phase I	NCT06909474	Recruiting						
CD70-specific CAR-NK cells	Phase I	NCT06696846	Not yet recruiting						
Oncolytic Virus									
Oncolytic Virus Injection (RT-01)	Phase I	NCT06508463	Unknown status						
Vesicular Stomatitis Virus (VSV)	Phase I	NCT05387226	Recruiting						
Vesicular Stomatitis Virus (VSV)	Phase I	NCT03017820	Recruiting						
Single Agent Immunomodulatory Drugs (IMiDs)									
Lenalidomide Monotherapy	Phase II	NCT01724177	Median: 2 (Range 1–4)	Total: 26 (All ATLL)	42%	19.2% (4 CR and 1 unconfirmed)	3.8 months	20.3 months	[228]
Lenalidomide Monotherapy	Phase II	NCT00322985	Median: 1 (range 0–5)	Total: 40	26% (10 of 39)	8%	4 months	12 months	[226]
Lenalidomide Monotherapy	Phase I	NCT01169298	Median: 1 (Range 1–3)	Total: 13 ATLL: 9 Other PTCL: 4	36% (4 of 11 evaluable)	0%	3.4 months	N/A	[271]

Table 2. *Cont.*

Regimen	Phase	Trial	Prior Lines of Therapy	No of Patients (TCL Cohort)	ORR	CR	Median PFS	OS	Reference
Lenalidomide Monotherapy	Phase II	NCT00655668 (EXPECT)	Median: 3 (Range 1–11)	Total: 54 AITL: 26 PTCL-NOS: 20 CTCL (MF): 3 sALCL: 3 pcALCL:1 ENKTL: 1	22% (12 of 54)	11%	2.5 months	N/A	[227]
Lenalidomide Monotherapy	Phase II	NCT01036399	Median: 4 (Range 2–7)	Total: 10 (All PTCL-NOS)	30%	30% (3 of 10)	N/A	N/A	[225]
Immunomodulatory Drugs (IMiDs) + Chemotherapy									
Chidamide plus prednisone, cyclophosphamide, and thalidomide (CPCT)	Phase II	NCT02879526	At least 1 prior line	Total: 45 AITL: 20 PTCL-NOS: 17 Other subtypes: 8	71.1% (32 of 45)	28.9% (13 of 45)	8.5 months	17.2 months	[232]
CHOP (cyclophosphamide, doxorubicin, vincristine, prednisone) vs. GDPT (gemcitabine, cisplatin, prednisone, thalidomide) in newly diagnosed PTCL patient	Phase IV	NCT01664975	0 (newly diagnosed cohort)	Total: 153 PTCL-NOS: 31 AITL: 37 ALCL: 49 Other subtypes: 36	66.3% (GDPT) versus 50.0% (CHOP)	42.9% (GDPT) vs. 27.6% (CHOP)	4-year PFS: 63.6% (GDPT) vs. 53.0% (CHOP)	4-year OS: 66.8% (GDPT) vs. 53.6% (CHOP	[233]
Lenalidomide in combination with vorinostat and dexamethasone	Phase I/II	NCT00972842	Median: 1 (Range 1–2)	Total: 8 AITL: 5 PTCL-NOS:1 ALCL: 1	25% (2 of 7 evaluable)	14.2% (1 of 7)	2.2 months	6.7 months	[272]
CHOP alone vs. CHOP plus thalidomide	N/A	N/A	N/A	Total: 46 NKTCL: 21 PTCL: 9 ALCL: 7 AITL: 4 Other subtypes: 5	79.2% (thalidomide group) vs. 63.6% (CHOP alone)	50% (thalidomide group) vs. 36.4% (CHOP alone)	12 months (thalidomide group) vs. 6 months in CHOP alone	Undefined (thalido-mide group) vs. 17 months in CHOP alone	[231]
Romidepsin, 5-azacitidine, Dexamethasone, plus Lenalidomide	Phase I	NCT04447027	Median: 2 (Range 1–8)	Total: 26 Nodal TCL: 16 MF: 6 ATLL: 4	56% (25 evaluable)	12%	1-year PFS: 14.9%	1-year OS: 63.3%	[273]

Table 2. *Cont.*

Regimen	Phase	Trial	Prior Lines of Therapy	No of Patients (TCL Cohort)	ORR	CR	Median PFS	OS	Reference
Lenalidomide plus CHOEP	Phase I/II	NCT02561273	0 (newly diagnosed)	Total: 39 PTCL-NOS: 19 AITL: 16 ALCL: 3	69%	49%	2-year PFS: 55%	2-year OS: 78%	[274]
Romidepsin and Lenalidomide	Phase II	NCT02232516	0 (newly diagnosed)	Total: 29 AITL: 16 PTCL-NOS: 10 ATLL: 2 EATL: 1	65.2%	26.1%	2-year PFS: 31.5%	2-year OS: 49.5%	[275]
Lenalidomide plus Gemcitabine	Phase I/II	NCT05105412	Terminated						
Bendamustine Combined With Chidamide and Lenalidomide	N/A	NCT07072221	Recruiting						
Chidamide Combination with Lenalidomide	Phase II	NCT04329130	Unknown status						
lenalidomide plus CHOP (L-CHOP) versus CHOP alone	Phase II	NCT04922567	Recruiting						
CHOP plus Lenalidomide	Phase II	NCT01553786	Completed						
Immunomodulatory Drugs (IMiDs) + Immunotherapy									
Lenalidomide + Sintilimab (anti-PD1)	Phase II	NCT04231370	Unknown status						
Anti-PD1 + Lenalidomide and azacytidine	Phase II	NCT05182957	Unknown status						
Lenalidomide, anti-PD1, Chidamide and Gemcitabine	Phase IV	NCT04040491	Unknown status						
Lenalidomide, anti-PD1, Chidamide and Etoposide	Phase IV	NCT04038411	Unknown status						
Durvalumab (anti-PDL1) with or without lenalidomide	Phase I/2	NCT03011814	Active, not recruiting						
	Phase II	NCT03054532	Unknown status						
Lenalidomide plus Brentuximab Vedotin	Phase I	NCT03302728	Completed						
	Phase II	NCT03409432	Completed						
Lenalidomide and Ipilimumab after Stem cell transplant	Phase II	NCT01919619	Completed						

Abbreviations: AITL, angioimmunoblastic T cell lymphoma; ALCL, anaplastic large cell lymphoma; ALK, anaplastic lymphoma kinase; ALK-, ALK-negative; ALK+, ALK-positive; ASCT, autologous stem cell transplantation; CR, complete response; DOR, duration of response; EATL, enteropathy-associated T cell lymphoma; ENKTL, extranodal natural killer/T cell lymphoma; HSTCL, hepatosplenic gamma delta T cell lymphoma; MEITL, monomorphic epitheliotropic intestinal T cell lymphoma; MF, mycosis fungoides; N/A, not applicable; NR, not reached; ORR, overall response rate; OS, overall survival; PCET, PD-1 antibody + chidamide + etoposide + thalidomide; PD, progressive disease; PD-L1, programmed death-ligand 1; PFS, progression-free survival; PTCL, peripheral T cell lymphoma; PTCL NOS, peripheral T cell lymphoma not otherwise specified; TCL, T cell lymphoma; TFH, T-follicular helper.

4. Biomarkers for Informing Management of PTCL

The heterogeneity of PTCL underscores the urgent need for robust biomarkers that can guide therapeutic choice and predict response to emerging immunotherapies. As discussed in the checkpoint inhibitor section, most of the biomarker literature to date comes from studies of PD-1/PD-L1 blockade, often extrapolated from non-PTCL contexts, and includes factors such as PD-L1 expression, EBV status, tumor mutational burden, and 9p24.1 structural variants. While these data provide important proof-of-concept, they remain incomplete and inconsistently predictive in PTCL. Moving beyond immune checkpoint therapy, additional modalities are beginning to yield important insights, including imaging biomarkers such as FDG-PET, genomic and circulating tumor DNA markers, immunohistochemical correlates, and gene expression-defined subtypes. Integrating these data into a coherent framework, though nascent, is essential for biomarker-driven stratification and personalized therapeutic strategies in PTCL.

4.1. Positron Emission Tomography

Functional imaging with 18F-FDG PET/CT is a cornerstone of response assessment across PTCLs. Baseline metabolic tumor volume, response kinetics during treatment, and end of treatment response all have prognostic implications in PTCLs [276–278]. Novel radiotracers targeting immune cell populations in an attempt to directly visualize the tumor microenvironment hold promise as potential biomarkers in PTCLs. For example, PD-1/PD-L1 axis radiotracers are currently under investigation as predictors of response to immune checkpoint inhibitor therapy, but data in PTCLs is currently lacking [279].

4.2. Genomics

Recent reports suggest that high pre-treatment circulating tumor DNA (ctDNA) levels predict lower response and survival rates in T and NK cell lymphomas [268]. In addition, the monitoring of somatic mutations over time has utility for predicting relapse [268,280]. Mutations of *RHOA*, *IDH2*, *TET2*, and *DNMT3A* are highly recurrent in nTFHL-AI and Tfh cell lymphomas and aid in diagnosis [270]. In nTFHL-AI particularly, *RHOA* and *IDH2* show promise as MRD markers because they are not present in pre-lymphoma clones [281]. The vast majority of patients reported by Kim et al. and Yannakou et al. were treated with conventional chemotherapy approaches as opposed to immunotherapies, however [280,281]. In a study of ctDNA in nTFHL-AI by Zhang et al., RHOA G17 codon mutations were significantly associated with genes involved in "PD-L1 expression and PD-1 checkpoint pathway in cancer" by pathway analysis, suggesting that patients harboring such mutations may respond more favorably to checkpoint inhibition [271].

4.3. Immunohistochemistry

CD30 is a key biomarker for treatment selection in the setting of PTCLs, as some degree of CD30 expression is required to justify treatment with brentuximab vedotin. In the ECHELON-2 study, a CD30 cut-off of 10% was used for patient eligibility, but there was no correlation between CD30 expression and clinical outcome [242].

ALK positivity is a key determinant of outcome in systemic ALCL; however, this does not predict response rates or survival outcomes post brentuximab vedotin in either the first-line or the relapsed setting [240,242]. The presence or absence of DUSP22 and TP63 rearrangements in ALK-negative ALCL is known to stratify patients by clinical outcome, with DUSP22 rearrangements having a positive impact and TP63 rearrangements having a negative impact on prognosis [272]. The utility of DUSP22 and TP63 rearrangements as biomarkers of response to BV is currently unknown given the low number of BV-treated patients described in the literature to date.

In ATLL, CCR4 mutations and immunohistochemistry (which is inversely correlated with mutation status) have been associated with superior mogamulizumab effect [273,274]. However, other reports assessing mogamulizumab for the treatment of T cell lymphoma have not demonstrated this correlation between CCR4 expression and clinical outcome [185].

4.4. Gene Expression

Huang et al. defined various molecular subtypes of PTCL using an integrated genomic and transcriptomic approach [11]. The "Tfh-like" subtype expressed higher levels of CRBN (Cereblon), TIGIT, and CD52, while increased expression of immune checkpoint genes such as PD-L1 and LAG3 was found in the "inflammatory" subtype. The "mesenchymal" subtype expressed higher levels of TNFRSF8 (CD30), IDO1, and TIM-3. Du et al. used spatial transcriptomics to show that CCL17 and CCL22, which encode the dominant ligands for CCR4, are upregulated within the tumor microenvironment of nTFHL-AI, suggesting that anti-CCR4 therapies such as mogamulizumab may have activity in this disease [275]. Such approaches provide tantalizing insights into how the heterogeneity of PTCL can be teased apart and provides a rationale for a more personalized approach to immunotherapy selection. However, at this time, correlation with clinical outcomes is lacking and further investigation is thus required.

4.5. Integrating Biomarkers

Collectively, these biomarker studies demonstrate both the progress and limitations of biomarker discovery in PTCL. As discussed in Section 3.1, PD-L1 expression and 9p24.1 amplification remain the best studied correlates of immune checkpoint sensitivity, but their predictive power is inconsistent across subtypes. EBV positivity may confer distinct immune–antigenic contexts relevant to both tumor biology and immunotherapy response, while TRBC restriction defines a potential avenue for selective CAR-T targeting. Quantitative and longitudinal ctDNA profiling offers a dynamic measure of disease burden and molecular response, and preliminary data suggest that circulating mutations such as RHOA G17V could enrich for immunotherapy-responsive phenotypes. TMB has been evaluated as a surrogate of neoantigenicity, but levels are typically low in PTCL and have not consistently correlated with response. Integration of these orthogonal biomarkers—genomic, transcriptomic, serologic, and microenvironmental—into cohesive, multi-omic frameworks will be critical to translate biological insight into clinically actionable stratification. However, existing approaches remain exploratory and lack prospective validation, underscoring the need for harmonized assays and correlative biomarker programs embedded within future clinical trials. At present, the clinical utility of these biomarkers remains limited, either individually or cumulatively considered.

5. Perspectives and Outlook on Immunotherapy in PTCL

Immunotherapy in PTCL remains an emerging frontier modality rather than an evidence-based standard. While isolated signals of activity have been observed across immune checkpoint blockade, antibody–drug conjugates, bispecific antibodies, and other immune-modulatory agents, these approaches are yet to consolidate into a coherent therapeutic framework. The absence of biomarker-directed patient selection and limited understanding of the tumor–microenvironment interface—particularly the immunologic consequences of key genomic and epigenomic alterations—continue to hinder rational treatment design. Without this biological foundation, it remains difficult to define evidence-based therapeutic sequencing strategies or identify synergistic combinations with cytotoxic, epigenetic, or targeted agents. These uncertainties are compounded by the intrinsic heterogeneity of

PTCL, especially within PTCL-NOS, where diverse cell-of-origin and transcriptional states dilute statistical power and cloud efficacy signals. Accordingly, immunotherapy in PTCL should be regarded as a field in early translation—with considerable promise but presently limited by incomplete biological insight and fragmented clinical evidence.

As the field progresses, genuine progress will require sophisticated frameworks that integrate multi-omic and spatial profiling to resolve the interplay between tumor-intrinsic drivers and the immune milieu. Such multi-dimensional analyses will be essential to systemically identify actionable immune vulnerabilities and redefine disease classification beyond the status quo histologic and lineage-based criteria. Ultimately, these advances may enable a shift from empirical immune modulation to biomarker-directed intervention, transforming immunotherapy in PTCLs from a theoretical concept into a precision discipline.

6. Conclusions

The therapeutic landscape of PTCLs is at an inflection point. While recent clinical trials demonstrate that immunotherapies can achieve responses in otherwise refractory disease, their efficacy is inconsistent and seldom durable. Current personalized strategies—such as PD-L1 immunohistochemistry, next-generation sequencing, or TRBC-restricted targeting—represent early steps toward a precision framework but require further validation and broader clinical application. The breadth of potential biomarkers reviewed herein attests to their potential utility in shaping the next generation of immunotherapy trials, yet their largely exploratory and poorly validated status highlights the parallel need for better validation and clinical integration in PTCL. Emerging technologies offer some promise to surmount many of the current limitations. Armored CAR-T cells engineered to secrete cytokines or resist checkpoint inhibition may overcome the issues of persistence and TME-mediated suppression. Allogeneic or gene-edited platforms could mitigate fratricide and reduce the risk of pan-T cell ablation, enabling safer and more scalable deployment. Bispecific antibodies and antibody-armed T cells may provide flexible, "off-the-shelf" alternatives that bypass manufacturing delays while still harnessing immune effectors in a controllable manner. Oncolytic viruses and immunomodulatory drugs add further opportunities to reshape the immune microenvironment, and biologically rational synergistic combinations of these modalities may ultimately generate deeper, more durable responses. Though the challenge posed by rare and heterogenous diseases like TCL is formidable, the next generation of trials must move beyond single-agent studies to adopt adaptive, biomarker-driven designs that incorporate ctDNA, immune-gene signatures, and TME characterization to directly test personalized strategies.

In summary, the future of PTCL therapy lies in a shift from empiricism toward precision. Achieving this will require coordinated efforts in translational research, adaptive trial design, and clinical implementation, but the growing complement of technologies outlined herein shows that such ambition will soon prove feasible. Personalized immunotherapy offers a compelling path forward for improving outcomes in this historically intractable disease.

Author Contributions: J.M.L.C. and X.J.O. contributed equally and share first authorship. J.Z., C.D., P.N. and H.M.P. share senior authorship. Conceptualization, J.M.L.C. and X.J.O.; writing—original draft preparation, J.M.L.C., X.J.O., C.v.d.W. and C.K.Y.; writing—review and editing, J.M.L.C., X.J.O., C.v.d.W., C.K.Y., J.Z., C.D., P.N. and H.M.P.; visualization, J.M.L.C. and X.J.O.; supervision, J.Z., C.D. and H.M.P. All authors have read and agreed to the published version of the manuscript.

Funding: This research received no external funding. C.D. is supported by a Victorian Cancer Agency fellowship (ECRF22015).

Institutional Review Board Statement: Not applicable.

Informed Consent Statement: Not applicable.

Data Availability Statement: No new data were created or analyzed in this study. Data sharing is not applicable to this article.

Conflicts of Interest: C.v.d.W is on the advisory board of Kyowa Kirin; H.M.P. is on advisory boards for Kyowa Kirin and MundiPharma and has received research funding from Kyowa Kirin. P.N. received research funding from Roche Genentech, BMS, MSD and ImmunOS. The remaining authors declare no conflicts of interest. The funders had no role in the study design; in the collection, analysis, and interpretation of the data; in the writing of the report, or the decision to submit the paper for publication.

Abbreviations

The following abbreviations are used in this manuscript:

ACT	Adoptive cell transfer
ADCC	Antibody-directed cellular cytotoxicity
AITL	Angioimmunoblastic T cell lymphoma
ALCL	Anaplastic large cell lymphoma
ALK	Anaplastic lymphoma kinase
allo-HSCT	Allogeneic hematopoietic stem cell transplantation
AML	Acute myeloid leukemia
ATLL	Adult T cell leukemia/lymphoma
auSCT	Autologous stem cell transplantation
BIA-ALCL	Breast-implant-associated anaplastic large cell lymphoma
BV	Brentuximab vedotin
BV-CHP	Brentuximab vedotin, cyclophosphamide, doxorubicin and prednisolone
c-FLIP	cellular FLICE inhibitory protein
CAR	Chimeric Antigen Receptor
CHOP	Cyclophosphamide, adriamycin, vincristine, and prednisone
CPCT	Chidamide, prednisone, cyclophosphamide, and thalidomide
CR	Complete response
CRBN	Cereblon
CRR	Complete response rate
CRS	Cytokine release syndrome
CTCL	Cutaneous T cell lymphoma
ctDNA	Circulating tumor DNA
dMMR	Deficient mismatch repair
EATL	Enteropathy-associated T cell lymphoma
EBV	Epstein–Barr Virus
EFS	Event free survival
EGFR	Epidermal Growth Factor Receptor
ENKTL	Extranodal NK/T cell lymphoma
FDC	Follicular dendritic cell
GvHD	Graft-versus-host disease
HDACi	Histone deacetylase inhibitor
HEV	High endothelial venule
HIF	Hypoxia-Inducible Factor
HL	Hodgkin lymphoma
HSTCL	Hepatosplenic gamma delta T cell lymphoma
HTLV-1	Human T lymphotropic virus 1
ICANS	Immune cell-associated neurotoxicity syndrome
ICE	Innate cell engager
ICI	Immune checkpoint inhibitor
ICOSL	Inducible T cell costimulator ligand

IMIDs	Immunomodulatory imide drugs
KIR	Killer Immunoglobulin-like Receptor
mDC	Myeloid dendritic cell
MDSC	Myeloid-derived suppressor cell
MEITL	Monomorphic epitheliotropic intestinal T cell lymphoma
MHC	Major Histocompatibility Complex
MRD	Minimal residual disease
MSI	Microsatellite instability
nTFHL	Nodal T-follicular helper cell lymphoma
nTFHL-AI	Nodal T-follicular helper cell lymphoma, angioimmunoblastic type
NHL	Non-Hodgkin lymphoma
NK	Natural Killer Cell
ORR	Overall response rate
PCET	PD-1 antibody + chidamide + etoposide + thalidomide
PD	Progressive disease
PFS	Progression-free survival
PMBCL	Primary mediastinal B cell lymphoma
PR	Partial response
PTCL	Peripheral T cell lymphomas
PTCL-NOS	Peripheral T cell lymphoma, not otherwise specified
r/r	relapsed/refractory
sALCL	Systemic ALCL
SD	Stable disease
SIRPα	Signal regulatory protein alpha
SS	Sezary Syndrome
T-ALL	T cell acute lymphoblastic leukemia
T-LBL	T cell lymphoblastic lymphoma
TAM	Tumor-associated macrophage
TCL	T cell lymphoma
TCR	T cell receptor
Tfh	T-follicular helper
Th1	T-helper 1
Th17	T-helper 17
Th2	T-helper 2
TIL	Tumor-infiltrating lymphocyte
TMB	Tumor mutational burden
TME	Tumor Microenvironment
TRAIL	TNF-related apoptosis-inducing ligand
Treg	Regulatory T cell
TTNT	Time to next treatment
VEGF	Vascular endothelial growth factor

References

1. Kwong, Y.-L.; Zhang, H.; Wang, X.; Tse, E. Epidemiology of mature T-cell and NK-cell neoplasms: East and west. *Lancet Reg. Health West. Pac.* **2025**, *62*, 101646. [CrossRef]
2. Brink, M.; Huisman, F.; Meeuwes, F.O.; van der Poel, M.W.M.; Kersten, M.J.; Wondergem, M.; Böhmer, L.; Woei-A-Jin, F.J.S.H.; Visser, O.; Oostvogels, R.; et al. Treatment strategies and outcome in relapsed peripheral T-cell lymphoma: Results from the Netherlands Cancer Registry. *Blood Adv.* **2024**, *8*, 3619–3628. [CrossRef]
3. Han, J.X.; Koh, M.J.; Boussi, L.; Sorial, M.; McCabe, S.M.; Peng, L.; Singh, S.; Eche-Ugwu, I.J.; Gabler, J.; Turizo, M.J.F.; et al. Global outcomes and prognosis for relapsed/refractory mature T-cell and NK-cell lymphomas: Results from the PETAL consortium. *Blood Adv.* **2024**, *9*, 583–602. [CrossRef] [PubMed]
4. Pizzi, M.; Margolskee, E.; Inghirami, G. Pathogenesis of Peripheral T Cell Lymphoma. *Annu. Rev. Pathol. Mech. Dis.* **2018**, *13*, 293–320. [CrossRef] [PubMed]

5. Fiore, D.; Cappelli, L.V.; Broccoli, A.; Zinzani, P.L.; Chan, W.C.; Inghirami, G. Peripheral T cell lymphomas: From the bench to the clinic. *Nat. Rev. Cancer* **2020**, *20*, 323–342. [CrossRef] [PubMed]
6. Swann, J.B.; Smyth, M.J. Immune surveillance of tumors. *J. Clin. Investig.* **2007**, *117*, 1137–1146. [CrossRef]
7. Anderson, N.M.; Simon, M.C. The tumor microenvironment. *Curr. Biol.* **2020**, *30*, R921–R925. [CrossRef]
8. Balkwill, F.R.; Capasso, M.; Hagemann, T. The tumor microenvironment at a glance. *J. Cell Sci.* **2012**, *125*, 5591–5596. [CrossRef]
9. Cornel, A.M.; Mimpen, I.L.; Nierkens, S. MHC Class I Downregulation in Cancer: Underlying Mechanisms and Potential Targets for Cancer Immunotherapy. *Cancers* **2020**, *12*, 1760. [CrossRef]
10. Watatani, Y.; Sato, Y.; Miyoshi, H.; Sakamoto, K.; Nishida, K.; Gion, Y.; Nagata, Y.; Shiraishi, Y.; Chiba, K.; Tanaka, H.; et al. Molecular heterogeneity in peripheral T-cell lymphoma, not otherwise specified revealed by comprehensive genetic profiling. *Leukemia* **2019**, *33*, 2867–2883. [CrossRef]
11. Huang, Y.-H.; Qiu, Y.-R.; Zhang, Q.-L.; Cai, M.-C.; Yu, H.; Zhang, J.-M.; Jiang, L.; Ji, M.-M.; Xu, P.-P.; Wang, L.; et al. Genomic and transcriptomic profiling of peripheral T cell lymphoma reveals distinct molecular and microenvironment subtypes. *Cell Rep. Med.* **2024**, *5*, 101416. [CrossRef]
12. Polprasert, C.; Takeuchi, Y.; Makishima, H.; Wudhikarn, K.; Kakiuchi, N.; Tangnuntachai, N.; Assanasen, T.; Sitthi, W.; Muhamad, H.; Lawasut, P.; et al. Frequent mutations in HLA and related genes in extranodal NK/T cell lymphomas. *Leuk. Lymphoma* **2021**, *62*, 95–103. [CrossRef] [PubMed]
13. Kataoka, K.; Nagata, Y.; Kitanaka, A.; Shiraishi, Y.; Shimamura, T.; Yasunaga, J.; Totoki, Y.; Chiba, K.; Sato-Otsubo, A.; Nagae, G.; et al. Integrated molecular analysis of adult T cell leukemia/lymphoma. *Nat. Genet.* **2015**, *47*, 1304–1315. [CrossRef] [PubMed]
14. Asano, N.; Miyoshi, H.; Kato, T.; Shimono, J.; Yoshida, N.; Kurita, D.; Sasaki, Y.; Kawamoto, K.; Ohshima, K.; Seto, M. Expression pattern of immunosurveillance-related antigen in adult T cell leukaemia/lymphoma. *Histopathology* **2018**, *72*, 945–954. [CrossRef] [PubMed]
15. Anfossi, N.; André, P.; Guia, S.; Falk, C.S.; Roetynck, S.; Stewart, C.A.; Breso, V.; Frassati, C.; Reviron, D.; Middleton, D.; et al. Human NK Cell Education by Inhibitory Receptors for MHC Class I. *Immunity* **2006**, *25*, 331–342. [CrossRef]
16. Cao, J.; Zhang, Y.; Yue, N.; Xiong, S.; Zhang, S.; Wu, C. A potential prognostic marker for hematologic neoplasms: CD58. *Front. Oncol.* **2025**, *15*, 1586842. [CrossRef]
17. Reina, M.; Espel, E. Role of LFA-1 and ICAM-1 in Cancer. *Cancers* **2017**, *9*, 153. [CrossRef]
18. Younes, S.; Zhao, S.; Bharadwaj, S.; Mosquera, A.P.; Libert, D.; Johnsrud, A.; Majzner, R.G.; Miklos, D.B.; Frank, M.J.; Natkunam, Y. Detection of Aberrant CD58 Expression in a Wide Spectrum of Lymphoma Subtypes: Implications for Treatment Resistance. *Mod. Pathol.* **2023**, *36*, 100256. [CrossRef]
19. Yoshida, N.; Karube, K.; Utsunomiya, A.; Tsukasaki, K.; Imaizumi, Y.; Taira, N.; Uike, N.; Umino, A.; Arita, K.; Suguro, M.; et al. Molecular Characterization of Chronic-type Adult T-cell Leukemia/Lymphoma. *Cancer Res.* **2014**, *74*, 6129–6138. [CrossRef]
20. Tanaka, Y.; Fukudome, K.; Hayashi, M.; Takagi, S.; Yoshie, O. Induction of ICAM-1 and LFA-3 by Tax1 of human T-cell leukemia virus type 1 and mechanism of down-regulation of ICAM-1 or LFA-1 in adult-T-cell-leukemia cell lines. *Int. J. Cancer* **1995**, *60*, 554–561. [CrossRef]
21. Majeti, R.; Chao, M.P.; Alizadeh, A.A.; Pang, W.W.; Jaiswal, S.; Gibbs, K.D.; Van Rooijen, N.; Weissman, I.L. CD47 Is an Adverse Prognostic Factor and Therapeutic Antibody Target on Human Acute Myeloid Leukemia Stem Cells. *Cell* **2009**, *138*, 286–299. [CrossRef] [PubMed]
22. Chao, M.P.; Alizadeh, A.A.; Tang, C.; Myklebust, J.H.; Varghese, B.; Gill, S.; Jan, M.; Cha, A.C.; Chan, C.K.; Tan, B.T.; et al. Anti-CD47 Antibody Synergizes with Rituximab to Promote Phagocytosis and Eradicate Non-Hodgkin Lymphoma. *Cell* **2010**, *142*, 699–713. [CrossRef] [PubMed]
23. Uger, R.; Johnson, L. Blockade of the CD47-SIRPα axis: A promising approach for cancer immunotherapy. *Expert Opin. Biol. Ther.* **2020**, *20*, 5–8. [CrossRef]
24. Logtenberg, M.E.W.; Scheeren, F.A.; Schumacher, T.N. The CD47-SIRPα Immune Checkpoint. *Immunity* **2020**, *52*, 742–752. [CrossRef]
25. Zhu, M.; Li, N.; Fan, L.; Wu, R.; Cao, L.; Ren, Y.; Lu, C.; Zhang, L.; Cai, Y.; Shi, Y.; et al. Single-cell transcriptomic and spatial analysis reveal the immunosuppressive microenvironment in relapsed/refractory angioimmunoblastic T-cell lymphoma. *Blood Cancer J.* **2024**, *14*, 218. [CrossRef]
26. de Leval, L.; Rickman, D.S.; Thielen, C.; de Reynies, A.; Huang, Y.-L.; Delsol, G.; Lamant, L.; Leroy, K.; Brière, J.; Molina, T.; et al. The gene expression profile of nodal peripheral T-cell lymphoma demonstrates a molecular link between angioimmunoblastic T-cell lymphoma (AITL) and follicular helper T (TFH) cells. *Blood* **2007**, *109*, 4952–4963. [CrossRef]
27. Jain, S.; Scoyk, A.V.; Morgan, E.A.; Matthews, A.; Stevenson, K.; Newton, G.; Powers, F.; Autio, A.; Louissaint, A.; Pontini, G.; et al. Targeted inhibition of CD47-SIRPα requires Fc-FcγR interactions to maximize activity in T-cell lymphomas. *Blood* **2019**, *134*, 1430–1440. [CrossRef]
28. Folkes, A.S.; Feng, M.; Zain, J.M.; Abdulla, F.; Rosen, S.T.; Querfeld, C. Targeting CD47 as a cancer therapeutic strategy: The cutaneous T-cell lymphoma experience. *Curr. Opin. Oncol.* **2018**, *30*, 332–337. [CrossRef]

29. Qin, L.; Li, Y.; Zeng, R.; He, Y.; Chen, X.; Xiao, L.; Zhou, H. A novel anti-CD47 antibody with therapeutic potential for NK/T-cell lymphoma. *Hum. Vaccines Immunother.* **2024**, *20*, 2408088. [CrossRef]
30. Johnson, L.D.S.; Banerjee, S.; Kruglov, O.; Viller, N.N.; Horwitz, S.M.; Lesokhin, A.; Zain, J.; Querfeld, C.; Chen, R.; Okada, C.; et al. Targeting CD47 in Sézary syndrome with SIRPαFc. *Blood Adv.* **2019**, *3*, 1145–1153. [CrossRef]
31. Ansell, S.M.; Maris, M.B.; Lesokhin, A.M.; Chen, R.W.; Flinn, I.W.; Sawas, A.; Minden, M.D.; Villa, D.; Percival, M.-E.M.; Advani, A.S.; et al. Phase I Study of the CD47 Blocker TTI-621 in Patients with Relapsed or Refractory Hematologic Malignancies. *Clin. Cancer Res.* **2021**, *27*, 2190–2199. [CrossRef]
32. Han, Z.; Wu, X.; Yuan, Y.-C.; Qin, H.; Su, C.; Zain, J.; Akilov, O.E.; Rosen, S.T.; Feng, M.; Querfeld, C. Blockade of the Immune Checkpoint CD47 By TTI-621 Potentiates the Response to Anti-PD-L1 in Cutaneous T Cell Lymphoma. *Blood* **2022**, *140*, 6376–6377. [CrossRef]
33. Wilde, L.; Kasner, M. Targeting CD47: Many misses; hopeful for a hit. *Blood* **2025**, *145*, 460–462. [CrossRef] [PubMed]
34. Shen, L.; Liang, A.C.T.; Lu, L.; Au, W.Y.; Kwong, Y.-L.; Liang, R.H.S.; Srivastava, G. Frequent Deletion of Fas Gene Sequences Encoding Death and Transmembrane Domains in Nasal Natural Killer/T-Cell Lymphoma. *Am. J. Pathol.* **2002**, *161*, 2123–2131. [CrossRef] [PubMed]
35. Takakuwa, T.; Dong, Z.; Nakatsuka, S.; Kojya, S.; Harabuchi, Y.; Yang, W.-I.; Nagata, S.; Aozasa, K. Frequent mutations of Fas gene in nasal NK/T cell lymphoma. *Oncogene* **2002**, *21*, 4702–4705. [CrossRef]
36. Hasegawa, H.; Yamada, Y.; Harasawa, H.; Tsuji, T.; Murata, K.; Sugahara, K.; Tsuruda, K.; Ikeda, S.; Imaizumi, Y.; Tomonaga, M.; et al. Sensitivity of adult T-cell leukaemia lymphoma cells to tumour necrosis factor-related apoptosis-inducing ligand. *Br. J. Haematol.* **2005**, *128*, 253–265. [CrossRef]
37. Zheng, Z.; Cheng, S.; Wu, W.; Wang, L.; Zhao, Y.; Shen, Y.; Janin, A.; Zhao, W.-L. c-FLIP is involved in tumor progression of peripheral T-cell lymphoma and targeted by histone deacetylase inhibitors. *J. Hematol. Oncol.* **2014**, *7*, 88. [CrossRef]
38. Spetz, J.; Presser, A.G.; Sarosiek, K.A. T Cells and Regulated Cell Death: Kill or Be Killed. *Int. Rev. Cell Mol. Biol.* **2018**, *342*, 27–71. [CrossRef]
39. Wang, T.; Feldman, A.L.; Wada, D.A.; Lu, Y.; Polk, A.; Briski, R.; Ristow, K.; Habermann, T.M.; Thomas, D.; Ziesmer, S.C.; et al. GATA-3 expression identifies a high-risk subset of PTCL, NOS with distinct molecular and clinical features. *Blood* **2014**, *123*, 3007–3015. [CrossRef]
40. Iqbal, J.; Wright, G.; Wang, C.; Rosenwald, A.; Gascoyne, R.D.; Weisenburger, D.D.; Greiner, T.C.; Smith, L.; Guo, S.; Wilcox, R.A.; et al. Gene expression signatures delineate biological and prognostic subgroups in peripheral T-cell lymphoma. *Blood* **2014**, *123*, 2915–2923. [CrossRef]
41. Alaggio, R.; Amador, C.; Anagnostopoulos, I.; Attygalle, A.D.; Araujo, I.B.O.; Berti, E.; Bhagat, G.; Borges, A.M.; Boyer, D.; Calaminici, M.; et al. The 5th edition of the World Health Organization Classification of Haematolymphoid Tumours: Lymphoid Neoplasms. *Leukemia* **2022**, *36*, 1720–1748. [CrossRef]
42. Dupuis, J.; Boye, K.; Martin, N.; Copie-Bergman, C.; Plonquet, A.; Fabiani, B.; Baglin, A.-C.; Haioun, C.; Delfau-Larue, M.-H.; Gaulard, P. Expression of CXCL13 by neoplastic cells in angioimmunoblastic T-cell lymphoma (AITL): A new diagnostic marker providing evidence that AITL derives from follicular helper T cells. *Am. J. Surg. Pathol.* **2006**, *30*, 490–494. [CrossRef] [PubMed]
43. Gaulard, P.; de Leval, L. The microenvironment in T-cell lymphomas: Emerging themes. *Semin. Cancer Biol.* **2014**, *24*, 49–60. [CrossRef] [PubMed]
44. Iqbal, J.; Weisenburger, D.D.; Greiner, T.C.; Vose, J.M.; McKeithan, T.; Kucuk, C.; Geng, H.; Deffenbacher, K.; Smith, L.; Dybkaer, K.; et al. Molecular signatures to improve diagnosis in peripheral T-cell lymphoma and prognostication in angioimmunoblastic T-cell lymphoma. *Blood* **2010**, *115*, 1026–1036. [CrossRef] [PubMed]
45. Karube, K.; Ohshima, K.; Tsuchiya, T.; Yamaguchi, T.; Kawano, R.; Suzumiya, J.; Utsunomiya, A.; Harada, M.; Kikuchi, M. Expression of FoxP3, a key molecule in CD4CD25 regulatory T cells, in adult T-cell leukaemia/lymphoma cells. *Br. J. Haematol.* **2004**, *126*, 81–84. [CrossRef]
46. Georgiev, P.; Charbonnier, L.-M.; Chatila, T.A. Regulatory T Cells: The Many Faces of Foxp3. *J. Clin. Immunol.* **2019**, *39*, 623–640. [CrossRef]
47. Amador, C.; Greiner, T.C.; Heavican, T.B.; Smith, L.M.; Galvis, K.T.; Lone, W.; Bouska, A.; D'Amore, F.; Pedersen, M.B.; Pileri, S.; et al. Reproducing the molecular subclassification of peripheral T-cell lymphoma–NOS by immunohistochemistry. *Blood* **2019**, *134*, 2159–2170. [CrossRef]
48. Amador, C.; Weisenburger, D.D.; Gomez, A.; Bouska, A.; Alshomrani, A.; Sharma, S.; Shah, A.R.; Greiner, T.C.; Vega, F.; Rosenwald, A.; et al. Refining Diagnostic Subtypes of Peripheral T-Cell Lymphoma Using a Multiparameter Approach. *Mod. Pathol.* **2025**, *38*, 100646. [CrossRef]
49. Heavican, T.B.; Bouska, A.; Yu, J.; Lone, W.; Amador, C.; Gong, Q.; Zhang, W.; Li, Y.; Dave, B.J.; Nairismägi, M.-L.; et al. Genetic drivers of oncogenic pathways in molecular subgroups of peripheral T-cell lymphoma. *Blood* **2019**, *133*, 1664–1676. [CrossRef]
50. Chiba, S.; Sakata-Yanagimoto, M. Advances in understanding of angioimmunoblastic T-cell lymphoma. *Leukemia* **2020**, *34*, 2592–2606. [CrossRef]

51. Pritchett, J.C.; Yang, Z.-Z.; Kim, H.J.; Villasboas, J.C.; Tang, X.; Jalali, S.; Cerhan, J.R.; Feldman, A.L.; Ansell, S.M. High-dimensional and single-cell transcriptome analysis of the tumor microenvironment in angioimmunoblastic T cell lymphoma (AITL). *Leukemia* **2022**, *36*, 165–176. [CrossRef] [PubMed]
52. Li, Y.; Luo, C.; Jiang, J.; He, S.; Liu, Y.; Yan, W.; Xia, Y.; Cui, Q.; Huang, Y.; Lim, J.Q.; et al. Single-Cell Analysis Reveals Malignant Cells Reshape the Cellular Landscape and Foster an Immunosuppressive Microenvironment of Extranodal NK/T-Cell Lymphoma. *Adv. Sci.* **2023**, *10*, 2303913. [CrossRef]
53. Feng, X.; Meng, M.; Li, H.; Gao, Y.; Song, W.; Di, R.; Li, Z.; Zhang, X.; Zhang, M. T-cell dysfunction in natural killer/T-cell lymphoma. *Oncoimmunology* **2023**, *12*, 2212532. [CrossRef] [PubMed]
54. Zhao, W.-L.; Mourah, S.; Mounier, N.; Leboeuf, C.; Daneshpouy, M.E.; Legrès, L.; Meignin, V.; Oksenhendler, E.; Maignin, C.L.; Calvo, F.; et al. Vascular endothelial growth factor-A is expressed both on lymphoma cells and endothelial cells in angioimmunoblastic T-cell lymphoma and related to lymphoma progression. *Lab. Investig.* **2004**, *84*, 1512–1519. [CrossRef] [PubMed]
55. Lunning, M.A.; Vose, J.M. Angioimmunoblastic T-cell lymphoma: The many-faced lymphoma. *Blood* **2017**, *129*, 1095–1102. [CrossRef]
56. Martinengo, C.; Poggio, T.; Menotti, M.; Scalzo, M.S.; Mastini, C.; Ambrogio, C.; Pellegrino, E.; Riera, L.; Piva, R.; Ribatti, D.; et al. ALK-Dependent Control of Hypoxia-Inducible Factors Mediates Tumor Growth and Metastasis. *Cancer Res.* **2014**, *74*, 6094–6106. [CrossRef]
57. Bruns, I.; Fox, F.; Reinecke, P.; Kobbe, G.; Kronenwett, R.; Jung, G.; Haas, R. Complete remission in a patient with relapsed angioimmunoblastic T-cell lymphoma following treatment with bevacizumab. *Leukemia* **2005**, *19*, 1993–1995. [CrossRef]
58. Cortes, J.R.; Ambesi-Impiombato, A.; Couronné, L.; Quinn, S.A.; Kim, C.S.; da Silva Almeida, A.C.; West, Z.; Belver, L.; Martin, M.S.; Scourzic, L.; et al. RHOA G17V Induces T Follicular Helper Cell Specification and Promotes Lymphomagenesis. *Cancer Cell* **2018**, *33*, 259–273.e7. [CrossRef]
59. Leca, J.; Lemonnier, F.; Meydan, C.; Foox, J.; Ghamrasni, S.E.; Mboumba, D.-L.; Duncan, G.S.; Fortin, J.; Sakamoto, T.; Tobin, C.; et al. IDH2 and TET2 mutations synergize to modulate T Follicular Helper cell functional interaction with the AITL microenvironment. *Cancer Cell* **2023**, *41*, 323–339.e10. [CrossRef]
60. Miyoshi, H.; Kiyasu, J.; Kato, T.; Yoshida, N.; Shimono, J.; Yokoyama, S.; Taniguchi, H.; Sasaki, Y.; Kurita, D.; Kawamoto, K.; et al. PD-L1 expression on neoplastic or stromal cells is respectively a poor or good prognostic factor for adult T-cell leukemia/lymphoma. *Blood* **2016**, *128*, 1374–1381. [CrossRef]
61. Takeuchi, M.; Miyoshi, H.; Nakashima, K.; Kawamoto, K.; Yamada, K.; Yanagida, E.; Muta, H.; Moritsubo, M.; Umeno, T.; Suzuki, T.; et al. Comprehensive immunohistochemical analysis of immune checkpoint molecules in adult T cell leukemia/lymphoma. *Ann. Hematol.* **2020**, *99*, 1093–1098. [CrossRef]
62. Wartewig, T.; Kurgyis, Z.; Keppler, S.; Pechloff, K.; Hameister, E.; Öllinger, R.; Maresch, R.; Buch, T.; Steiger, K.; Winter, C.; et al. PD-1 is a haploinsufficient suppressor of T cell lymphomagenesis. *Nature* **2017**, *552*, 121–125. [CrossRef]
63. Ratner, L.; Waldmann, T.A.; Janakiram, M.; Brammer, J.E. Rapid Progression of Adult T-Cell Leukemia–Lymphoma after PD-1 Inhibitor Therapy. *N. Engl. J. Med.* **2018**, *378*, 1947–1948. [CrossRef] [PubMed]
64. Rauch, D.A.; Conlon, K.C.; Janakiram, M.; Brammer, J.E.; Harding, J.C.; Ye, B.H.; Zang, X.; Ren, X.; Olson, S.; Cheng, X.; et al. Rapid progression of adult T-cell leukemia/lymphoma as tumor-infiltrating Tregs after PD-1 blockade. *Blood* **2019**, *134*, 1406–1414. [CrossRef] [PubMed]
65. Ishitsuka, K.; Utsunomiya, A.; Ishida, T. PD-1 Inhibitor Therapy in Adult T-Cell Leukemia–Lymphoma. *N. Engl. J. Med.* **2018**, *379*, 695–697. [CrossRef]
66. Ahearne, M.J.; Gaskell, C.; Jackson, A.E.; Morland, C.; Hopkins, L.; Nawaz, N.; Timmins, M.A.; Fox, C.P.; Collins, G.P.; Davies, A.; et al. AVAIL-T: A Phase 2a Trial of Avelumab, and Anti-PD-L1 Antibody, in Relapsed and Refractory Peripheral T-Cell Lymphoma (PTCL). *Blood* **2020**, *136*, 18–19. [CrossRef]
67. Barta, S.K.; Zain, J.; MacFarlane, A.W.; Smith, S.M.; Ruan, J.; Fung, H.C.; Tan, C.R.; Yang, Y.; Alpaugh, R.K.; Dulaimi, E.; et al. Phase II Study of the PD-1 Inhibitor Pembrolizumab for the Treatment of Relapsed or Refractory Mature T-cell Lymphoma. *Clin. Lymphoma Myeloma Leuk.* **2019**, *19*, 356–364.e3. [CrossRef]
68. Lesokhin, A.M.; Ansell, S.M.; Armand, P.; Scott, E.C.; Halwani, A.; Gutierrez, M.; Millenson, M.M.; Cohen, A.D.; Schuster, S.J.; Lebovic, D.; et al. Nivolumab in Patients with Relapsed or Refractory Hematologic Malignancy: Preliminary Results of a Phase Ib Study. *J. Clin. Oncol.* **2016**, *34*, 2698–2704. [CrossRef]
69. Shi, Y.; Wu, J.; Wang, Z.; Zhang, L.; Wang, Z.; Zhang, M.; Cen, H.; Peng, Z.; Li, Y.; Fan, L.; et al. Efficacy and safety of geptanolimab (GB226) for relapsed or refractory peripheral T cell lymphoma: An open-label phase 2 study (Gxplore-002). *J. Hematol. Oncol.* **2021**, *14*, 12. [CrossRef]
70. Saba, R.; Mehta-Shah, N.; Ghobadi, A.; DiPersio, J.F.; Cashen, A.F.; Wu, N. Phase II Trial of Duvelisib Maintenance after Autologous Stem Cell Transplant in T-Cell and B-Cell Non-Hodgkin Lymphomas: Results of Safety Lead in. *Blood* **2023**, *142*, 6245. [CrossRef]

71. Merrill, M.H.; Dahi, P.B.; Redd, R.A.; McDonough, M.M.; Chen, Y.-B.; DeFilipp, Z.; Herrera, A.F.; Fisher, D.C.; LaCasce, A.S.; Odejide, O.O.; et al. A phase 2 study of pembrolizumab after autologous stem cell transplantation in patients with T-cell non-Hodgkin lymphoma. *Blood* **2023**, *142*, 621–628. [CrossRef]
72. Kwong, Y.-L.; Chan, T.S.Y.; Tan, D.; Kim, S.J.; Poon, L.-M.; Mow, B.; Khong, P.-L.; Loong, F.; Au-Yeung, R.; Iqbal, J.; et al. PD1 blockade with pembrolizumab is highly effective in relapsed or refractory NK/T-cell lymphoma failing l-asparaginase. *Blood* **2017**, *129*, 2437–2442. [CrossRef]
73. Chan, T.; Tse, E. Pembrolizumab in Relapsed/Refractory Extranodal NK/T Cell Lymphoma and Mature T Cell Lymphoma: o A Prospective Phase II Study. *Blood* **2023**, *142*, 1726. [CrossRef]
74. Li, X.; Cheng, Y.; Zhang, M.; Yan, J.; Li, L.; Fu, X.; Zhang, X.; Chang, Y.; Sun, Z.; Yu, H.; et al. Activity of pembrolizumab in relapsed/refractory NK/T-cell lymphoma. *J. Hematol. Oncol.* **2018**, *11*, 15. [CrossRef]
75. Kim, S.-J.; Hyeon, J.; Cho, I.; Ko, Y.H.; Kim, W.S. Comparison of Efficacy of Pembrolizumab between Epstein-Barr Virus—Positive and —Negative Relapsed or Refractory Non-Hodgkin Lymphomas. *Cancer Res. Treat.* **2018**, *51*, 611–622. [CrossRef]
76. Tao, R.; Fan, L.; Song, Y.; Hu, Y.; Zhang, W.; Wang, Y.; Xu, W.; Li, J. Sintilimab for relapsed/refractory extranodal NK/T cell lymphoma: A multicenter, single-arm, phase 2 trial (ORIENT-4). *Signal Transduct. Target. Ther.* **2021**, *6*, 365. [CrossRef]
77. Huang, H.; Tao, R.; Zou, L.; Cen, H.; Guo, Y.; Huang, Y.; Qian, W.; Zhang, L.; Zhou, H.; Yang, Y.; et al. Preliminary Results from a Multicenter, Single-Arm, Phase 2 Study of CS1001, an Anti-Programmed Death-Ligand 1 (PD-L1) Human Monoclonal Antibody (mAb), in Patients (pts) with Relapsed or Refractory Extranodal Natural Killer/T Cell Lymphoma (rr-ENKTL). *Blood* **2019**, *134*, 2833. [CrossRef]
78. Kim, S.J.; Lim, J.Q.; Laurensia, Y.; Cho, J.; Yoon, S.E.; Lee, J.Y.; Ryu, K.J.; Ko, Y.H.; Koh, Y.; Cho, D.; et al. Avelumab for the treatment of relapsed or refractory extranodal NK/T-cell lymphoma: An open-label phase 2 study. *Blood* **2020**, *136*, 2754–2763. [CrossRef] [PubMed]
79. Luo, Y.; Liu, Y.; Wang, C.; Gan, R. Signaling pathways of EBV-induced oncogenesis. *Cancer Cell Int.* **2021**, *21*, 93. [CrossRef] [PubMed]
80. Green, M.R.; Rodig, S.; Juszczynski, P.; Ouyang, J.; Sinha, P.; O'Donnell, E.; Neuberg, D.; Shipp, M.A. Constitutive AP-1 Activity and EBV Infection Induce PD-L1 in Hodgkin Lymphomas and Posttransplant Lymphoproliferative Disorders: Implications for Targeted Therapy. *Clin. Cancer Res.* **2012**, *18*, 1611–1618. [CrossRef]
81. Wang, J.; Ge, J.; Wang, Y.; Xiong, F.; Guo, J.; Jiang, X.; Zhang, L.; Deng, X.; Gong, Z.; Zhang, S.; et al. EBV miRNAs BART11 and BART17-3p promote immune escape through the enhancer-mediated transcription of PD-L1. *Nat. Commun.* **2022**, *13*, 866. [CrossRef] [PubMed]
82. Mpakali, A.; Stratikos, E. The Role of Antigen Processing and Presentation in Cancer and the Efficacy of Immune Checkpoint Inhibitor Immunotherapy. *Cancers* **2021**, *13*, 134. [CrossRef] [PubMed]
83. Mahoney, K.M.; Atkins, M.B. Prognostic and predictive markers for the new immunotherapies. *Oncology* **2014**, *28* (Suppl. S3), 39–48. [PubMed]
84. Goodman, A.M.; Kato, S.; Bazhenova, L.; Patel, S.P.; Frampton, G.M.; Miller, V.; Stephens, P.J.; Daniels, G.A.; Kurzrock, R. Tumor Mutational Burden as an Independent Predictor of Response to Immunotherapy in Diverse Cancers. *Mol. Cancer Ther.* **2017**, *16*, 2598–2608. [CrossRef]
85. Rizvi, H.; Sanchez-Vega, F.; La, K.; Chatila, W.; Jonsson, P.; Halpenny, D.; Plodkowski, A.; Long, N.; Sauter, J.L.; Rekhtman, N.; et al. Molecular Determinants of Response to Anti-Programmed Cell Death (PD)-1 and Anti–Programmed Death-Ligand (PD-L)-Ligand 1 Blockade in Patients With Non–Small-Cell Lung Cancer Profiled With Targeted Next-Generation Sequencing. *J. Clin. Oncol.* **2018**, *36*, 633–641. [CrossRef]
86. Yarchoan, M.; Hopkins, A.; Jaffee, E.M. Tumor Mutational Burden and Response Rate to PD-1 Inhibition. *N. Engl. J. Med.* **2017**, *377*, 2500–2501. [CrossRef]
87. Wirth, T.C.; Kühnel, F. Neoantigen Targeting—Dawn of a New Era in Cancer Immunotherapy? *Front. Immunol.* **2017**, *8*, 1848. [CrossRef]
88. Galanina, N.; Bejar, R.; Choi, M.; Goodman, A.; Wieduwilt, M.; Mulroney, C.; Kim, L.; Yeerna, H.; Tamayo, P.; Vergilio, J.-A.; et al. Comprehensive Genomic Profiling Reveals Diverse but Actionable Molecular Portfolios across Hematologic Malignancies: Implications for Next Generation Clinical Trials. *Cancers* **2018**, *11*, 11. [CrossRef]
89. Thomas, S.D.; Jeong, A.-R.; Sakowski, P.J.; Sokol, E.S.; Kurzrock, R.; Goodman, A.M. Tumor Mutational Burden and PD-L1 Expression in Hematologic Malignancies. *Blood* **2020**, *136*, 15–17. [CrossRef]
90. Griffin, R.; Wenzl, K.; Sarangi, V.; Rimsza, L.M.; King, R.; Feldman, A.L.; Maurer, M.J.; Nowakowski, G.S.; Link, B.K.; Habermann, T.M.; et al. Tumor Mutational Burden as a Prognostic Factor in Diffuse Large B-Cell Lymphoma. *Blood* **2023**, *142*, 1633. [CrossRef]
91. Cho, J.; Yoon, S.E.; Kim, S.J.; Ko, Y.H.; Kim, W.S. Comparison of tumor mutation burden of 300 various non-Hodgkin lymphomas using panel based massively parallel sequencing. *BMC Cancer* **2021**, *21*, 972. [CrossRef]

92. McGrail, D.J.; Pilié, P.G.; Rashid, N.U.; Voorwerk, L.; Slagter, M.; Kok, M.; Jonasch, E.; Khasraw, M.; Heimberger, A.B.; Lim, B.; et al. High tumor mutation burden fails to predict immune checkpoint blockade response across all cancer types. *Ann. Oncol.* **2021**, *32*, 661–672. [CrossRef] [PubMed]
93. Thibodeau, S.N.; Bren, G.; Schaid, D. Microsatellite Instability in Cancer of the Proximal Colon. *Science* **1993**, *260*, 816–819. [CrossRef] [PubMed]
94. Le, D.T.; Durham, J.N.; Smith, K.N.; Wang, H.; Bartlett, B.R.; Aulakh, L.K.; Lu, S.; Kemberling, H.; Wilt, C.; Luber, B.S.; et al. Mismatch repair deficiency predicts response of solid tumors to PD-1 blockade. *Science* **2017**, *357*, 409–413. [CrossRef] [PubMed]
95. Zhao, P.; Li, L.; Jiang, X.; Li, Q. Mismatch repair deficiency/microsatellite instability-high as a predictor for anti-PD-1/PD-L1 immunotherapy efficacy. *J. Hematol. Oncol.* **2019**, *12*, 54. [CrossRef]
96. Chapuy, B.; Stewart, C.; Dunford, A.J.; Kim, J.; Kamburov, A.; Redd, R.A.; Lawrence, M.S.; Roemer, M.G.M.; Li, A.J.; Ziepert, M.; et al. Molecular subtypes of diffuse large B cell lymphoma are associated with distinct pathogenic mechanisms and outcomes. *Nat. Med.* **2018**, *24*, 679–690. [CrossRef]
97. Tian, T.; Li, J.; Xue, T.; Yu, B.; Li, X.; Zhou, X. Microsatellite instability and its associations with the clinicopathologic characteristics of diffuse large B-cell lymphoma. *Cancer Med.* **2020**, *9*, 2330–2342. [CrossRef]
98. Xu-Monette, Z.Y.; Yu, L.; Luo, C.; Li, Y.; Bhagat, G.; Tzankov, A.; Visco, C.; Fan, X.; Fang, X.; Dybkaer, K.; et al. Diffuse Large B-Cell Lymphoma Has a Low Frequency of dMMR and High Frequencies of DNA Mismatch Repair Protein High Expression Associated with Lower T-Cell Infiltration. *Blood* **2023**, *142*, 6079. [CrossRef]
99. Veloza, L.; Fischer, A.; Vallois, D.; Rattina, V.; Lefort, K.; Bisig, B.; Gaulard, P.; Siebert, R.; de Leval, L.; Missiaglia, E. TCL-473 Role of Microsatellite Instability in the Oncogenesis of Primary Intestinal T-Cell Lymphomas. *Clin. Lymphoma Myeloma Leuk.* **2023**, *23*, S471. [CrossRef]
100. Miyashita, K.; Fujii, K.; Taguchi, K.; Shimokawa, M.; Yoshida, M.A.; Abe, Y.; Okamura, J.; Oda, S.; Uike, N. A specific mode of microsatellite instability is a crucial biomarker in adult T-cell leukaemia/lymphoma patients. *J. Cancer Res. Clin. Oncol.* **2017**, *143*, 399–408. [CrossRef]
101. Roemer, M.G.M.; Advani, R.H.; Ligon, A.H.; Natkunam, Y.; Redd, R.A.; Homer, H.; Connelly, C.F.; Sun, H.H.; Daadi, S.E.; Freeman, G.J.; et al. PD-L1 and PD-L2 Genetic Alterations Define Classical Hodgkin Lymphoma and Predict Outcome. *J. Clin. Oncol.* **2016**, *34*, 2690–2697. [CrossRef]
102. Younes, A.; Santoro, A.; Shipp, M.; Zinzani, P.L.; Timmerman, J.M.; Ansell, S.; Armand, P.; Fanale, M.; Ratanatharathorn, V.; Kuruvilla, J.; et al. Nivolumab for classical Hodgkin's lymphoma after failure of both autologous stem-cell transplantation and brentuximab vedotin: A multicentre, multicohort, single-arm phase 2 trial. *Lancet Oncol.* **2016**, *17*, 1283–1294. [CrossRef]
103. Ansell, S.M.; Lesokhin, A.M.; Borrello, I.; Halwani, A.; Scott, E.C.; Gutierrez, M.; Schuster, S.J.; Millenson, M.M.; Cattry, D.; Freeman, G.J.; et al. PD-1 Blockade with Nivolumab in Relapsed or Refractory Hodgkin's Lymphoma. *N. Engl. J. Med.* **2015**, *372*, 311–319. [CrossRef]
104. Chen, R.; Zinzani, P.L.; Fanale, M.A.; Armand, P.; Johnson, N.A.; Brice, P.; Radford, J.; Ribrag, V.; Molin, D.; Vassilakopoulos, T.P.; et al. Phase II Study of the Efficacy and Safety of Pembrolizumab for Relapsed/Refractory Classic Hodgkin Lymphoma. *J. Clin. Oncol.* **2017**, *35*, 2125–2132. [CrossRef] [PubMed]
105. Green, M.R.; Monti, S.; Rodig, S.J.; Juszczynski, P.; Currie, T.; O'Donnell, E.; Chapuy, B.; Takeyama, K.; Neuberg, D.; Golub, T.R.; et al. Integrative analysis reveals selective 9p24.1 amplification, increased PD-1 ligand expression, and further induction via JAK2 in nodular sclerosing Hodgkin lymphoma and primary mediastinal large B-cell lymphoma. *Blood* **2010**, *116*, 3268–3277. [CrossRef] [PubMed]
106. Armand, P.; Rodig, S.; Melnichenko, V.; Thieblemont, C.; Bouabdallah, K.; Tumyan, G.; Özcan, M.; Portino, S.; Fogliatto, L.; Caballero, M.D.; et al. Pembrolizumab in Relapsed or Refractory Primary Mediastinal Large B-Cell Lymphoma. *J. Clin. Oncol.* **2019**, *37*, 3291–3299. [CrossRef]
107. Kataoka, K.; Miyoshi, H.; Sakata, S.; Dobashi, A.; Couronné, L.; Kogure, Y.; Sato, Y.; Nishida, K.; Gion, Y.; Shiraishi, Y.; et al. Frequent structural variations involving programmed death ligands in Epstein-Barr virus-associated lymphomas. *Leukemia* **2019**, *33*, 1687–1699. [CrossRef]
108. Ng, S.-B.; Chung, T.-H.; Kato, S.; Nakamura, S.; Takahashi, E.; Ko, Y.-H.; Khoury, J.D.; Yin, C.C.; Soong, R.; Jeyasekharan, A.D.; et al. Epstein-Barr virus-associated primary nodal T/NK-cell lymphoma shows a distinct molecular signature and copy number changes. *Haematologica* **2018**, *103*, 278–287. [CrossRef]
109. Beygi, S.; Fernandez-Pol, S.; Duran, G.; Wang, E.B.; Stehr, H.; Zehnder, J.L.; Ramchurren, N.; Fling, S.P.; Cheever, M.A.; Weng, W.-K.; et al. Pembrolizumab in mycosis fungoides with PD-L1 structural variants. *Blood Adv.* **2021**, *5*, 771–774. [CrossRef]
110. Sakihama, S.; Morichika, K.; Saito, R.; Miyara, M.; Miyagi, T.; Hayashi, M.; Uchihara, J.; Tomoyose, T.; Ohshiro, K.; Nakayama, S.; et al. Genetic profile of adult T-cell leukemia/lymphoma in Okinawa: Association with prognosis, ethnicity, and HTLV-1 strains. *Cancer Sci.* **2021**, *112*, 1300–1309. [CrossRef]

111. Kataoka, K.; Iwanaga, M.; Yasunaga, J.; Nagata, Y.; Kitanaka, A.; Kameda, T.; Yoshimitsu, M.; Shiraishi, Y.; Sato-Otsubo, A.; Sanada, M.; et al. Prognostic relevance of integrated genetic profiling in adult T-cell leukemia/lymphoma. *Blood* **2018**, *131*, 215–225. [CrossRef] [PubMed]
112. Nair, R.; Duenas, D.E.; Liu, J.; Prakash, R.; Zhou, C.; Koksoy, A.A.; Xu, J.; McAllen, S.A.; Malpica, L.; Luthra, R.; et al. An Integrated Spatial, Codex, and Genomic Analysis Predicts Responsiveness and Survival in the Phase II Combination of Pembrolizumab and Romidepsin in PTCL. *Blood* **2024**, *144*, 455. [CrossRef]
113. Roberts, N.; Lister, J.; Bennani, N.N.; Jain, S.; Battaglia, T.; Ayers, E.C.; Portell, C.A.; Williams, M.E.; Batchala, P.; Pal, I.; et al. Pembrolizumab in Combination with Epigenetic Therapy Is Safe and Active in Heavily Treated Patients with Peripheral T-Cell Lymphoma (PTCL) and Cutaneous T-Cell Lymphoma (CTCL): Preliminary Results from the Embolden Trial. *Blood* **2022**, *140*, 9425–9426. [CrossRef]
114. Du, L.; Zhang, L.; Li, L.; Li, X.; Yan, J.; Wang, X.; Fu, X.; Sun, Z.; Zhang, X.; Li, Z.; et al. Effective Treatment with PD-1 Antibody, Chidamide, Etoposide, and Thalidomide (PCET) for Relapsed/Refractory Natural Killer/T-Cell Lymphoma: A Report of Three Cases. *OncoTargets Ther.* **2020**, *13*, 7189–7197. [CrossRef]
115. Bhabha, F.K.; Weyden, C.V.D.; Casan, J.M.L.; Campbell, B.A.; McCormack, C.; Prince, H.M. Immune pathways, current and potential therapies in Mycosis fungoides and Sezary syndrome. *Expert Rev. Clin. Immunol.* **2025**, *21*, 1003–1018. [CrossRef]
116. Lou, N.; Yang, M.; Xie, Z.; Gao, R.; Zhang, L.; Tang, L.; Yao, J.; Han, X.; Shi, Y. JAK3 A573V and JAK3 M511I mutations in peripheral T-cell lymphoma mediating resistance to anti-PD-1 therapy through the STAT3/PD-L1 pathway. *J. Immunother. Cancer* **2025**, *13*, e010783. [CrossRef]
117. Berdeja, J.G.; Madduri, D.; Usmani, S.Z.; Jakubowiak, A.; Agha, M.; Cohen, A.D.; Stewart, A.K.; Hari, P.; Htut, M.; Lesokhin, A.; et al. Ciltacabtagene autoleucel, a B-cell maturation antigen-directed chimeric antigen receptor T-cell therapy in patients with relapsed or refractory multiple myeloma (CARTITUDE-1): A phase 1b/2 open-label study. *Lancet* **2021**, *398*, 314–324. [CrossRef]
118. Maude, S.L.; Laetsch, T.W.; Buechner, J.; Rives, S.; Boyer, M.; Bittencourt, H.; Bader, P.; Verneris, M.R.; Stefanski, H.E.; Myers, G.D.; et al. Tisagenlecleucel in Children and Young Adults with B-Cell Lymphoblastic Leukemia. *N. Engl. J. Med.* **2018**, *378*, 439–448. [CrossRef]
119. Neelapu, S.S.; Locke, F.L.; Bartlett, N.L.; Lekakis, L.J.; Miklos, D.B.; Jacobson, C.A.; Braunschweig, I.; Oluwole, O.O.; Siddiqi, T.; Lin, Y.; et al. Axicabtagene Ciloleucel CAR T-Cell Therapy in Refractory Large B-Cell Lymphoma. *N. Engl. J. Med.* **2017**, *377*, 2531–2544. [CrossRef]
120. June, C.H.; O'Connor, R.S.; Kawalekar, O.U.; Ghassemi, S.; Milone, M.C. CAR T cell immunotherapy for human cancer. *Science* **2018**, *359*, 1361–1365. [CrossRef]
121. Uppal, S.S.; Verma, S.; Dhot, P.S. Normal values of CD4 and CD8 lymphocyte subsets in healthy indian adults and the effects of sex, age, ethnicity, and smoking. *Cytom. B Clin. Cytom.* **2003**, *52B*, 32–36. [CrossRef]
122. Luckheeram, R.V.; Zhou, R.; Verma, A.D.; Xia, B. CD4+T Cells: Differentiation and Functions. *J. Immunol. Res.* **2012**, *2012*, 925135. [CrossRef]
123. Pu, Q.; Qiao, J.; Liu, Y.; Cao, X.; Tan, R.; Yan, D.; Wang, X.; Li, J.; Yue, B. Differential diagnosis and identification of prognostic markers for peripheral T-cell lymphoma subtypes based on flow cytometry immunophenotype profiles. *Front. Immunol.* **2022**, *13*, 1008695. [CrossRef]
124. Pinz, K.; Liu, H.; Golightly, M.; Jares, A.; Lan, F.; Zieve, G.W.; Hagag, N.; Schuster, M.; Firor, A.E.; Jiang, X.; et al. Preclinical targeting of human T-cell malignancies using CD4-specific chimeric antigen receptor (CAR)-engineered T cells. *Leukemia* **2016**, *30*, 701–707. [CrossRef] [PubMed]
125. Ma, G.; Shen, J.; Pinz, K.; Wada, M.; Park, J.; Kim, S.; Togano, T.; Tse, W. Targeting T Cell Malignancies Using CD4CAR T-Cells and Implementing a Natural Safety Switch. *Stem Cell Rev. Rep.* **2019**, *15*, 443–447. [CrossRef] [PubMed]
126. Feng, J.; Xu, H.; Cinquina, A.; Wu, Z.; Zhang, W.; Sun, L.; Chen, Q.; Tian, L.; Song, L.; Pinz, K.G.; et al. Treatment of aggressive T-cell lymphoma/leukemia with anti-CD4 CAR T cells. *Front. Immunol.* **2022**, *13*, 997482. [CrossRef]
127. Mamonkin, M.; Rouce, R.H.; Tashiro, H.; Brenner, M.K. A T-cell–directed chimeric antigen receptor for the selective treatment of T-cell malignancies. *Blood* **2015**, *126*, 983–992. [CrossRef]
128. Herndler-Brandstetter, D.; Brunner, S.; Weiskopf, D.; van Rijn, R.; Landgraf, K.; Dejaco, C.; Duftner, C.; Schirmer, M.; Kloss, F.; Gassner, R.; et al. Post-thymic regulation of CD5 levels in human memory T cells is inversely associated with the strength of responsiveness to interleukin-15. *Hum. Immunol.* **2011**, *72*, 627–631. [CrossRef]
129. Elghawy, O.; Cao, M.; Xu, J.; Landsburg, D.J.; Svoboda, J.; Nasta, S.D.; Chong, E.A.; Schuster, S.J.; Thomas, C.J.; Carter, J.S.; et al. Prevalence and Prognostication of CD5+ Mature T-Cell Lymphomas. *Cancers* **2024**, *16*, 3430. [CrossRef]
130. Patel, R.P.; Ghilardi, G.; Zhang, Y.; Chiang, Y.-H.; Xie, W.; Guruprasad, P.; Kim, K.H.; Chun, I.; Angelos, M.G.; Pajarillo, R.; et al. CD5 deletion enhances the antitumor activity of adoptive T cell therapies. *Sci. Immunol.* **2024**, *9*, eadn6509. [CrossRef]
131. Wada, M.; Zhang, H.; Fang, L.; Feng, J.; Tse, C.O.; Zhang, W.; Chen, Q.; Sha, S.; Cao, Y.; Chen, K.H.; et al. Characterization of an Anti-CD5 Directed CAR T-Cell against T-Cell Malignancies. *Stem Cell Rev. Rep.* **2020**, *16*, 369–384. [CrossRef]

132. Lin, H.; Cheng, J.; Zhu, L.; Zeng, Y.; Dai, Z.; Zhang, Y.; Zhu, X.; Mu, W. Anti-CD5 CAR-T cells with a tEGFR safety switch exhibit potent toxicity control. *Blood Cancer J.* **2024**, *14*, 98. [CrossRef] [PubMed]
133. Hill, L.C.; Rouce, R.H.; Wu, M.J.; Wang, T.; Ma, R.; Zhang, H.; Mehta, B.; Lapteva, N.; Mei, Z.; Smith, T.S.; et al. Antitumor efficacy and safety of unedited autologous CD5.CAR T cells in relapsed/refractory mature T-cell lymphomas. *Blood* **2024**, *143*, 1231–1241. [CrossRef] [PubMed]
134. Mu, W.; Zhang, M.; Hu, G.; Han, Y.; Mao, X.; Chen, C.; Shen, K.; Dai, Z.; Zhu, X.; Zhou, X.; et al. Case report: Differential diagnosis of highly amplified anti-CD5 CAR T cells and relapsed lymphoma cells in a patient with refractory ALK positive anaplastic large cell lymphoma. *Front. Immunol.* **2023**, *14*, 1280007. [CrossRef]
135. Feng, J.; Xu, H.; Cinquina, A.; Wu, Z.; Chen, Q.; Zhang, P.; Wang, X.; Shan, H.; Xu, L.; Zhang, Q.; et al. Treatment of Aggressive T Cell Lymphoblastic Lymphoma/leukemia Using Anti-CD5 CAR T Cells. *Stem Cell Rev. Rep.* **2021**, *17*, 652–661. [CrossRef]
136. Pan, J.; Tan, Y.; Shan, L.; Seery, S.; Deng, B.; Ling, Z.; Xu, J.; Duan, J.; Wang, Z.; Wang, K.; et al. Allogeneic CD5-specific CAR-T therapy for relapsed/refractory T-ALL: A phase 1 trial. *Nat. Med.* **2025**, *31*, 126–136. [CrossRef]
137. Haynes, B.F.; Eisenbarth, G.S.; Fauci, A.S. Human lymphocyte antigens: Production of a monoclonal antibody that defines functional thymus-derived lymphocyte subsets. *Proc. Natl. Acad. Sci. USA* **1979**, *76*, 5829–5833. [CrossRef]
138. Png, Y.T.; Vinanica, N.; Kamiya, T.; Shimasaki, N.; Coustan-Smith, E.; Campana, D. Blockade of CD7 expression in T cells for effective chimeric antigen receptor targeting of T-cell malignancies. *Blood Adv.* **2017**, *1*, 2348–2360. [CrossRef]
139. Karube, K.; Aoki, R.; Nomura, Y.; Yamamoto, K.; Shimizu, K.; Yoshida, S.; Komatani, H.; Sugita, Y.; Ohshima, K. Usefulness of flow cytometry for differential diagnosis of precursor and peripheral T-cell and NK-cell lymphomas: Analysis of 490 cases. *Pathol. Int.* **2008**, *58*, 89–97. [CrossRef]
140. Gomes-Silva, D.; Srinivasan, M.; Sharma, S.; Lee, C.M.; Wagner, D.L.; Davis, T.H.; Rouce, R.H.; Bao, G.; Brenner, M.K.; Mamonkin, M. CD7-edited T cells expressing a CD7-specific CAR for the therapy of T-cell malignancies. *Blood* **2017**, *130*, 285–296. [CrossRef]
141. Watanabe, N.; Mo, F.; Zheng, R.; Ma, R.; Bray, V.C.; van Leeuwen, D.G.; Sritabal-Ramirez, J.; Hu, H.; Wang, S.; Mehta, B.; et al. Feasibility and preclinical efficacy of CD7-unedited CD7 CAR T cells for T cell malignancies. *Mol. Ther.* **2023**, *31*, 24–34. [CrossRef] [PubMed]
142. Lu, P.; Liu, Y.; Yang, J.; Zhang, X.; Yang, X.; Wang, H.; Wang, L.; Wang, Q.; Jin, D.; Li, J.; et al. Naturally selected CD7 CAR-T therapy without genetic manipulations for T-ALL/LBL: First-in-human phase 1 clinical trial. *Blood* **2022**, *140*, 321–334. [CrossRef] [PubMed]
143. Yang, J.; Zhang, X.; Li, J.; Qiu, L.; Wang, L.; Lu, P. CD7-Targeted CAR-T Cell Therapy Shows Promising Efficacy and Safety in Treating Refractory/Relapsed Peripheral T-Cell Lymphoma: Phase I Clinical Trial. *Blood* **2024**, *144*, 2075. [CrossRef]
144. Tan, Y.; Shan, L.; Zhao, L.; Deng, B.; Ling, Z.; Zhang, Y.; Peng, S.; Xu, J.; Duan, J.; Wang, Z.; et al. Long-term follow-up of donor-derived CD7 CAR T-cell therapy in patients with T-cell acute lymphoblastic leukemia. *J. Hematol. Oncol.* **2023**, *16*, 34. [CrossRef]
145. Went, P.; Agostinelli, C.; Gallamini, A.; Piccaluga, P.P.; Ascani, S.; Sabattini, E.; Bacci, F.; Falini, B.; Motta, T.; Paulli, M.; et al. Marker Expression in Peripheral T-Cell Lymphoma: A Proposed Clinical-Pathologic Prognostic Score. *J. Clin. Oncol.* **2006**, *24*, 2472–2479. [CrossRef]
146. Maciocia, P.M.; Wawrzyniecka, P.A.; Philip, B.; Ricciardelli, I.; Akarca, A.U.; Onuoha, S.C.; Legut, M.; Cole, D.K.; Sewell, A.K.; Gritti, G.; et al. Targeting the T cell receptor β-chain constant region for immunotherapy of T cell malignancies. *Nat. Med.* **2017**, *23*, 1416–1423. [CrossRef]
147. Berg, H.; Otteson, G.E.; Corley, H.; Shi, M.; Horna, P.; Jevremovic, D.; Olteanu, H. Flow cytometric evaluation of TRBC1 expression in tissue specimens and body fluids is a novel and specific method for assessment of T-cell clonality and diagnosis of T-cell neoplasms. *Cytom. B Clin. Cytom.* **2021**, *100*, 361–369. [CrossRef]
148. Horna, P.; Weybright, M.J.; Ferrari, M.; Jungherz, D.; Peng, Y.; Akbar, Z.; Ilca, F.T.; Otteson, G.E.; Seheult, J.N.; Ortmann, J.; et al. Dual T-cell constant β chain (TRBC)1 and TRBC2 staining for the identification of T-cell neoplasms by flow cytometry. *Blood Cancer J.* **2024**, *14*, 34. [CrossRef]
149. Cwynarski, K.; Iacoboni, G.; Tholouli, E.; Menne, T.F.; Irvine, D.A.; Balasubramaniam, N.; Wood, L.; Shang, J.; Zhang, Y.; Basilico, S.; et al. First in Human Study of AUTO4, a TRBC1-Targeting CAR T-Cell Therapy in Relapsed/Refractory TRBC1-Positive Peripheral T-Cell Lymphoma. *Blood* **2022**, *140*, 10316–10317. [CrossRef]
150. Nichakawade, T.D.; Ge, J.; Mog, B.J.; Lee, B.S.; Pearlman, A.H.; Hwang, M.S.; DiNapoli, S.R.; Wyhs, N.; Marcou, N.; Glavaris, S.; et al. TRBC1-targeting antibody–drug conjugates for the treatment of T cell cancers. *Nature* **2024**, *628*, 416–423. [CrossRef]
151. Baguet, C.; Larghero, J.; Mebarki, M. Early predictive factors of failure in autologous CAR T-cell manufacturing and/or efficacy in hematologic malignancies. *Blood Adv.* **2023**, *8*, 337–342. [CrossRef]
152. Ferrari, M.; Baldan, V.; Ghongane, P.; Nicholson, A.; Bughda, R.; Akbar, Z.; Wawrzyniecka, P.; Maciocia, P.; Cordoba, S.; Thomas, S.; et al. Abstract 2183: Targeting TRBC1 and 2 for the treatment of T cell lymphomas. *Cancer Res.* **2020**, *80*, 2183. [CrossRef]

153. Stein, H.; Mason, D.Y.; Gerdes, J.; O'Connor, N.; Wainscoat, J.; Pallesen, G.; Gatter, K.; Falini, B.; Delsol, G.; Lemke, H.; et al. The Expression of the Hodgkin's Disease Associated Antigen Ki-1 in Reactive and Neoplastic Lymphoid Tissue: Evidence That Reed-Sternberg Cells and Histiocytic Malignancies Are Derived from Activated Lymphoid Cells. *Blood* **1985**, *66*, 848–858. [CrossRef]
154. van der Weyden, C.A.; Pileri, S.A.; Feldman, A.L.; Whisstock, J.; Prince, H.M. Understanding CD30 biology and therapeutic targeting: A historical perspective providing insight into future directions. *Blood Cancer J.* **2017**, *7*, e603. [CrossRef] [PubMed]
155. Bossard, C.; Dobay, M.P.; Parrens, M.; Lamant, L.; Missiaglia, E.; Haioun, C.; Martin, A.; Fabiani, B.; Delarue, R.; Tournilhac, O.; et al. Immunohistochemistry as a valuable tool to assess CD30 expression in peripheral T-cell lymphomas: High correlation with mRNA levels. *Blood* **2014**, *124*, 2983–2986. [CrossRef] [PubMed]
156. Sabattini, E.; Pizzi, M.; Tabanelli, V.; Baldin, P.; Sacchetti, C.S.; Agostinelli, C.; Zinzani, P.L.; Pileri, S.A. CD30 expression in peripheral T-cell lymphomas. *Haematologica* **2013**, *98*, e81–e82. [CrossRef]
157. Prince, H.M.; Kim, Y.H.; Horwitz, S.M.; Dummer, R.; Scarisbrick, J.; Quaglino, P.; Zinzani, P.L.; Wolter, P.; Sanches, J.A.; Ortiz-Romero, P.L.; et al. Brentuximab vedotin or physician's choice in CD30-positive cutaneous T-cell lymphoma (ALCANZA): An international, open-label, randomised, phase 3, multicentre trial. *Lancet* **2017**, *390*, 555–566. [CrossRef]
158. Horwitz, S.; O'Connor, O.A.; Pro, B.; Illidge, T.; Fanale, M.; Advani, R.; Bartlett, N.L.; Christensen, J.H.; Morschhauser, F.; Domingo-Domenech, E.; et al. Brentuximab vedotin with chemotherapy for CD30-positive peripheral T-cell lymphoma (ECHELON-2): A global, double-blind, randomised, phase 3 trial. *Lancet* **2019**, *393*, 229–240. [CrossRef]
159. Bradley, A.M.; Devine, M.; DeRemer, D. Brentuximab vedotin: An anti-CD30 antibody–drug conjugate. *Am. J. Health Syst. Pharm.* **2013**, *70*, 589–597. [CrossRef]
160. Kim, Y.H.; Tavallaee, M.; Sundram, U.; Salva, K.A.; Wood, G.S.; Li, S.; Rozati, S.; Nagpal, S.; Krathen, M.; Reddy, S.; et al. Phase II Investigator-Initiated Study of Brentuximab Vedotin in Mycosis Fungoides and Sézary Syndrome with Variable CD30 Expression Level: A Multi-Institution Collaborative Project. *J. Clin. Oncol.* **2015**, *33*, 3750–3758. [CrossRef]
161. Melenhorst, J.J.; Chen, G.M.; Wang, M.; Porter, D.L.; Chen, C.; Collins, M.A.; Gao, P.; Bandyopadhyay, S.; Sun, H.; Zhao, Z.; et al. Decade-long leukaemia remissions with persistence of CD4+ CAR T cells. *Nature* **2022**, *602*, 503–509. [CrossRef] [PubMed]
162. Voorhees, T.J.; Ghosh, N.; Grover, N.; Block, J.; Cheng, C.; Morrison, K.; Ivanova, A.; Dotti, G.; Serody, J.; Savoldo, B.; et al. Long-term remission in multiply relapsed enteropathy-associated T-cell lymphoma following CD30 CAR T-cell therapy. *Blood Adv.* **2020**, *4*, 5925–5928. [CrossRef] [PubMed]
163. Ramos, C.A.; Ballard, B.; Zhang, H.; Dakhova, O.; Gee, A.P.; Mei, Z.; Bilgi, M.; Wu, M.-F.; Liu, H.; Grilley, B.; et al. Clinical and immunological responses after CD30-specific chimeric antigen receptor–redirected lymphocytes. *J. Clin. Investig.* **2017**, *127*, 3462–3471. [CrossRef]
164. Wang, D.; Zeng, C.; Xu, B.; Xu, J.-H.; Wang, J.; Jiang, L.-J.; Wang, Q.-X.; Li, C.-R.; Wang, N.; Huang, L.; et al. Anti-CD30 chimeric antigen receptor T cell therapy for relapsed/refractory CD30+ lymphoma patients. *Blood Cancer J.* **2020**, *10*, 8. [CrossRef]
165. Grover, N.S.; Hucks, G.; Riches, M.L.; Ivanova, A.; Moore, D.T.; Shea, T.C.; Seegars, M.B.; Armistead, P.M.; Kasow, K.A.; Beaven, A.W.; et al. Anti-CD30 CAR T cells as consolidation after autologous haematopoietic stem-cell transplantation in patients with high-risk CD30+ lymphoma: A phase 1 study. *Lancet Haematol.* **2024**, *11*, e358–e367. [CrossRef]
166. O'Neill, R.E.; Du, W.; Mohammadpour, H.; Alqassim, E.; Qiu, J.; Chen, G.; McCarthy, P.L.; Lee, K.P.; Cao, X. T Cell–Derived CD70 Delivers an Immune Checkpoint Function in Inflammatory T Cell Responses. *J. Immunol.* **2017**, *199*, 3700–3710. [CrossRef]
167. Tesselaar, K.; Xiao, Y.; Arens, R.; van Schijndel, G.M.; Schuurhuis, D.H.; Mebius, R.E.; Borst, J.; van Lier, R.A. Expression of the Murine CD27 Ligand CD70 In Vitro and In Vivo. *J. Immunol.* **2003**, *170*, 33–40. [CrossRef]
168. Flieswasser, T.; den Eynde, A.V.; Audenaerde, J.V.; Waele, J.D.; Lardon, F.; Riether, C.; de Haard, H.; Smits, E.; Pauwels, P.; Jacobs, J. The CD70-CD27 axis in oncology: The new kids on the block. *J. Exp. Clin. Cancer Res.* **2022**, *41*, 12. [CrossRef]
169. Masamoto, I.; Yoshimitsu, M.; Kuroki, A.; Horai, S.; Ezinne, C.C.; Kozako, T.; Hachiman, M.; Kamada, Y.; Baba, M.; Arima, N. Clinical significance of CD70 expression on T cells in human T-lymphotropic virus type-1 carriers and adult T cell leukemia/lymphoma patients. *Leuk. Lymphoma* **2016**, *57*, 685–691. [CrossRef]
170. Marques-Piubelli, M.L.; Soto, L.S.; Iyer, S.P.; Sagert, J.; Pham, M.T.; Tipton, K.; Lu, W.; Khan, K.B.; Zorrilla, L.G.H.; Chapman, J.R.; et al. CD70 Expression in Mature T-Cell Lymphomas. *Blood* **2021**, *138*, 4493. [CrossRef]
171. Wu, C.-H.; Wang, L.; Yang, C.-Y.; Wen, K.W.; Hinds, B.R.; Gill, R.; McCormick, F.; Moasser, M.; Pincus, L.; Ai, W.Z. Targeting CD70 in cutaneous T-cell lymphoma using an antibody-drug conjugate in patient-derived xenograft models. *Blood Adv.* **2021**, *6*, 2290–2302. [CrossRef]
172. Leupin, N.; Zinzani, P.L.; Morschhauser, F.; Dalle, S.; Maerevoet, M.; Michot, J.; Ribrag, V.; Offner, F.; Beylot-Barry, M.; Moins-Teisserenc, H.; et al. Cusatuzumab for treatment of CD70-positive relapsed or refractory cutaneous T-cell lymphoma. *Cancer* **2022**, *128*, 1004–1014. [CrossRef]
173. Iyer, S.P.; Sica, R.A.; Ho, P.J.; Prica, A.; Zain, J.; Foss, F.M.; Hu, B.; Beitinjaneh, A.; Weng, W.-K.; Kim, Y.H.; et al. Safety and activity of CTX130, a CD70-targeted allogeneic CRISPR-Cas9-engineered CAR T-cell therapy, in patients with relapsed or refractory

T-cell malignancies (COBALT-LYM): A single-arm, open-label, phase 1, dose-escalation study. *Lancet Oncol.* **2024**, *26*, 110–122. [CrossRef] [PubMed]
174. Wang, L.; Wang, Y.; He, X.; Mo, Z.; Zhao, M.; Liang, X.; Hu, K.; Wang, K.; Yue, Y.; Mo, G.; et al. CD70-targeted iPSC-derived CAR-NK cells display potent function against tumors and alloreactive T cells. *Cell Rep. Med.* **2025**, *6*, 101889. [CrossRef] [PubMed]
175. Ferenczi, K.; Fuhlbrigge, R.C.; Kupper, T.S.; Pinkus, J.L.; Pinkus, G.S. Increased CCR4 Expression in Cutaneous T Cell Lymphoma. *J. Investig. Dermatol.* **2002**, *119*, 1405–1410. [CrossRef]
176. Ishida, T.; Utsunomiya, A.; Iida, S.; Inagaki, H.; Takatsuka, Y.; Kusumoto, S.; Takeuchi, G.; Shimizu, S.; Ito, M.; Komatsu, H.; et al. Clinical significance of CCR4 expression in adult T-cell leukemia/lymphoma: Its close association with skin involvement and unfavorable outcome. *Clin. Cancer Res.* **2003**, *9*, 3625–3634.
177. Ishida, T.; Inagaki, H.; Utsunomiya, A.; Takatsuka, Y.; Komatsu, H.; Iida, S.; Takeuchi, G.; Eimoto, T.; Nakamura, S.; Ueda, R. CXC Chemokine Receptor 3 and CC Chemokine Receptor 4 Expression in T-Cell and NK-Cell Lymphomas with Special Reference to Clinicopathological Significance for Peripheral T-Cell Lymphoma, Unspecified. *Clin. Cancer Res.* **2004**, *10*, 5494–5500. [CrossRef]
178. Asano, N.; Suzuki, R.; Ohshima, K.; Kagami, Y.; Ishida, F.; Yoshino, T.; Ogawa, H.; Morishima, Y.; Nakamura, S. Linkage of expression of chemokine receptors (CXCR3 and CCR4) and cytotoxic molecules in peripheral T cell lymphoma, not otherwise specified and ALK-negative anaplastic large cell lymphoma. *Int. J. Hematol.* **2010**, *91*, 426–435. [CrossRef]
179. Geller, S.; Hollmann, T.J.; Horwitz, S.M.; Myskowski, P.L.; Pulitzer, M. C-C chemokine receptor 4 expression in CD8+ cutaneous T-cell lymphomas and lymphoproliferative disorders, and its implications for diagnosis and treatment. *Histopathology* **2020**, *76*, 222–232. [CrossRef]
180. Shono, Y.; Suga, H.; Kamijo, H.; Fujii, H.; Oka, T.; Miyagaki, T.; Shishido-Takahashi, N.; Sugaya, M.; Sato, S. Expression of CCR3 and CCR4 Suggests a Poor Prognosis in Mycosis Fungoides and Sézary Syndrome. *Acta Derm. Venereol.* **2019**, *99*, 809–812. [CrossRef]
181. Duvic, M.; Pinter-Brown, L.C.; Foss, F.M.; Sokol, L.; Jorgensen, J.L.; Challagundla, P.; Dwyer, K.M.; Zhang, X.; Kurman, M.R.; Ballerini, R.; et al. Phase 1/2 study of mogamulizumab, a defucosylated anti-CCR4 antibody, in previously treated patients with cutaneous T-cell lymphoma. *Blood* **2015**, *125*, 1883–1889. [CrossRef]
182. Kim, Y.H.; Bagot, M.; Pinter-Brown, L.; Rook, A.H.; Porcu, P.; Horwitz, S.M.; Whittaker, S.; Tokura, Y.; Vermeer, M.; Zinzani, P.L.; et al. Mogamulizumab versus vorinostat in previously treated cutaneous T-cell lymphoma (MAVORIC): An international, open-label, randomised, controlled phase 3 trial. *Lancet Oncol.* **2018**, *19*, 1192–1204. [CrossRef]
183. Ishida, T.; Jo, T.; Takemoto, S.; Suzushima, H.; Uozumi, K.; Yamamoto, K.; Uike, N.; Saburi, Y.; Nosaka, K.; Utsunomiya, A.; et al. Dose-intensified chemotherapy alone or in combination with mogamulizumab in newly diagnosed aggressive adult T-cell leukaemia-lymphoma: A randomized phase II study. *Br. J. Haematol.* **2015**, *169*, 672–682. [CrossRef] [PubMed]
184. Ishida, T.; Joh, T.; Uike, N.; Yamamoto, K.; Utsunomiya, A.; Yoshida, S.; Saburi, Y.; Miyamoto, T.; Takemoto, S.; Suzushima, H.; et al. Defucosylated Anti-CCR4 Monoclonal Antibody (KW-0761) for Relapsed Adult T-Cell Leukemia-Lymphoma: A Multicenter Phase II Study. *J. Clin. Oncol.* **2012**, *30*, 837–842. [CrossRef] [PubMed]
185. Ogura, M.; Ishida, T.; Hatake, K.; Taniwaki, M.; Ando, K.; Tobinai, K.; Fujimoto, K.; Yamamoto, K.; Miyamoto, T.; Uike, N.; et al. Multicenter Phase II Study of Mogamulizumab (KW-0761), a Defucosylated Anti-CC Chemokine Receptor 4 Antibody, in Patients With Relapsed Peripheral T-Cell Lymphoma and Cutaneous T-Cell Lymphoma. *J. Clin. Oncol.* **2014**, *32*, 1157–1163. [CrossRef]
186. Perera, L.P.; Zhang, M.; Nakagawa, M.; Petrus, M.N.; Maeda, M.; Kadin, M.E.; Waldmann, T.A.; Perera, P. Chimeric antigen receptor modified T cells that target chemokine receptor CCR4 as a therapeutic modality for T-cell malignancies. *Am. J. Hematol.* **2017**, *92*, 892–901. [CrossRef]
187. Watanabe, K.; Gomez, A.M.; Kuramitsu, S.; Siurala, M.; Da, T.; Agarwal, S.; Song, D.; Scholler, J.; Rotolo, A.; Posey, A.D.; et al. Identifying highly active anti-CCR4-CAR T cells for the treatment of T-cell lymphoma. *Blood Adv.* **2023**, *7*, 3416–3430. [CrossRef]
188. Ni, X.; Jorgensen, J.L.; Goswami, M.; Challagundla, P.; Decker, W.K.; Kim, Y.H.; Duvic, M.A. Reduction of Regulatory T Cells by Mogamulizumab, a Defucosylated Anti-CC Chemokine Receptor 4 Antibody, in Patients with Aggressive/Refractory Mycosis Fungoides and Sézary Syndrome. *Clin. Cancer Res.* **2015**, *21*, 274–285. [CrossRef]
189. Chen, K.H.; Wada, M.; Firor, A.E.; Pinz, K.G.; Jares, A.; Liu, H.; Salman, H.; Golightly, M.; Lan, F.; Jiang, X.; et al. Novel anti-CD3 chimeric antigen receptor targeting of aggressive T cell malignancies. *Oncotarget* **2016**, *7*, 56219–56232. [CrossRef]
190. Kobayashi, E.; Kamihara, Y.; Arai, M.; Wada, A.; Kikuchi, S.; Hatano, R.; Iwao, N.; Susukida, T.; Ozawa, T.; Adachi, Y.; et al. Development of a Novel CD26-Targeted Chimeric Antigen Receptor T-Cell Therapy for CD26-Expressing T-Cell Malignancies. *Cells* **2023**, *12*, 2059. [CrossRef]
191. Zi, Z.; Zhao, H.; Wang, H.; Ma, X.; Wei, F. B7-H3 Chimeric Antigen Receptor Redirected T Cells Target Anaplastic Lymphoma Kinase-Positive Anaplastic Large Cell Lymphoma. *Cancers* **2020**, *12*, 3815. [CrossRef] [PubMed]
192. Zheng, D.; Wang, X.; Cheng, L.; Qin, L.; Jiang, Z.; Zhao, R.; Li, Y.; Shi, J.; Wu, Q.; Long, Y.; et al. The Chemokine Receptor CCR8 Is a Target of Chimeric Antigen T Cells for Treating T Cell Malignancies. *Front. Immunol.* **2022**, *13*, 808347. [CrossRef]

193. Frigault, M.J.; Graham, C.E.; Berger, T.R.; Ritchey, J.; Horick, N.K.; El-Jawahri, A.; Scarfò, I.; Schmidts, A.; Haradhvala, N.J.; Wehrli, M.; et al. Phase 1 study of CAR-37 T cells in patients with relapsed or refractory CD37+ lymphoid malignancies. *Blood* **2024**, *144*, 1153–1167. [CrossRef]
194. Acker, H.H.V.; Capsomidis, A.; Smits, E.L.; Tendeloo, V.F.V. CD56 in the Immune System: More Than a Marker for Cytotoxicity? *Front. Immunol.* **2017**, *8*, 892. [CrossRef]
195. Dalle, I.A.; Dulery, R.; Moukalled, N.; Ricard, L.; Stocker, N.; El-Cheikh, J.; Mohty, M.; Bazarbachi, A. Bi- and Tri-specific antibodies in non-Hodgkin lymphoma: Current data and perspectives. *Blood Cancer J.* **2024**, *14*, 23. [CrossRef]
196. Paul, S.; Pearlman, A.H.; Douglass, J.; Mog, B.J.; Hsiue, E.H.-C.; Hwang, M.S.; DiNapoli, S.R.; Konig, M.F.; Brown, P.A.; Wright, K.M.; et al. TCR β chain–directed bispecific antibodies for the treatment of T cell cancers. *Sci. Transl. Med.* **2021**, *13*, eabd3595. [CrossRef]
197. Kerbauy, L.N.; Marin, N.D.; Kaplan, M.; Banerjee, P.P.; Berrien-Elliott, M.M.; Becker-Hapak, M.; Basar, R.; Foster, M.; Melo, L.G.; Neal, C.C.; et al. Combining AFM13, a Bispecific CD30/CD16 Antibody, with Cytokine-Activated Blood and Cord Blood–Derived NK Cells Facilitates CAR-like Responses Against CD30+ Malignancies. *Clin. Cancer Res.* **2021**, *27*, 3744–3756. [CrossRef]
198. Rothe, A.; Sasse, S.; Topp, M.S.; Eichenauer, D.A.; Hummel, H.; Reiners, K.S.; Dietlein, M.; Kuhnert, G.; Kessler, J.; Buerkle, C.; et al. A phase 1 study of the bispecific anti-CD30/CD16A antibody construct AFM13 in patients with relapsed or refractory Hodgkin lymphoma. *Blood* **2015**, *125*, 4024–4031. [CrossRef]
199. Sawas, A.; Chen, P.-H.; Lipschitz, M.; Rodig, S.; Vlad, G. Title: Clinical and Biological Evaluation of the Novel CD30/CD16A Tetravalent Bispecific Antibody (AFM13) in Relapsed or Refractory CD30-Positive Lymphoma with Cutaneous Presentation: A Biomarker Phase Ib/IIa Study (NCT03192202). *Blood* **2020**, *136*, 25–26. [CrossRef]
200. Bartlett, N.L.; Herrera, A.F.; Domingo-Domenech, E.; Mehta, A.; Forero-Torres, A.; Garcia-Sanz, R.; Armand, P.; Devata, S.; Izquierdo, A.R.; Lossos, I.S.; et al. A phase 1b study of AFM13 in combination with pembrolizumab in patients with relapsed or refractory Hodgkin lymphoma. *Blood* **2020**, *136*, 2401–2409. [CrossRef]
201. Kim, W.S.; Shortt, J.; Zinzani, P.L.; Mikhailova, N.; Radeski, D.; Ribrag, V.; Domenech, E.D.; Sawas, A.; Alexis, K.; Emig, M.; et al. A Phase II Study of Acimtamig (AFM13) in Patients with CD30-Positive, Relapsed, or Refractory Peripheral T-cell Lymphomas. *Clin. Cancer Res.* **2025**, *31*, 65–73. [CrossRef] [PubMed]
202. Nieto, Y.; Banerjee, P.; Kaur, I.; Basar, R.; Li, Y.; Daher, M.; Rafei, H.; Kerbauy, L.N.; Kaplan, M.; Marin, D.; et al. Allogeneic NK cells with a bispecific innate cell engager in refractory relapsed lymphoma: A phase 1 trial. *Nat. Med.* **2025**, *31*, 1987–1993. [CrossRef] [PubMed]
203. Taylor, N.P. Genmab Axes 3 Programs to Focus on Plumped-Up Pivotal Pipeline. 2024. Available online: https://www.fiercebiotech.com/bic axes-3-programs-focus-plumped-pivotal-pipeline (accessed on 25 September 2025).
204. Chikada, T.; Asano, H.; Terashima, M.; Tsuchiya, T.; Kabumoto, Y.; Okita, G.; Takahashi, T.; Nakakubo, H.; Mieno, R.; Ito, Y.; et al. Bispecific T Cell Engager with Trbc-Targeting Antibody Against Effector T Cells for the Treatment of T Cell Malignancy. *Blood* **2024**, *144*, 2060. [CrossRef]
205. Wang, J.; Qi, J.; Li, W.; Zhai, Z.; Li, P.; Zou, W.; Ding, M.; Yang, X.; Wang, R.; Guo, W.; et al. GNC-038, a tetra-specific antibody, in patients with R/R non-Hodgkin lymphoma or acute lymphoblastic leukemia: A phase 1 study design and rationale. *J. Clin. Oncol.* **2023**, *41*, TPS2668. [CrossRef]
206. Tateshita, N.; Watanabe, N.; Shimbo, T.; Morimoto, A.; Takeda, K.; Tanihiro, T. Abstract 7324: ONO-4685: A novel PD-1/CD3 bispecific T-cell engager (TCE) for the treatment of T-cell malignancies. *Cancer Res.* **2025**, *85*, 7324. [CrossRef]
207. Park, J.A.; Santich, B.H.; Xu, H.; Lum, L.G.; Cheung, N.-K.V. Potent ex vivo armed T cells using recombinant bispecific antibodies for adoptive immunotherapy with reduced cytokine release. *J. Immunother. Cancer* **2021**, *9*, e002222. [CrossRef]
208. Fukuhara, H.; Ino, Y.; Todo, T. Oncolytic virus therapy: A new era of cancer treatment at dawn. *Cancer Sci.* **2016**, *107*, 1373–1379. [CrossRef]
209. Macedo, N.; Miller, D.M.; Haq, R.; Kaufman, H.L. Clinical landscape of oncolytic virus research in 2020. *J. Immunother. Cancer* **2020**, *8*, e001486. [CrossRef]
210. Pasin, F.; Calveri, M.M.; Pizzarelli, G.; Calabrese, A.; Andreoli, M.; Bongiovanni, I.; Cattaneo, C.; Rignanese, G. Oncolytic effect of SARS-CoV2 in a patient with NK lymphoma. *Acta Biomed.* **2020**, *91*, 2531–6745. [CrossRef]
211. Snowden, C.; Ng, S.; Choi, J. Partial remission of advanced untreated Sézary syndrome after COVID-19. *JAAD Case Rep.* **2022**, *21*, 165–168. [CrossRef]
212. Ohadi, L.; Hosseinzadeh, F.; Dadkhahfar, S.; Nasiri, S. Oncolytic effect of SARS-CoV-2 in a patient with mycosis fungoides: A case report. *Clin. Case Rep.* **2022**, *10*, e05682. [CrossRef]
213. Heinzerling, L.; Künzi, V.; Oberholzer, P.A.; Kündig, T.; Naim, H.; Dummer, R. Oncolytic measles virus in cutaneous T-cell lymphomas mounts antitumor immune responses in vivo and targets interferon-resistant tumor cells. *Blood* **2005**, *106*, 2287–2294. [CrossRef] [PubMed]

214. Cook, J.; Peng, K.W.W.; Witzig, T.E.; Broski, S.M.; Villasboas, J.C.; Paludo, J.; Patnaik, M.M.; Rajkumar, V.; Dispenzieri, A.; Leung, N.; et al. Clinical Activity of Single Dose Systemic Oncolytic VSV Virotherapy in Patients with Relapsed Refractory T-Cell Lymphoma. *Blood Adv.* **2022**, *6*, 3268–3279. [CrossRef] [PubMed]
215. Angelova, A.; Barf, M.; Just, A.; Leuchs, B.; Rommelaere, J.; Ungerechts, G. H-1 Parvovirus-Induced Oncolysis and Tumor Microenvironment Immune Modulation in a Novel Heterotypic Spheroid Model of Cutaneous T-Cell Lymphoma. *Cancers* **2024**, *16*, 2711. [CrossRef]
216. Chesney, J.; Puzanov, I.; Collichio, F.; Singh, P.; Milhem, M.M.; Glaspy, J.; Hamid, O.; Ross, M.; Friedlander, P.; Garbe, C.; et al. Randomized, Open-Label Phase II Study Evaluating the Efficacy and Safety of Talimogene Laherparepvec in Combination With Ipilimumab Versus Ipilimumab Alone in Patients With Advanced, Unresectable Melanoma. *J. Clin. Oncol.* **2017**, *36*, 1658–1667. [CrossRef] [PubMed]
217. Quach, H.; Ritchie, D.; Stewart, A.K.; Neeson, P.; Harrison, S.; Smyth, M.J.; Prince, H.M. Mechanism of action of immunomodulatory drugs (IMiDS) in multiple myeloma. *Leukemia* **2010**, *24*, 22–32. [CrossRef]
218. Colley, A.; Brauns, T.; Sluder, A.E.; Poznansky, M.C.; Gemechu, Y. Immunomodulatory drugs: A promising clinical ally for cancer immunotherapy. *Trends Mol. Med.* **2024**, *30*, 765–780. [CrossRef]
219. Zinzani, P.L.; Pellegrini, C.; Broccoli, A.; Stefoni, V.; Gandolfi, L.; Quirini, F.; Argnani, L.; Berti, E.; Derenzini, E.; Pileri, S.; et al. Lenalidomide monotherapy for relapsed/refractory peripheral T-cell lymphoma not otherwise specified. *Leuk. Lymphoma* **2011**, *52*, 1585–1588. [CrossRef]
220. Toumishey, E.; Prasad, A.; Dueck, G.; Chua, N.; Finch, D.; Johnston, J.; van der Jagt, R.; Stewart, D.; White, D.; Belch, A.; et al. Final report of a phase 2 clinical trial of lenalidomide monotherapy for patients with T-cell lymphoma. *Cancer* **2015**, *121*, 716–723. [CrossRef]
221. Morschhauser, F.; Fitoussi, O.; Haioun, C.; Thieblemont, C.; Quach, H.; Delarue, R.; Glaisner, S.; Gabarre, J.; Bosly, A.; Lister, J.; et al. A phase 2, multicentre, single-arm, open-label study to evaluate the safety and efficacy of single-agent lenalidomide (Revlimid®) in subjects with relapsed or refractory peripheral T-cell non-Hodgkin lymphoma: The EXPECT trial. *Eur. J. Cancer.* **2013**, *49*, 2869–2876. [CrossRef]
222. Ishida, T.; Fujiwara, H.; Nosaka, K.; Taira, N.; Abe, Y.; Imaizumi, Y.; Moriuchi, Y.; Jo, T.; Ishizawa, K.; Tobinai, K.; et al. Multicenter Phase II Study of Lenalidomide in Relapsed or Recurrent Adult T-Cell Leukemia/Lymphoma: ATLL-002. *J. Clin. Oncol.* **2016**, *34*, 4086–4093. [CrossRef]
223. Dogan, A.; Ngu, L.S.P.; Ng, S.H.; Cervi, P.L. Pathology and clinical features of angioimmunoblastic T-cell lymphoma after successful treatment with thalidomide. *Leukemia* **2005**, *19*, 873–875. [CrossRef] [PubMed]
224. Gottardi, M.; Danesin, C.; Canal, F.; Tos, A.P.D.; Stefani, P.M.; Calistri, E.; Salvadori, U.; Gherlinzoni, F. Complete remission induced by thalidomide in a case of angioimmunoblastic T-cell lymphoma refractory to autologous stem cell transplantation. *Leuk. Lymphoma* **2008**, *49*, 1836–1838. [CrossRef] [PubMed]
225. Wu, H.; Zhao, C.; Gu, K.; Jiao, Y.; Hao, J.; Sun, G. Thalidomide plus chemotherapy exhibit enhanced efficacy in the clinical treatment of T-cell non-Hodgkin's lymphoma: A prospective study of 46 cases. *Mol. Clin. Oncol.* **2014**, *2*, 695–700. [CrossRef] [PubMed]
226. Liang, J.; Wang, L.; Wang, X.; Cui, G.; Zhou, J.; Xing, T.; Du, K.; Xu, J.; Wang, L.; Liang, R.; et al. Chidamide plus prednisone, cyclophosphamide, and thalidomide for relapsed or refractory peripheral T-cell lymphoma: A multicenter phase II trial. *Chin. Med. J.* **2024**, *137*, 1576–1582. [CrossRef]
227. Sun, Y.; Li, L.; Li, X.; Zhang, L.; Wang, X.; Fu, X.; Sun, Z.; Zhang, X.; Li, Z.; Wu, J.; et al. Outcomes of GDPT (gemcitabine, cisplatin, prednisone, thalidomide) versus CHOP in newly diagnosed peripheral T-cell lymphoma patients. *Ther. Adv. Med. Oncol.* **2020**, *12*, 1758835920923829. [CrossRef]
228. Querfeld, C.; Chen, L.; Wu, X.; Han, Z.; Su, C.; Banez, M.; Quach, J.; Barnhizer, T.; Crisan, L.; Rosen, S.T.; et al. Preliminary Analysis Demonstrates Durvalumab (Anti-PD-L1) & Lenalidomide Is Superior to Single-Agent Durvalumab (anti-PD-L1) in Refractory/Advanced Cutaneous T Cell Lymphoma in a Randomized Phase 2 Trial. *Blood* **2023**, *142*, 3077. [CrossRef]
229. Usmani, S.Z.; Schjesvold, F.; Oriol, A.; Karlin, L.; Cavo, M.; Rifkin, R.M.; Yimer, H.A.; LeBlanc, R.; Takezako, N.; McCroskey, R.D.; et al. Pembrolizumab plus lenalidomide and dexamethasone for patients with treatment-naive multiple myeloma (KEYNOTE-185): A randomised, open-label, phase 3 trial. *Lancet Haematol.* **2019**, *6*, e448–e458. [CrossRef]
230. Mateos, M.-V.; Blacklock, H.; Schjesvold, F.; Oriol, A.; Simpson, D.; George, A.; Goldschmidt, H.; Larocca, A.; Chanan-Khan, A.; Sherbenou, D.; et al. Pembrolizumab plus pomalidomide and dexamethasone for patients with relapsed or refractory multiple myeloma (KEYNOTE-183): A randomised, open-label, phase 3 trial. *Lancet Haematol.* **2019**, *6*, e459–e469. [CrossRef]
231. Leonard, J.P.; Trneny, M.; Izutsu, K.; Fowler, N.H.; Hong, X.; Zhu, J.; Zhang, H.; Offner, F.; Scheliga, A.; Nowakowski, G.S.; et al. AUGMENT: A Phase III Study of Lenalidomide Plus Rituximab Versus Placebo Plus Rituximab in Relapsed or Refractory Indolent Lymphoma. *J. Clin. Oncol.* **2019**, *37*, 1188–1199. [CrossRef]

232. van der Weyden, C.; Bressel, M.; Khot, A.; Prince, H.M.; Dickinson, M. Assessment of the Tolerability and Optimal Dosing of the Combination of Brentuximab Vedotin and Lenalidomide in Patients with Relapsed or Refractory T-cell Lymphoma: Results of a Single-centre Phase 1 Dose-escalation Study. *EJHaem* **2025**, *6*, e70033. [CrossRef] [PubMed]
233. Reneau, J.C.; Huang, Y.; Hanel, W.; Brammer, J.E.; Chung, C.; William, B. Final Results of a Phase II Study of Brentuximab Vedotin and Lenalidomide in Relapsed and Refractory T-Cell Lymphomas. *Blood* **2024**, *144*, 4438. [CrossRef]
234. Prince, H.M.; Duvic, M.; Martin, A.; Sterry, W.; Assaf, C.; Sun, Y.; Straus, D.; Acosta, M.; Negro-Vilar, A. Phase III Placebo-Controlled Trial of Denileukin Diftitox for Patients with Cutaneous T-Cell Lymphoma. *J. Clin. Oncol.* **2010**, *28*, 1870–1877. [CrossRef] [PubMed]
235. Foss, F.M.; Kim, Y.H.; Prince, H.M.; Akilov, O.E.; Querfeld, C.; Seminario-Vidal, L.; Fisher, D.C.; Kuzel, T.M.; Yannakou, C.K.; Geskin, L.J.; et al. Efficacy and Safety of Denileukin Diftitox-Cxdl, an Improved Purity Formulation of Denileukin Diftitox, in Patients with Relapsed or Refractory Cutaneous T-Cell Lymphoma. *J. Clin. Oncol.* **2025**, *43*, 1198–1209. [CrossRef]
236. Foss, F.M.; Sjak-Shie, N.; Goy, A.; Jacobsen, E.; Advani, R.; Smith, M.R.; Komrokji, R.; Pendergrass, K.; Bolejack, V. A multicenter phase II trial to determine the safety and efficacy of combination therapy with denileukin diftitox and cyclophosphamide, doxorubicin, vincristine and prednisone in untreated peripheral T-cell lymphoma: The CONCEPT study. *Leuk. Lymphoma* **2013**, *54*, 1373–1379. [CrossRef]
237. Younes, A.; Bartlett, N.L.; Leonard, J.P.; Kennedy, D.A.; Lynch, C.M.; Sievers, E.L.; Forero-Torres, A. Brentuximab vedotin (SGN-35) for relapsed CD30-positive lymphomas. *N. Engl. J. Med.* **2010**, *363*, 1812–1821. [CrossRef]
238. Pro, B.; Advani, R.; Brice, P.; Bartlett, N.L.; Rosenblatt, J.D.; Illidge, T.; Matous, J.; Ramchandren, R.; Fanale, M.; Connors, J.M.; et al. Brentuximab Vedotin (SGN-35) in Patients with Relapsed or Refractory Systemic Anaplastic Large-Cell Lymphoma: Results of a Phase II Study. *J. Clin. Oncol.* **2012**, *30*, 2190–2196. [CrossRef]
239. Duvic, M.; Tetzlaff, M.T.; Gangar, P.; Clos, A.L.; Sui, D.; Talpur, R. Results of a Phase II Trial of Brentuximab Vedotin for CD30+ Cutaneous T-Cell Lymphoma and Lymphomatoid Papulosis. *J. Clin. Oncol.* **2015**, *33*, 3759–3765. [CrossRef]
240. Pro, B.; Advani, R.; Brice, P.; Bartlett, N.L.; Rosenblatt, J.D.; Illidge, T.; Matous, J.; Ramchandren, R.; Fanale, M.; Connors, J.M.; et al. Five-year results of brentuximab vedotin in patients with relapsed or refractory systemic anaplastic large cell lymphoma. *Blood* **2017**, *130*, 2709–2717. [CrossRef]
241. Horwitz, S.M.; Advani, R.H.; Bartlett, N.L.; Jacobsen, E.D.; Sharman, J.P.; O'Connor, O.A.; Siddiqi, T.; Kennedy, D.A.; Oki, Y. Objective responses in relapsed T-cell lymphomas with single-agent brentuximab vedotin. *Blood* **2014**, *123*, 3095–3100. [CrossRef]
242. Horwitz, S.; O'Connor, O.A.; Pro, B.; Trümper, L.; Iyer, S.; Advani, R.; Bartlett, N.L.; Christensen, J.H.; Morschhauser, F.; Domingo-Domenech, E.; et al. The ECHELON-2 Trial: 5-year results of a randomized, phase III study of brentuximab vedotin with chemotherapy for CD30-positive peripheral T-cell lymphoma. *Ann. Oncol.* **2022**, *33*, 288–298. [CrossRef]
243. Horwitz, S.M.; Scarisbrick, J.J.; Dummer, R.; Whittaker, S.; Duvic, M.; Kim, Y.H.; Quaglino, P.; Zinzani, P.L.; Bechter, O.; Eradat, H.; et al. Randomized phase 3 ALCANZA study of brentuximab vedotin vs physician's choice in cutaneous T-cell lymphoma: Final data. *Blood Adv.* **2021**, *5*, 5098–5106. [CrossRef]
244. Marie-Cardine, A.; Viaud, N.; Thonnart, N.; Joly, R.; Chanteux, S.; Gauthier, L.; Bonnafous, C.; Rossi, B.; Bléry, M.; Paturel, C.; et al. IPH4102, a Humanized KIR3DL2 Antibody with Potent Activity against Cutaneous T-cell Lymphoma. *Cancer Res.* **2014**, *74*, 6060–6070. [CrossRef]
245. Ortonne, N.; Gouvello, S.L.; Tabak, R.; Marie-Cardine, A.; Setiao, J.; Berrehar, F.; Nghe-Tang, A.; Martin, N.; Bagot, M.; Bensussan, A. CD158k/KIR3DL2 and NKp46 are frequently expressed in transformed mycosis fungoides. *Exp. Dermatol.* **2012**, *21*, 461–463. [CrossRef] [PubMed]
246. Thonnart, N.; Caudron, A.; Legaz, I.; Bagot, M.; Bensussan, A.; Marie-Cardine, A. KIR3DL2 is a coinhibitory receptor on Sézary syndrome malignant T cells that promotes resistance to activation-induced cell death. *Blood* **2014**, *124*, 3330–3332. [CrossRef] [PubMed]
247. Battistella, M.; Janin, A.; Jean-Louis, F.; Collomb, C.; Leboeuf, C.; Sicard, H.; Bonnafous, C.; Dujardin, A.; Ram-Wolff, C.; Kadin, M.E.; et al. KIR3DL2 (CD158k) is a potential therapeutic target in primary cutaneous anaplastic large-cell lymphoma. *Br. J. Dermatol.* **2016**, *175*, 325–333. [CrossRef] [PubMed]
248. Battistella, M.; Leboeuf, C.; Ram-Wolff, C.; Hurabielle, C.; Bonnafous, C.; Sicard, H.; Bensussan, A.; Bagot, M.; Janin, A. KIR3DL2 expression in cutaneous T-cell lymphomas: Expanding the spectrum for KIR3DL2 targeting. *Blood* **2017**, *130*, 2900–2902. [CrossRef]
249. Ghazi, B.; Thonnart, N.; Bagot, M.; Bensussan, A.; Marie-Cardine, A. KIR3DL2/CpG ODN Interaction Mediates Sézary Syndrome Malignant T Cell Apoptosis. *J. Investig. Dermatol.* **2015**, *135*, 229–237. [CrossRef]
250. Bagot, M.; Porcu, P.; Ram-Wolff, C.; Khodadoust, M.; Basem, W.; Battistella, M.; Marie-Cardine, A.; Vermeer, M.; Mathieu, S.; Whittaker, S.; et al. Phase I Study of IPH4102, Anti-KIR3DL2 Mab, in Relapsed/Refractory Cutaneous T-Cell Lymphomas (CTCL): Dose-escalation Safety, Biomarker and Clinical Activity Results. *Hematol. Oncol.* **2017**, *35*, 48–49. [CrossRef]
251. Bagot, M.; Kim, Y.; Zinzani, P.L.; Dalle, S.; Beylot-Barry, M.; Ortiz-Romero, P.L.; Cambalia, A.; Dereure, O.; Mortier, L.; Jacobsen, E.; et al. Tre-O2-07 Lacutamab in patients (pts) with advanced mycosis fungoides (MF) according to KIR3DL2 expression: Early results from the TELLOMAK phase 2 trial. *Eur. J. Cancer.* **2021**, *156*, S20–S21. [CrossRef]

252. Porcu, P.; Bagot, M.; Kim, Y.H.; Ram-Wolff, C.; Geskin, L.J.; Ortiz-Romero, P.L.; Kim, E.J.; Mehta-Shah, N.; Dereure, O.; Ingen-Housz-Oro, S.; et al. Lacutamab in patients with relapsed and refractory Sézary syndrome: Long term follow-up from the TELLOMAK phase 2 trial. *J. Clin. Oncol.* **2025**, *43*, 2522. [CrossRef]
253. Decroos, A.; Cheminant, M.; Bruneau, J.; Carras, S.; Parinet, V.; Pelletier, L.; Lacroix, L.; Martin, N.; Giustiniani, J.; Lhermitte, L.; et al. KIR3DL2 may represent a novel therapeutic target in aggressive systemic peripheral T-cell lymphoma. *Haematologica* **2023**, *108*, 2830–2836. [CrossRef] [PubMed]
254. Iyer, S.P.; Ayyappan, S.R.; Greenwell, I.B.; Kim, W.S.; Lee, S.T.; Kim, J.S.; Lee, W.-S.; Jeon, Y.; Johnson, W.; Dave, U.P.; et al. Strategies to Develop Anti-KIR Mab Lacutamab in Patients with Peripheral T-Cell Lymphoma: Preliminary Monotherapy Clinical Data and Pre-Clinical Combinability Data. *Blood* **2023**, *142*, 3072. [CrossRef]
255. Iyer, S.P.; Greenwell, I.B.; Shea, L.K.; Lee, J.-H.; Muller, M. 647TiP A multi-center phase Ib trial evaluating the safety and efficacy of lacutamab in patients with relapsed/refractory peripheral T-cell lymphoma that express KIR3DL2. *Ann. Oncol.* **2022**, *33*, S837. [CrossRef]
256. Bratulic, A. Innate Pulls Back on Lacutumab Monotherapy for PTCL After Efficacy Loss. 2024. Available online: https://firstwordpharma.com/story/5839110 (accessed on 20 September 2025).
257. Cheminant, M.; Carras, S.; Bruneau, J.; Lemonnier, F.; Bachy, E.; Herbaux, C.; Feugier, P.; Daguindau, N.; Gastinne, T.; Guillermin, Y.; et al. Kilt: A randomized non-comparative phase II LYSA study of lacutamab with gemox versus gemox in relapsed/refractory peripheral t-cell lymphoma. *Hematol. Oncol.* **2023**, *41*, 838–839. [CrossRef]
258. Cowan, R.A.; Scarisbrick, J.J.; Zinzani, P.L.; Nicolay, J.P.; Sokol, L.; Pinter-Brown, L.; Quaglino, P.; Iversen, L.; Dummer, R.; Musiek, A.; et al. Efficacy and safety of mogamulizumab by patient baseline blood tumour burden: A post hoc analysis of the MAVORIC trial. *J. Eur. Acad. Dermatol. Venereol.* **2021**, *35*, 2225–2238. [CrossRef]
259. Zinzani, P.L.; Karlin, L.; Radford, J.; Caballero, D.; Fields, P.; Chamuleau, M.E.D.; d'Amore, F.; Haioun, C.; Thieblemont, C.; González-Barca, E.; et al. European phase II study of mogamulizumab, an anti-CCR4 monoclonal antibody, in relapsed/refractory peripheral T-cell lymphoma. *Haematologica* **2016**, *101*, e407–e410. [CrossRef]
260. Ishitsuka, K.; Yasukawa, T.; Tsuji, Y. Safety and effectiveness of mogamulizumab in relapsed or refractory CC chemokine receptor 4-positive peripheral T-cell lymphoma and relapsed or refractory cutaneous T-cell lymphoma: A post-marketing surveillance in Japan. *Hematol. Oncol.* **2024**, *42*, e3292. [CrossRef]
261. Cordover, E.; Pradhan, K.; Townsend, L.; Goldfinger, M.; Mantzaris, I.; Shah, N.; Shastri, A.; Kornblum, N.; Cooper, D.; Gupta, R.; et al. Efficacy and manageable toxicity of mogamulizumab in a real-world North American cohort of adult T-cell leukemia/lymphoma (ATLL). *J. Clin. Oncol.* **2025**, *43*, e18603. [CrossRef]
262. Yonekura, K.; Kusumoto, S.; Choi, I.; Nakano, N.; Ito, A.; Suehiro, Y.; Imaizumi, Y.; Yoshimitsu, M.; Nosaka, K.; Ohtsuka, E.; et al. Mogamulizumab for adult T-cell leukemia-lymphoma: A multicenter prospective observational study. *Blood Adv.* **2020**, *4*, 5133–5145. [CrossRef]
263. Satake, A.; Azuma, Y.; Tsubokura, Y.; Yoshimura, H.; Hotta, M.; Nakanishi, T.; Fujita, S.; Nakaya, A.; Ito, T.; Ishii, K.; et al. Clinical Impact of Mogamulizumab Against Aggressive ATL: A Single-Center Retrospective Analysis. *Blood* **2017**, *130*, 4092. Available online: https://ashpublications.org/blood/article/130/Supplement%201/4092/73007/Clinical-Impact-of-Mogamulizumab-Against (accessed on 11 November 2025).
264. Phillips, A.A.; Fields, P.A.; Hermine, O.; Ramos, J.C.; Beltran, B.E.; Pereira, J.; Wandroo, F.; Feldman, T.; Taylor, G.P.; Sawas, A.; et al. Mogamulizumab versus investigator's choice of chemotherapy regimen in relapsed/refractory adult T-cell leukemia/lymphoma. *Haematologica* **2019**, *104*, 993–1003. [CrossRef] [PubMed]
265. Choi, I.; Yoshimitsu, M.; Kusumoto, S.; Shimokawa, M.; Utsunomiya, A.; Suehiro, Y.; Hidaka, T.; Nosaka, K.; Sasaki, H.; Rai, S.; et al. A phase 2 trial of CHOP with anti-CCR4 antibody mogamulizumab for elderly patients with CCR4-positive adult T-cell leukemia/lymphoma. *J. Clin. Oncol.* **2023**, *41*, 7504. [CrossRef]
266. Edner, N.M.; Carlesso, G.; Rush, J.S.; Walker, L.S.K. Targeting co-stimulatory molecules in autoimmune disease. *Nat. Rev. Drug Discov.* **2020**, *19*, 860–883. [CrossRef]
267. Chavez, J.C.; Foss, F.M.; William, B.M.; Brammer, J.E.; Smith, S.M.; Prica, A.; Zain, J.M.; Tuscano, J.M.; Shah, H.; Mehta-Shah, N.; et al. Targeting the Inducible T-cell Costimulator (ICOS) in Patients with Relapsed/Refractory T-follicular Helper Phenotype Peripheral T-cell and Angioimmunoblastic T-cell Lymphoma. *Clin. Cancer Res.* **2023**, *29*, 1869–1878. [CrossRef]
268. Wei, C.; Wang, W.; Zhang, Y.; Zhao, D.; Zhang, W.; Zhou, D. Mutation profiling, tumour burden assessment, outcome prediction and disease monitoring by circulating tumour DNA in peripheral T-cell lymphoma. *Br. J. Haematol.* **2023**, *202*, 86–95. [CrossRef]
269. Zhang, M.; Fu, X.; Meng, H.; Wang, M.; Wang, Y.; Zhang, L.; Li, L.; Li, X.; Wang, X.; Sun, Z.; et al. A Single-Arm, Open-Label, Pilot Trial of Autologous CD7-CAR-T Cells for CD7 Positive Relapsed and Refractory T-Lymphoblastic Leukemia/Lymphoma. *Blood* **2021**, *138*, 3829. [CrossRef]
270. Palomero, T.; Couronné, L.; Khiabanian, H.; Kim, M.-Y.; Ambesi-Impiombato, A.; Perez-Garcia, A.; Carpenter, Z.; Abate, F.; Allegretta, M.; Haydu, J.E.; et al. Recurrent mutations in epigenetic regulators, RHOA and FYN kinase in peripheral T cell lymphomas. *Nat. Genet.* **2014**, *46*, 166–170. [CrossRef]

271. Zhang, C.; Mou, B.; Xu, J.; Wang, J.; Liu, Q.; Yang, Y.; Tang, W.; Zhong, X.; Xu, C. Angioimmunoblastic T-cell lymphoma: Novel recurrent mutations and prognostic biomarkers by cell-free DNA profiling. *Br. J. Haematol.* **2023**, *203*, 807–819. [CrossRef]
272. Sibon, D.; Bisig, B.; Bonnet, C.; Poullot, E.; Bachy, E.; Cavalieri, D.; Fataccioli, V.; Bregnard, C.; Drieux, F.; Bruneau, J.; et al. ALK-negative anaplastic large cell lymphoma with DUSP22 rearrangement has distinctive disease characteristics with better progression-free survival: A LYSA study. *Haematologica* **2022**, *108*, 1590–1603. [CrossRef]
273. Sakamoto, Y.; Ishida, T.; Masaki, A.; Murase, T.; Yonekura, K.; Tashiro, Y.; Tokunaga, M.; Utsunomiya, A.; Ito, A.; Kusumoto, S.; et al. CCR4 mutations associated with superior outcome of adult T-cell leukemia/lymphoma under mogamulizumab treatment. *Blood* **2018**, *132*, 758–761. [CrossRef] [PubMed]
274. Fujii, K.; Sakamoto, Y.; Masaki, A.; Murase, T.; Tashiro, Y.; Yonekura, K.; Utsunomiya, A.; Ito, A.; Kusumoto, S.; Iida, S.; et al. Immunohistochemistry for CCR4 C-terminus predicts CCR4 mutations and mogamulizumab efficacy in adult T-cell leukemia/lymphoma. *J. Pathol. Clin. Res.* **2021**, *7*, 52–60. [CrossRef] [PubMed]
275. Du, J.; Qiu, C.; Li, W.-S.; Wang, B.; Han, X.-L.; Lin, S.-W.; Fu, X.-H.; Hou, J.; Huang, Z.-F. Spatial Transcriptomics Analysis Reveals that CCL17 and CCL22 are Robust Indicators of a Suppressive Immune Environment in Angioimmunoblastic T Cell Lymphoma (AITL). *Front. Biosci. Landmark* **2022**, *27*, 270. [CrossRef] [PubMed]
276. Gleeson, M.; Arias, C.G.; Cunningham, D.; Peckitt, C.; Thomas, K.; Du, Y.; Hujairi, N.; To, Y.M.; Chen, H.C.; Patel, S.; et al. The role of PET/CT in peripheral T-cell lymphoma: Results from the PET/CT substudy of the UK NCRI phase 2 CHEMO-T trial. *Br. J. Haematol.* **2025**, *207*, 407–416. [CrossRef]
277. Pellegrini, C.; Argnani, L.; Broccoli, A.; Stefoni, V.; Derenzini, E.; Gandolfi, L.; Casadei, B.; Maglie, R.; Pileri, S.; Zinzani, P.L. Prognostic Value of Interim Positron Emission Tomography in Patients with Peripheral T-Cell Lymphoma. *Oncologist* **2014**, *19*, 746–750. [CrossRef]
278. Song, G.-Y.; Jung, S.-H.; Ahn, S.-Y.; Kim, M.; Ahn, J.-S.; Lee, J.-J.; Kim, H.-J.; Moon, J.B.; Yoo, S.W.; Kwon, S.Y.; et al. Prognostic Significance Of Sequential 18f-fdg Pet/Ct During Frontline Treatment of Peripheral T Cell Lymphomas. *Korean J. Intern. Med.* **2024**, *39*, 327–337. [CrossRef]
279. Krutzek, F.; Kopka, K.; Stadlbauer, S. Development of Radiotracers for Imaging of the PD-1/PD-L1 Axis. *Pharmaceuticals* **2022**, *15*, 747. [CrossRef]
280. Kim, S.J.; Kim, Y.J.; Yoon, S.E.; Ryu, K.J.; Park, B.; Park, D.; Cho, D.; Kim, H.-Y.; Cho, J.; Ko, Y.H.; et al. Circulating Tumor DNA-Based Genotyping and Monitoring for Predicting Disease Relapses of Patients with Peripheral T-Cell Lymphomas. *Cancer Res. Treat.* **2022**, *55*, 291–303. [CrossRef]
281. Yannakou, C.K.; Wu, S.; Rajah, K.; Abeyakoon, C.; Nguyen-Ngo, C.; Yap, Y.Z.; Sheldon, J.; Blombery, P.; Prince, H.M. Circulating Tumour DNA Is a Biomarker of Response in Angioimmunoblastic T-Cell Lymphoma. *Int. J. Mol. Sci.* **2025**, *26*, 6719. [CrossRef]

Journal of
Personalized Medicine

MDPI

Review

Personalizing DNA Cancer Vaccines

Annie A. Wu [1], Kaiqi Peng [1], Melanie Vukovich [1], Michelle Zhu [1], Yuki Lin [1], Arindam Bagga [1], TC Wu [1,2,3,4] and Chien-Fu Hung [1,2,3,*]

1 Department of Pathology, Johns Hopkins School of Medicine, Baltimore, MD 21205, USA; awu20@jhmi.edu (A.A.W.); kpeng15@alumni.jh.edu (K.P.); mvukovi1@jh.edu (M.V.); mzhu3605@sas.upenn.edu (M.Z.); ylin155@jh.edu (Y.L.); abagga1@jh.edu (A.B.); wutc@jhmi.edu (T.W.)
2 Department of Oncology, Johns Hopkins School of Medicine, Baltimore, MD 21205, USA
3 Department of Obstetrics and Gynecology, Johns Hopkins School of Medicine, Baltimore, MD 21287, USA
4 Department of Molecular Microbiology and Immunology, Bloomberg School of Public Health, Johns Hopkins School of Medicine, Baltimore, MD 21205, USA
* Correspondence: chung2@jhmi.edu; Tel.: +1-410-502-8215; Fax: +1-442-287-4295

Abstract: Recent progress in tumor immunotherapy highlights the important role of the immune system in combating various cancers. Traditionally designed to protect against infectious diseases, vaccines are now being adapted to stimulate immune responses against tumor-specific neoantigens. Both preclinical studies and clinical trials have explored innovative approaches for identifying neoantigens and optimizing vaccine design, advancing the field of personalized oncology. Among these, DNA-based vaccines have become a particularly attractive approach for cancer immunotherapy. This evolution has been driven by improvements in molecular biology techniques, including more precise methods for detecting tumor-specific mutations, computational tools for predicting immunogenic antigens, and novel platforms for delivering nucleic acid vaccines. Personalized DNA vaccines are typically developed through a complex, multi-step process that involves sequencing a patient's tumor, computational analysis to identify potential targets, and custom vaccine production. In this review, we examine the use of both shared tumor antigens and individualized neoantigens in cancer vaccine development. We outline strategies for neoantigen identification that provide insights into tumor-specific alterations. Furthermore, we highlight recent advances in DNA vaccine technologies, address the current limitations facing cancer vaccines, propose strategies to overcome these challenges, and consider key clinical and technical factors for successful implementation.

Keywords: cancer vaccine; DNA; neoantigens; tumor antigens; clinical trial

1. Introduction

Cancer vaccines are gaining increasing attention in oncology due to their ability to activate the immune system to destroy tumor cells without harming normal tissues. Designing such vaccines requires careful selection of target antigens that can trigger precise immune responses [1]. Among these, neoantigens—novel peptides arising from tumor-specific somatic mutations or mutation-independent cancer-specific changes—are particularly promising, as they are not found in healthy cells and are uniquely presented on cancer cells. Neoantigen-based vaccines are often given in combination with immune checkpoint inhibitors (ICIs), a type of immunotherapy that reinvigorates cytotoxic T cells by blocking inhibitory receptors. ICIs have shown notable success in cancers that have a high mutational burden [2,3].

Neoantigens serve as prime candidates for personalized cancer immunotherapy as they are uniquely expressed in each patient's tumor. Inputting the terms "neoantigens" and "vaccines" into the search engine of clinicaltrials.gov reveals over 100 clinical trials, highlighting the growing interest in this field. While many trials have yet to demonstrate clear therapeutic benefits, some DNA vaccines have shown encouraging results, including extended recurrence-free survival (RFS) [4,5]. These positive outcomes are supported by technological advances in personalized oncology [6]. Notably, next-generation sequencing (NGS) has enabled comprehensive characterization of tumor genomes, providing insights into mutational profiles, transcriptomic changes, and epigenetic alterations. This information facilitates the individualized identification of immunologically relevant targets.

Selecting suitable delivery systems is also essential in vaccine design. Various platforms exist for delivering neoantigens, such as dendritic cell vaccines, tumor cell preparations, viral vectors, peptides, messenger RNA (mRNA), and DNA-based systems. Among these, DNA-based platforms have gained considerable attention. DNA vaccines offer practical benefits, including rapid production, stability, scalability, and strong safety profiles, though improving their delivery efficiency remains a challenge [7].

This review focuses on DNA-based therapeutic cancer vaccines and their role in enhancing antigen presentation and eliciting immunologic responses to tumors. We will discuss first, the classification and use of shared and personalized tumor antigens; second, approaches for identifying highly immunogenic neoantigens for personalized vaccines; third, the range of vaccine delivery platforms with an emphasis on DNA-based technologies; fourth, current challenges and potential strategies to address them; and fifth, clinical considerations for using personalized vaccines in an adjuvant setting in early stage cancers and in the maintenance setting in advanced disease.

2. Classes of Tumor Antigens

Tumor antigens can be divided into two categories—shared and personalized—based on how frequently they are expressed among patients [8]. Shared antigens are commonly found in multiple individuals and represent a potential avenue for developing universal, off-the-shelf cancer immunotherapies. In contrast, personalized antigens are unique to an individual's tumor, offering a more tailored approach that may enhance immune responsiveness. This section outlines the major classes of tumor antigens and reviews their progress in clinical vaccine development.

2.1. Shared Antigens

Shared antigens have been extensively studied for their relevance in oncology and include both tumor-associated antigens (TAAs) and tumor-specific antigens (TSAs). TAAs are typically present at elevated levels in cancer cells relative to normal tissue, while TSAs are uniquely expressed by malignant cells [9]. These features make them attractive, though not always ideal, targets for immunotherapy.

TAAs, such as cancer-testis antigens (CTAs), human telomerase reverse transcriptase (hTERT), and lineage-restricted markers like prostate-specific antigen (PSA) or prostate-specific membrane antigen (PSMA), have been widely investigated in vaccine development [10–24]. CTAs (e.g., NY-ESO-1, MAGE family proteins) are notable for their limited expression in immunologically privileged sites (ex. testis) and lack of expression in lymphoid tissues, making them potentially highly immunogenic [10]. hTERT is a catalytic subunit of the enzyme telomerase that is upregulated in various tumor types such as glioblastomas, hepatocellular carcinoma, and bladder cancer. Notable examples of vaccines targeting TAAs include the personalized dendritic cell (CD)-based vaccine Sipuleucel-T (Dendreon Corporation, LLC, Seal Beach, CA, USA), which received FDA approval for prostate cancer [25–28], and options targeting HER2, HER3, or IGFBP2 [29–33]. However, because TAAs are often expressed at low levels in normal tissues raising the risk of autoimmunity, and clinical benefit from single-antigen TAA vaccines has generally been modest [9,34,35].

TSAs may be of viral origin (e.g., HPV E6/E7, EBV, HBV), representing highly specific and immunogenic targets, or non-viral "public" neoantigens, such as recurrent mutations in Kirsten rat sarcoma virus (KRAS), Wilm's tumor 1 (WT1), or tumor protein p53 [36–47]. Vaccines against viral oncoproteins, specifically E6 and E7, are in active clinical development, with multiple candidates advancing for HPV-related cancers [40–46]. The broader applicability of shared antigens makes them attractive, but their limited specificity and immunogenicity remain major barriers.

2.2. Personalized Neoantigens

Personalized cancer vaccines can bolster immune responses against neoantigens that arise from each patient's distinctive tumor profile. These may be mutation-dependent (e.g., single nucleotide variants, insertions and deletions, structural variants, gene fusions) or mutation-independent, originating from cryptic translation events, splicing, or post-translational modifications [48–80]. Single nucleotide variants (SNVs) are the most extensively studied but neoantigens derived from SNVs often resemble normal peptides, limiting their immunogenic potential. In contrast, mutation derived frameshift or fusion neoantigens often display strong immunogenicity while cryptic antigens from the "dark proteome" represent a promising but still underexplored resource in cancer vaccine development [81].

Early approaches using autologous or allogeneic tumor lysates (e.g., M-Vax [AVAX Technologies, Philadelphia, PA, USA] and Melacine [Corixa Corporation, Seattle, WA, USA]) achieved limited success [82–85]. Advances in next-generation sequencing and bioinformatics now allow systematic identification of high-affinity patient-specific neoantigens, enabling vaccine formulations tailored to individual HLA backgrounds. These strategies aim to overcome tumor heterogeneity and immune escape while maximizing antitumor immunity.

3. Identification of Neoantigens

With the increasing need to discover antigens capable of provoking strong immune responses, the identification of novel, clinically relevant neoantigens has become a key objective in advancing personalized cancer vaccine development.

The general workflow for neoantigen discovery consists of three main stages: identifying potential targets, predicting which candidates may be immunogenic, and validating their biological relevance. Once validated, selected neoantigens are incorporated into vaccines using different technological platforms.

To pinpoint relevant neoantigens—whether they originate from genetic mutations or non-mutational mechanisms—the biological process of antigen creation, processing, and presentation should be considered. This cascade includes: (1) DNA transcription into messenger RNA, (2) RNA translation into protein, (3) protein breakdown into peptides by proteasomes, (4) peptide loading onto MHCs, (5) T cell receptor recognition of peptide-MHC complexes, and (6) T cell activation to initiate an immune response [54]. Each of these steps can be modeled or predicted using computational tools, which are critical for narrowing down the vast pool of potential neoantigens to a practical list for experimental validation [54,86].

This section will begin by outlining current strategies for identifying mutation-derived neoantigens, followed by approaches used to detect non-mutational neoantigen candidates.

We will then discuss how immunogenicity can be enhanced through predictive modeling and optimization techniques.

3.1. Neoantigen Identification and Sources

Identifying genetic alterations in tumors is the initial step in uncovering mutation-based neoantigens. This is commonly achieved using computational tools, including variant calling algorithms, which compare tumor DNA to a reference either through whole genome sequencing (WGS), whole exome sequencing (WES) [87], or targeted sequencing panels. Additionally, RNA sequencing (RNA-seq) can be employed to analyze tumor tissue and matched normal tissues, typically using peripheral blood mononuclear cells (PBMCs) as the normal reference [87–99]. Variant calling algorithms compare tumor and matched normal DNA, often peripheral blood mononuclear cells, to identify single nucleotide variants (SNVs), insertions and deletions (indels), and structural variants. While multiple variant callers achieve high sensitivity and precision in pure tumor samples [89,90], performance is often compromised by tumor heterogeneity, stromal admixture, and limited sample quality [88]. Formalin-fixed, paraffin-embedded (FFPE) samples, valuable for their ability to maintain tissue architecture and molecular stability, remain widely available for research and clinical use, but fixation introduces chemical alterations to nucleotides that complicate analysis [92–94]. Ensemble calling techniques and neural network-based algorithms have helped mitigate these issues [95,96].

RNA sequencing offers both expression profiles and mutation detection, and when aligned wither to the genome or transcriptome, can identify tumor-specific splice variants. Although sensitivity can exceed 85% under optimal conditions, false-positive rates in SNV calling are strongly influenced by read length [97,98]. More recently, single-cell RNA-seq has enabled variant detection at the cellular level, with encouraging sensitivity but ongoing challenges related to dropout effects and low transcript coverage [99]. Large-scale proteogenomic efforts, such as the Clinical Proteomic Tumor Analysis Consortium (CPTAC), have integrated WGS, WES, and proteomic data to connect genetic variants to actual protein products, helping prioritize functionally relevant neoantigens for cancer vaccine development [100].

To uncover tumor neoantigens that do not arise from genetic mutations, it is crucial to apply advanced methods that analyze high-throughput sequencing data. Ribosome profiling (RiboSeq) is a powerful technique that captures fragments of mRNA protected by ribosomes, thereby providing a genome-wide snapshot of active translation in both tumor and normal tissues [101,102]. This allows researchers to examine the actual protein products being synthesized, including those not linked to known mutations. Immunopeptidomics, based on mass spectrometry, directly detects peptides presented by MHC class I on tumor cells [72,103]. Unlike predictive methods that infer potential antigens from DNA or RNA data, immunopeptidomics offers direct evidence of peptide presentation, capturing the antigenic landscape as it exists on the surface of tumor cells. The combined used of RiboSeq and immunopeptidomics enables the identification of novel translation products—particularly those originating from non-canonical or cryptic sources—that may act as immunogenic targets for therapeutic vaccine development.

3.2. Antigen Processing, MHC Presentation, and Immunogenicity Prediction

Following antigen creation, peptides must be processed, transported, and loaded onto MHC molecules for recognition by T cells. Determining an individual's human leukocyte antigen (HLA) genotype is instrumental for neoantigen prediction, since each allele has unique binding preferences. Computational tools such as Opitype, ArcasHLA, ATHLATES, and seq2HLA can infer MHC class I and II alleles from sequencing data, although short-read sequencing often struggles to fully resolve polymorphisms; targeted sequencing remains the gold standard [104–110].

Over time, numerous computational models have been created for predicting the likelihood of specific peptides to bind to MHC molecules. Earlier algorithms relied on position-specific scoring matrices, whereas more recent models have adopted machine learning approaches such as neural networks trained on large experimental datasets. NetMHC-4.0 and NetMHCpan-4.0 remain widely used for class I binding [111–113], while NetMHCIIpan-2.0 and NetMHCIIpan-3.1 provide improved predictions for class II peptides, which are longer and more structurally diverse [114–118]. Incorporation of large-scale peptide elution datasets from mass spectrometry has further improved predictive accuracy [119]. Proprietary platforms such as EDGE and BigMHC integrate deep learning with ligand data to refine prediction across diverse HLA alleles [120,121].

Predicting T cell receptor (TCR) interactions adds another layer of complexity, as recognition depends on peptide sequence, MHC allele, and both TCR α and β chains. Databases including VDJdb, McPAS-TCR, and the Immune Epitope Database (IEDB) [122–126] provide valuable training data, and high-throughput methods such as single-cell TCR sequencing have expanded available datasets [127–129]. While benchmarking studies exist [130], most models struggle with generalizability due to the enormous diversity of potential TCR and pMHC pairings [131,132]. Emerging technologies such as single-cell TCR sequencing from platforms like 10× Genomics have the potential to generate expansive, high-throughput datasets, making them promising resources for enhancing future prediction models [133].

Clonality is an important factor in determining the immunogenic potential of neoantigens. Based on their distribution within the tumor, neoantigens can be classified as either clonal or subclonal. Clonal neoantigens are found uniformly across all tumor cells, whereas subclonal neoantigens are restricted to specific subsets of the tumor. Research indicates that clonal neoantigens are more strongly associated with positive responses to immunotherapies, making them attractive targets for vaccine development and other immune-based treatment [134]. However, targeting clonal driver mutations can be challenging, as tumors may evolve mechanisms for evading detection by the immune system, including down-regulating the antigen or altering antigen presentation pathways [135,136]. This form of immune escape may explain the limited success of some therapies directed at commonly shared tumor antigens, such as EGFRvIII, which failed to show clinical benefit in late-stage trials [137,138]. Personalized cancer vaccines offer a potential solution by incorporating a diverse repertoire of neoantigens, including both clonal and subclonal targets, to minimize the risk of immune evasion [135]. Numerous computational tools have been developed to estimate clonality using bulk tumor sequencing data [139]. These include FastClone (University of Michigan School of Medicine, Ann Arbor, MI, USA) [140], PyClone (Shah Lab, BC Cancer Agency, Vancouver, BC, Canada) [141], and sciClone (Shattuck Lab, Washington University, St. Louis) [142]. For greater resolution, single-cell sequencing enables the identification of specific tumor cell populations harboring distinct mutations, providing deeper insights into clonal architecture. Additionally, spatial transcriptomics is emerging as a powerful technique to complement single-cell analyses by mapping gene expression in the spatial context of the tumor. Spatial transcriptomics can shed light on the functional relationships between tumor cells and the microenvironment, including immune cell infiltrates. This means spatial transcriptomics provide insight into cell–cell proximity and contact, helping to distinguish between potential and functional interactions. Additionally, it enables the identification of spatial niches within the tumor microenvironment, revealing how cellular composition, density, and localization contribute to interactions between tumor cells and surrounding stromal and immune populations.

3.3. Prioritization and Validation of Candidate Neoantigens

With thousands of candidates generated per tumor, ranking and selection are necessary to focus validation efforts. With numerous prediction tools available, each focusing on identifying top-ranking neoantigens based on metrics such as MHC affinity or TCR recognition, a major challenge is how to unify these outputs into a coherent framework for selecting a manageable number of candidates for experimental testing. Open-source pipelines such as pVACtools (Griffith Lab, Washington University School of Medicine, MS, USA) and OpenVax (Icahn School of Medicine at Mount Sinai, New York, NY, USA) integrate outputs from multiple prediction models and apply scoring thresholds to nominate high-confidence epitopes [143–146]. Still, computational predictions require experimental validation, since many candidates fail to stimulate effective T cell responses.

Validation typically involves patient-derived T cells, obtained from PBMCs or TILs, cocultured with antigen-presenting cells (APCs) pulsed with candidate peptides. Functional assays, including enzyme-linked immunosorbent spot (ELISpot) and intracellular cytokine staining, assess interferon gamma (IFN-γ) production and T cell activation [147–150]. Functional killing assays have been developed to assess the cytotoxic ability of T cells [150–152]. Expanded approaches such as targeted TCR sequencing, single-cell profiling (e.g., TCR-sqe and scRNA-seq), and the mutation-associated neoantigen functional expansion of specific T cells (MANAFEST) assay allow sensitive detection of neoantigen-reactive T cells, even when rare [153–157].

Preclinical testing in standard and humanized mouse models remains important for assessing in vivo immunogenicity and antitumor efficacy [158,159]. However, resource intensity and limited predictive power constrain their widespread use. Challenges also persist in translating predictions into effective immunity. These include antigens that are poorly cross-presented, unstable, or rapidly degraded; others suppressed within the tumor microenvironment [62,63,160–164]. Naïve T cell priming often depends on higher levels of peptide-MHC complexes than tumors naturally provide, a limitation that can be mitigated through strong adjuvants and well-designed vaccine platforms [165]. While neoantigen peptides are highly promising targets for cancer immunotherapy, comprehensive strategies must be employed to avoid missing potentially effective epitopes.

4. DNA-Based Vaccine Platforms

DNA vaccines have been used in fewer clinical studies compared to RNA-based platforms. One of the key challenges is that DNA must reach the cell nucleus to be transcribed, requiring it to cross the plasma membrane and the nuclear envelope [166,167]. However, DNA vaccines offer several unique benefits, and improvements in delivery methods could enhance their future application. Figure 1 displays the diverse DNA vaccine delivery strategies and types of DNA-based constructs in current vaccine development.

The DNA vaccine safety profile has been evaluated in multiple clinical trials [168–170]. Research has shown that there is an extremely low likelihood of DNA integrating into the host genome, less than that of naturally occurring spontaneous mutations [167,171]. Additionally, DNA vaccines are inherently more stable than RNA, allowing them to be administered in unformulated or "naked" form, which often results in reduced adverse reactions [172–174]. RNA vaccines, however, often entail delivery via lipid nanoparticles (LNPs) containing polyethylene glycol (PEG), a component that has been linked to hypersensitivity reactions in some individuals. The ability to administer DNA without LNPs also contributes to lower manufacturing costs and facilitates easier large-scale production [167,175]. Another advantage of DNA vaccines is their prolonged intracellular persistence. Once inside the nucleus, DNA can remain intact and transcriptionally active for several months without integrating into the genome. This contrasts with RNA molecules, which are more transient and rapidly degraded in the cytoplasm [176].

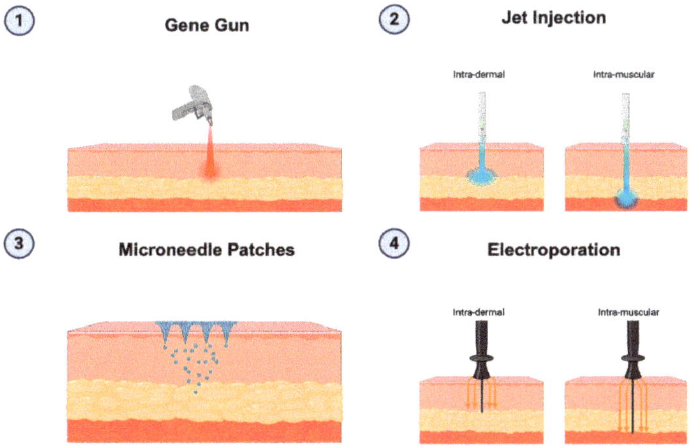

Figure 1. Delivery of DNA vaccines. Outside of conventional intramuscular injection, there are four common strategies used to deliver DNA vaccines. 1. Gene gun, which propels DNA-coated particles into the epidermis. 2. Jet injection, which delivers DNA into the intradermal or intramuscular compartments using high-pressured liquid streams. 3. Microneedle patches, which create microchannels in the skin to release DNA into the dermis. 4. Electroporation, which uses brief electrical pulses that enhances DNA uptake by increasing cell membrane permeability after intradermal or intramuscular injection [4,5]. Created in BioRender. Wu, T. (2025) https://BioRender.com/h276moj (Accessed on 26 July 2025).

Various strategies have been developed to improve the delivery efficiency of DNA vaccines, as summarized in Figure 1. Because DNA must traverse the cell membrane and nuclear envelope to initiate transcription, intramuscular (I.M.) injection of unformulated DNA often results in poor cellular uptake. To overcome this, electroporation is commonly used, which temporarily increases cell membrane permeability and significantly enhances DNA entry and immune activation. However, the reliance on specialized electroporation devices presents practical challenges for widespread vaccine distribution, as highlighted during the coronavirus disease-2019 (COVID-19) pandemic [177]. Alternative delivery methods are under investigation to broaden the applicability of DNA vaccines. These include physical techniques, such as the gene gun, which propels DNA-coated metal particles into tissue; jet injection, which delivers DNA using a high-velocity fluid stream without needles; and microneedle patches, which use tiny projections to penetrate the skin. These methods are delivered intradermally (I.D.), which has demonstrated improved immune responses compared to traditional I.M. routes. This enhancement is likely due to the fact that the skin has a high density of APCs, enabling more efficient DNA uptake and subsequent antigen presentation [178,179]. Several clinical trials have employed these delivery techniques. In a phase I study (NCT00199849), the gene gun was utilized for the delivery of a DNA vaccine encoding NY-ESO-1 antigen (pPJV7611). Among 15 individuals with no baseline immune response, 33% showed CD8+ T cell responses and 93% exhibited CD4+ T cell responses after vaccination. Despite these promising results, the durability of the immune response was limited, possibly due to suppression by regulatory T cells [13]. Another example is GNOS-PV02 (NCT04251117), a personalized DNA vaccine delivered intradermally followed by electroporation, which led to CD4+ and CD8+ neoantigen-specific T cell responses in 86.4% of patients enrolled in the ongoing phase I/IIa trial [5].

Various alternative strategies have been explored to enhance DNA vaccine immunogenicity by targeting APCs, especially DCs. One approach involves encoding the antigen in fusion with heat shock protein 70 (HSP70), which interacts with specific receptors on DCs, promoting uptake and facilitating cross-presentation [180]. The pNGVL4a-Sig/E7(detox)/HSP70 DNA vaccine, which encodes HPV-16 E7 fused to HSP70, was given to patients with HPV16-positive cervical intraepithelial neoplasia in a phase I/II clinical trial (NCT00121173) [181]. Higher vaccine doses were associated with greater T cell responses. Although not statistically significant, in the highest dose cohort (3 mg), compete histologic regression occurred in 33% (3/9) of participants, slightly higher than the approximately 25% expected in unvaccinated cohorts. Another strategy uses fms-like tyrosine kinase 3 ligand (FLT3L), which binds receptors on DCs stimulating their growth and development. A DNA vaccine, GX-188E, incorporating FLT3L and HPV16/18 E6 and E7 genes, was assessed in a phase II clinical trial (NCT02139267) for HPV-related cervical lesions [182,183]. The trial had promising results. At 20 weeks, histopathologic regression was observed in 52% (33/64) patients, and 73% of those with regression demonstrated HPV clearance. At 36 weeks regression increased to 67% (35/52) with HPV clearance in 77% of regressors. Additionally, fusing target antigens to calreticulin (CRT) can enhance DC-mediated antigen processing. CRT provides a signal to "eat-me", encouraging DCs to engulf and present the encoded antigens. The pNGVL4a-CRT/E7(detox) vaccine, designed for HPV-positive head and neck carcinomas, was tested in a phase I clinical trial (NCT01493154) [184]. However, the trial was terminated, and no results were posted.

To further increase DNA vaccine stability and delivery efficiency, preventing degradation by nucleases is crucial. Encapsulating DNA within synthetic carriers can improve protection and facilitate cellular uptake. An example is Amolimogene (ZYC101a), which uses poly-lactide-co-glycolide microparticles to deliver a DNA plasmid that encodes HPV-16 and HPV-18 E6/E7 epitopes. This formulation was evaluated for patients with HPV-positive cervical dysplasia in a phase II/III trial (NCT00264732) [185,186]. Results showed that histologic resolution was observed in 43% of vaccinated patients as opposed to 27% of the placebo patients; this difference in resolution was not significant. However, in women under 25 years of age there was a significant difference between treatment arms with vaccinated patients experiencing a resolution of 70% compared to 23% in unvaccinated patients. Furthermore, nuclear localization signals (NLS) can be attached to the DNA vector to enhance transport through the nuclear pore complex into the nucleus, improving transcription efficiency [187–189].

Recent advances in DNA vector design have introduced alternative platforms such as doggybone DNA (dbDNA), minicircle DNA (mcDNA), and nanoplasmid DNA, which offer distinct advantages over conventional plasmid DNA (pDNA). Traditional pDNA contains bacterial elements and antibiotic resistance genes, which can induce unwanted immune responses and raise safety concerns due to the potential contribution to antibiotic resistance [190]. In contrast, these newer constructs are engineered to remove such prokaryotic components, reducing the risk of inflammation and improving safety. Moreover, the reduced size of their backbones facilitates more efficient cellular uptake and gene expression [191,192]. Minicircle DNA was first developed in 1997 [193]. It is produced by inserting a plasmid into bacterial cells, where a site-specific recombinase removes the bacterial backbone, leaving only the expression cassette which contains the gene of interest and its regulatory sequences [194,195]. Although mcDNA demonstrates improved transfection performance, its production process is complex and costly, and residual bacterial sequences may still be present after processing. Nanoplasmid DNA, introduced in the early 2000s, addressed some of these challenges by incorporating an antibiotic-free selection mechanism. Plasmids can be selected without antibiotic resistance genes by relying on antisense RNA (RNA-OUT) to silence the expression of a toxic gene (sacB) [196,197]. Although a small portion of the bacterial sequence remains, nanoplasmids have demonstrated significantly enhanced gene delivery, with some studies reporting an increase in transfection efficient up to a tenfold compared to standard pDNA [192,198]. The most recent innovation, dbDNA, was developed in 2017. This approach completely removes the need for bacterial propagation by using a cell-free, enzyme-driven method. Enzymes such as Phi29 DNA polymerase and protelomerase are used to synthesize a covalently closed linear DNA molecule in vitro [199]. This process allows for rapid, large-scale production of simplified DNA constructs, positioning dbDNA as a promising gene therapy vector for vaccine development.

Personalized DNA Vaccine for Cancer Immunotherapy

Recent progress in personalized cancer vaccine development has emphasized identifying individual tumor mutations to design neoantigen-based therapies tailored to each patient. Interestingly, tumors with high TMB are considered more suitable for such approaches due to the increased likelihood of producing immunogenic neoantigens [200–202]. The developmental pipeline of personalized cancer vaccines, starting from the acquisition of a sample to the production of the vaccine is summarized (Figure 2). Numerous vaccine platforms are currently advancing through clinical trials, with companies including Moderna, Merck, BioNTech, and Genentech leading late-stage development efforts in phase II and III clinical studies.

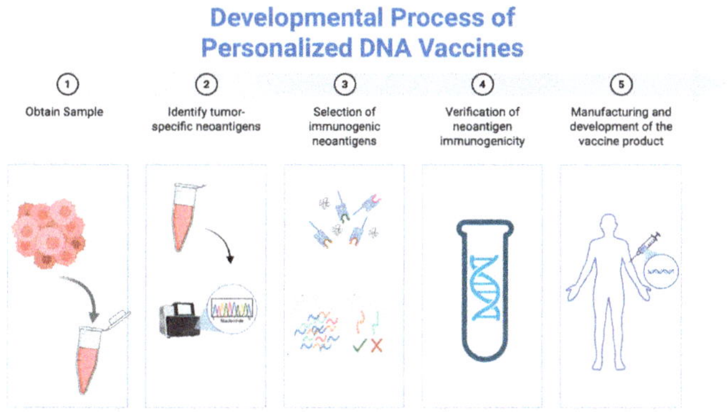

Figure 2. Pipeline for Personalized Cancer Vaccine Development. 1. Obtain Sample. Tumor tissue or blood is collected from the patient with PBMCs or matched normal tissues as germline controls—the source of genetic material. 2. Identify tumor-specific neoantigens. Subsequently, sequencing and bioinformatics analyses are performed to detect somatic mutations and generate a list of potential neoantigen candidates. Mutation-dependent neoantigens can be detected using variant callers while mutation-independent neoantigens are detected using RiboSeq or immunopeptidomics. 3. Selection of immunogenic neoantigens. Computational tools prioritize neoantigen candidates based on predicted MHC binding, TCR recognition, clonality, and dissimilarity to self. 4. Verification of neoantigen immunogenicity After potential neoantigen candidates are identified, possible peptides are experimentally validated for their ability to activate T cells using TCR activation assays or T cell killing assays. 5. Manufacturing and development of the vaccine product. The selected neoantigens are encoded into a DNA vaccine platform and administered back to the patient. Created in BioRender. Wu, T. (2025) https://BioRender.com/uefdnut (Accessed on 26 July 2025).

Key clinical trials involving DNA vaccines developed for personalized therapies is summarized (Table 1). These vaccines are usually injected via intradermal (I.D.) or intramuscular (I.M.) injection, often with special devices including electroporation or needle-free injection to enhance delivery. Each study varies in vaccine design, combination treatments (like checkpoint inhibitors or cytokines), and route of administration, with DNA vaccines tested in various cancer stages and tumor types. While a few have reported promising initial data, many remain ongoing or have yet to publish clinical results.

Table 1. DNA Vaccines targeting Personalized Neoantigens.

Organ System	Vaccine Name	Vaccine Target	Target Disease	Delivery Method	Combination	Phase	Status	Outcome	NCT Number
Lymphatic System	scFv-CCL20 plasmid DNA vaccine	MIP3α-fused lymphoma idiotype	Lympho-plasmacytic lymphoma	DNA plasmid via I.D. injection with a needle-free bioinjector		I	Active, not recruiting	No results posted	NCT01209871 [203,204]
Breast	Personalized polyepitope DNA vaccine	4–20 patient specific neoantigens	TNBC	DNA plasmid via I.M. injection and electroporation	-	I	Complete	36-month recurrence-free survival: 87.5%	NCT02348320 [4]
Pancreas	Neoantigen DNA vaccine	Personalized neoantigen DNA vaccine	Pancreatic Cancer—surgically resected with adjuvant chemotherapy without evidence of recurrent disease	DNA plasmid via I.M. injection and electroporation	Chemotherapy	I	Terminated due to loss of funding	Treatment-related adverse events grade $\leq$ 3: 7/7	NCT03122106 [203]
Skin, Lung, Kidney, Bladder, Head and Neck, Breast, Cervix, Anus, Stomach/ Esophagus, Colon	VB10.NEO	Up to 40 patient-specific neoantigens	Solid tumors	DNA plasmid via I.M. injection with a needle-free bioinjector	Atezolizumab—CPI (anti-PD-1 or anti-PD-L1), Bempe-galdesleukin	I II/III	Complete	Stable disease: 34.8% (8/23) Neoantigen-specific response in stable disease patients: 100% (8/8)	NCT03548467 NCT05018273 [204]
Prostate	Neoantigen DNA vaccine	Patient-specific neoantigens	Prostate cancer	DNA plasmid via I.M. injection and electroporation	Nivolumab (anti-PD-1), Ipilimumab (anti-CTLA-4), PROSTVAC (PSA vaccine)	I	Complete	Treatment-related adverse events: Grade 3—13.3% (2/15) Grade $\leq$ 2: 86.7% (13/15)	NCT03532217 [205]
Liver	GNOS-PV02	Up to 40 patient-specific neoantigens	Hepatocellular carcinoma	DNA plasmid via I.D. injection and electroporation	INO-9012 and pem-brolizumab	I/II	Active, not recruiting	Objective response: 30.6% (11/36) Complete response: 8.3% (3/36)	NCT04251117 [5]
Brain/ Meninges	GNOS-PV01	Up to 30 antigens (27 TSA and 3 patient-specific)	Unmethylated glioblastoma	DNA plasmid via I.M. injection and electroporation	INO-9012 (plasmid encoding IL-12)	I	Active, not recruiting	No results posted	NCT04015700 [206]
	Personalized neoantigen DNA vaccine	Patient-specific neoantigens	Glioblastoma	DNA plasmid via I.M. injection and electroporation	Retifanlimab	I	Recruiting	No results posted	NCT05743595 [207]
	Personalized neoantigen DNA vaccine	Patient-specific neoantigens	Brain tumors	DNA plasmid via I.M. injection and electroporation	-	I	Recruiting	No results posted	NCT03988283 [208]
Kidney	Neoantigen DNA vaccine	Personalized neoantigen	Metastatic/ advanced (inoperable) RCC	DNA plasmid via I.M. injection and electroporation	Durvalumab and tremelimumab	II	Withdrawn, FDA contin-gencies unresolved	No results posted	NCT03598816 [209]
Lungs	Neoantigen DNA vaccine	Patient-specific neoantigens	SCLC	DNA plasmid via I.M. injection and electroporation	Durvalumab, (and Carboplatin, Etoposide)	II	Active, not recruiting	No results posted	NCT04397003 [210]
Skin	EVX-02	13 neoantigens	Melanoma	I.M. injection	Nivolumab (anti-PD-1)	I/IIa	Terminated	No results posted	NCT04455503 [211]

One of the earliest trials using DNA vaccines for personalized medicine focused on cancers of the lymphatic system. A phase I clinical study (NCT01209871) published by Thomas et al. in BMC Cancer [212], tested a DNA vaccine designed for patients with untreated asymptomatic lymphoplasmacytic lymphoma (LPL) [212]. This vaccine consisted of a recombinant plasmid DNA encoding a chemokine called MIP3α, which was fused to autologous lymphoma LPL-derived Ig single chain variable fragment (scFv), an endocytic surface receptor on APCs to improve targeting to dendritic cells. It was delivered intradermally using a needle-free injector at three time points (weeks 0, 4, and 8). The trial showed that this approach was capable of stimulating an immune response, providing early evidence that personalized vaccines could work in blood cancers. A follow-up analysis published in Nature Communications confirmed durable immune activation, while also revealing a dichotomous response: the vaccine significantly reduced clonal B-cell subpopulations but had limited impact on plasma cell-like tumor clones, indicating a potential mechanism of immune resistance [213].

Subsequently, DNA vaccines have been tested for solid tumors in clinical trials. A clinical trial (NCT02348320) tested a personalized polyepitope DNA vaccine for triple-negative breast cancer (TNBC), particularly in patients with persistent disease following neoadjuvant chemotherapy [4]. Published by Zhang et al. in Genome Medicine, the study showed that most patients developed T cell responses to one or more of their vaccine-targeted tumor antigens [4]. In a phase I clinical trial, 14/18 vaccinated participants had detectable neoantigen-specific responses and 87.5% of vaccinated patients were recurrence free at 36 months as opposed to 49% of unvaccinated patients. This trial also highlighted the role of computer-based tools in selecting which neoantigens to include, as candidate neoantigens ranked highly by prediction models were more likely to trigger immune responses.

In pancreatic cancer, there has been a phase 1 clinical trial (NCT03122106) testing a personalized neoantigen DNA vaccine for surgically resected pancreatic cancer with adjuvant chemotherapy. There was at least one patient with widely metastatic PDAC who had complete remission following the personalized neoantigen DNA vaccine [214].

Researchers have also explored personalized DNA vaccines in prostate cancers. A trial in prostate cancer (NCT03532217) combined personalized DNA vaccines with a shared prostate cancer vaccine (PROSTVAC) and two checkpoint inhibitors (nivolumab and ipilimumab). According to an abstract by Shah et al., 79% of participants with hormone-sensitive prostate cancer that had metastasized were given the personalized DNA vaccine, and the treatment was well tolerated [205]. Preliminary results showing upregulation of activation, co-stimulatory, and co-inhibitory markers post-treatment suggested immune priming, even in a tumor with low TMB such as prostate cancer.

In liver cancer, the GNOS-PV02 trial (NCT04251117) tested a personalized DNA vaccine for hepatocellular carcinoma (HCC). This vaccine includes up to 40 tumor-specific neoantigens and was given with interleukin-12 (IL-12) to boost T cell activity and pembrolizumab, a PD-1 inhibitor. An early report published in Nature Medicine by Yarchoan et al. showed that these DNA vaccines could activate CD4+ and CD8+ effector T cells in HCC patients [5], and 86.4% of the patients evaluated had neoantigen-specific T cells responses. Clinically, 30.6% (11/36) patients had an objective response, including 8.3% (3/36) of patients with a complete response. A subset of patients had tumor infiltration of T cells. These findings suggest that DNA vaccines could help convert advanced liver tumors, often resistant to immunotherapy due to low T cell infiltration, into more responsive ones.

For skin cancers, EVX-02 is a personalized DNA plasmid that targets neoantigens given with anti-PD1 to patients with complete resection of late stage melanoma in a phase I/II clinical trial (NCT04455503). Results demonstrated increases in T cell responses that were long-lasting, with CD4+ and CD8+ T cells reactive to vaccine antigens [211].

More recent clinical trials are exploring how personalized DNA vaccines might benefit brain cancers. One ongoing study (NCT04015700), nearing completion, is testing a neoantigen DNA vaccine (GNOS-PV01) for newly diagnosed, unmethylated glioblastoma. The personalized DNA vaccine is delivered with IL-12 using an electroporation device. Preliminary results of a subset of patients showed detectable responses, with 6 out of 7 patients with a sustained T cell response against cancer neoantigens after treatment [215].

Efforts are also underway to apply DNA vaccine technology to treat lung cancers. A phase II clinical trial (NCT04397003) tested a neoantigen DNA vaccine with the programmed death-ligand 1 (PD-L1) inhibitor durvalumab for extensive-stage small cell lung cancer (ES-SCLC). Although still in early stages, with just a few patients enrolled so far, the clinical trial is expected to run through 2029. The long timeline reflects the complexity of making personalized vaccines and the need for extended follow-up in aggressive cancers. Taken together, these trials show how DNA vaccines are gradually becoming a key part of personalized cancer treatment.

Combining DNA vaccine therapies with other treatment methods has proven to reduce immunosuppressive processes, thereby augmenting the functional capacity of immune cells [216]. Some of these treatment methods include chemotherapy, radiation therapies, and the use of immune checkpoint inhibitors. Combination of DNA vaccines with chemotherapy has been shown to increase tumor antigen release, promotes T-cell activity, reduces immunosuppression, and has shown improved survival in preclinical models [217]. Additionally, in preclinical trials, vaccine and radiation therapies has enhanced tumor antigen release and cancer cell damage, and decreased tumor size [218]. Immune checkpoint inhibitors, such as CTLA-4 and PD-1 blockade augments antigen-specific T-cell activation, suppresses inhibitory cytokines including IL-10 and TGF-ß, and has demonstrated delayed tumor progression in preclinical and clinical studies [219,220].

DNA vaccines generally exhibit a favorable safety profile compared with alternative therapies as a result of their specificity and limited normal cell toxicity. Reported adverse events in early-phase clinical trials have primarily been mild (grade 1–2), such as injection site reactions or flu-like symptoms [203,205]. Grade 3 events have been uncommon and occurred in only a small number of participants. The safety profile of DNA vaccines in combination regimes varies depending on the partner therapy [216]. When combined with chemotherapy or radiation, side effects are typically attributable to the partnered treatment rather than the vaccine itself. The addition of immune checkpoint inhibitors may result in immune-related events, most of which are mild (grade 1–2) though severe events (grade 3–4) occasionally occur. Combining vaccine therapy with cytokine use may augment systemic reactogenicity, leading to more pronounced flu-like symptoms.

As research continues, these DNA vaccine therapies may offer new hope for patients by tailoring treatment to their unique tumor makeup and training their immune systems to respond more effectively.

5. Limitations in DNA Vaccine Effectiveness and Solutions

Several barriers may limit the therapeutic impact of DNA vaccines despite their successful clinical application. These challenges can be grouped into factors that impair the function of vaccine-induced T cells and barriers arising from the tumor microenvironment.

A hurdle for DNA vaccines includes immune tolerance, especially since tumor antigens utilized in DNA vaccines may be self-antigens typically bypassed by the immune system. A way to enhance the immunogenicity of DNA vaccines is to overcome immune tolerance. One method is to use xenogeneic version of antigens, which are homologous genes from another species to avoid tolerance and induce stronger immune responses. In a study where mice encoded human p53 gene, vaccination with a xenogeneic hp53 DNA construct delivered intramuscularly with electroporation generated a strong antibody response and promoted proliferation and activation of murine p53-specific CD8+ T cells. These CD8+ T cells were identified as the primary mediators of both prophylactic and therapeutic antitumor effects in murine colon cancer models. This demonstrates how xenogeneic antigens can overcome immune tolerance and enhance vaccine efficacy [221]. Another method involves encoding tumor antigens as fusion protein, such as linking them to immunoglobulin domains or forming single-chain trimers (SCTs) by utilizing MHC class I components. This method bypasses antigen-processing pathways by directly presenting peptides to CD8+ cytotoxic T cells while the IgG domain increases dendritic cell uptake and priming. In preclinical melanoma models, an SCT fused to tyrosinase related protein 2 (Trp2) enhanced CD8+ t cell responses and antitumor effects, demonstrating their potential to overcome tolerance to endogenous antigens [222]. These strategies allow for stable and direct antigen presentation to cytotoxic T cells.

Another hurdle is MHC class I downregulation by tumor cells, which allows tumors to evade CTL recognition. This reduction in MHC class I expression can result from a variety of mechanisms, including mutations, transcriptional silencing, epigenetic changes, disruptions in translation, and post-transcriptional or post-translational interference [223]. A key strategy to counteract this involves boosting MHC class I expression levels through treatments with pro-inflammatory cytokines, including IL-1, type I/II interferons, and tumor necrosis factor (TNF), or through the use of stimulator of interferon genes [224] or toll-like receptor (TLR) agonists [225]. Propper et al. showed that administering low doses of IFN-γ could elevate MHC class I and II levels in metastatic melanoma tissue [226]. Another approach involves the use of chemotherapy or radiotherapy to enhance antigen presentation, as these treatments can increase MHC class I expression. However, they may simultaneously promote an immunosuppressive environment, which could reduce overall treatment efficacy [227–229]. As a result, determining an optimal dosing strategy for such treatments remains an important area for further investigation. More recently, efforts have focused on small-molecule inhibitors aimed at restoring proper antigen presentation by targeting specific components of the regulatory pathways that suppress MHC expression [230]. However, identifying appropriate molecular targets would likely require genome-wide screening to uncover novel regulators involved in antigen processing and presentation [230].

An additional challenge that must be considered is the impact extrachromosomal DNA (ecDNA) has on the treatment process. ecDNA consists of large, circular DNA that can integrate into or separate from a chromosome, contributing to genomic remodeling through enhancer hijacking or disruption of tumor suppressor genes. They are often enriched in oncogenes and regulatory elements, and their circular structure leads to an open chromatin state that promotes high oncogene expression and novel gene-enhancer interactions [231–233]. Because ecDNA lacks centromeres, they segregate randomly during cell division, fueling tumor heterogeneity and accelerating clonal evolution. Their abundance can also change drastically under treatment pressure, with some ecDNAs expanding or disappearing to enable drug resistance [232,233]. Clinically, ecDNAs are now recognized as common across tumor types, and using data from the 100,000 Genomes Project, it is estimated that they can be found in approximately 17.1% of tumors, where their presence is associated with poor prognosis and unfavorable outcomes [231]. For DNA vaccines, this presents a significant problem. ecDNAs may alter antigen expression patterns and generate heterogeneity within the tumor, making it difficult to achieve effective immune control [234]. Conversely, their tumor-specific presence and role in shaping novel regulatory interactions may provide opportunities for vaccine targeting if ecDNA-derived neoantigens can be identified [235,236].

Another key challenge to the success of DNA vaccines and other immunotherapies is the immunosuppressive nature of the tumor microenvironment, which undergoes constant remodeling to support tumor progression [237]. This remodeling affects cancer cells as well as the surrounding blood vessels and stromal components such as cancer-associated fibroblasts, ultimately creating conditions that suppress immune cell activity [238,239]. One aspect of this suppression is the formation of physical barriers that limit immune cell infiltration. An example is the dense stromal architecture of PDAC that restricts T cell infiltration into and movement within the tumor tissue [240,241]. Several signaling pathways, including Hippo, TGFβ, and Wnt/β-catenin, have been implicated in the establishment of such barriers, and targeting these pathways has been explored to improve immune access [242–244]. Furthermore, impaired vasculature, commonly observed in tumors including PDAC, can reduce the efficiency of T cell trafficking into the tumor [245]. This insufficient vascularization is often accompanied by low levels of chemokines such as CCL4, CCL5, and CCL20, which are essential for recruiting dendritic cells to the tumor site for effective antigen presentation [246,247]. The use of chemotherapy or radiotherapy to enhance vessel permeability are ways to overcome these vascular limitations. In a notable study, Olive et al. demonstrated that inhibiting the hedgehog pathway could decrease stromal fibroblasts and improve blood vessel formation [248].

An additional limitation that must be taken into consideration is the variability of immune responses between individuals, which can be influenced by MHC class I diversity. Humans express a minimum of three and up to six HLA class I alleles, each with a distinct peptide-binding preferences. If the epitopes encoded by the vaccine, such as HPV E7-derived peptides, cannot be efficiently presented by a patient's HLA molecules, then CD8+ T cell activation and subsequent antitumor immunity may be limited [234,249]. To address this, DNA vaccine constructs can be designed to include multiple epitopes from the same antigen or from several antigens, thereby increasing the likelihood of coverage across diverse HLA types [250]. Another approach is to focus on epitopes presented by common HLA alleles to maximize population-level effectiveness [251]. Importantly, personalized DNA vaccines tailor epitope selection to an individual's HLA profile which offers a promising strategy to overcome this hurdle and optimize immune responses [252,253].

Beyond structural barriers, the tumor microenvironment contains immunosuppressive cells that interfere with T cell function. These immunosuppressive cells include fibroblasts associated with tumors, M2-polarized macrophages, regulatory T cells, and myeloid-derived suppressor cells [254,255]. One mechanism of T cell inhibition involves PD-1 on T cells interacting with its ligand PD-L1 present on tumor cells or macrophages in the tumor environment [256,257]. Additionally, immunosuppressive cytokines like IL-10 and TGFβ, and metabolic enzymes including indoleamine 2,3-dioxygenase (IDO), can hinder the activity and expansion of vaccine-induced T cells [258–260].

Another potential solution consists of adjusting the immune microenvironment to improve DNA vaccine potency. DNA plasmids co-administered with immunostimulatory molecules, such as IL-2, GM-CSF, or ligands for toll-like receptors (TLRs), can enhance dendritic cell activations and T cell priming [222]. CpG motifs in plasmid DNA can activate TLR9, while cytosolic DNA sensors can engage STING/TBK1 pathways leading to the production of type 1 interferons, which are crucial for effective immune responses [261]. Furthermore, stronger effector T cell responses can be accomplished by depleting regulatory T cells, allowing for unrestrained and enhanced immune activation [222].

On a broader scale, conditions such as acidic extracellular pH, hypoxia, and increased interstitial pressure within the tumor can suppress immune function [262]. Due to the evolving nature of the tumor microenvironment, addressing these immunosuppressive elements remains a significant obstacle. Current approaches include drugs that selectively target hypoxic regions and inhibitors that block immunosuppressive metabolites [263–265].

Elevated tumor burden and hypoxic conditions can contribute to T cell exhaustion, ultimately impairing the effectiveness of cancer vaccines [237]. Exhausted T cells show reduced functional capacity, diminished proliferation, elevated levels of inhibitory receptors, and an increased likelihood of cell death [266]. This dysfunctional state is primarily caused by prolonged exposure to tumor antigens, which leads to chronic TCR activation and subsequent metabolic stress, further exacerbated by the oxygen-deprived tumor microenvironment. To prevent or reverse exhaustion in vaccine-induced T cells, several strategies are being explored. These strategies include neoantigen vaccines combined with immune checkpoint inhibitors to restore T cell activity, targeting DNA methyltransferases such as DNMT1, DNMT3A, and DNMT3B that promote exhaustion-related epigenetic modifications, or attenuating hyperactive TCR signaling by inhibiting kinases that function downstream and are involved in chronic activation [267,268]. Additionally, modulating T cell metabolism, either by promoting the oxidation of fatty acids to favor memory T cell formation or by suppressing excessive glycolysis, may also enhance vaccine-induced responses. Another potential strategy involves combining vaccines with adoptive T cell transfer to increase therapeutic impact.

In cases of advanced or metastatic disease, neoantigen vaccines may be less effective on their own due to the larger tumor burden, heterogeneity of tumors, and evolving nature of metastatic lesions. As tumors spread, immune escape mechanisms such as epitope loss and clonal selection may arise, diminishing the ability of the immune system to identify vaccine-targeted antigens [269]. Moreover, distinct tumor microenvironments in metastatic sites can present further immunological barriers. In such scenarios, integrating neoantigen vaccines with other therapeutic approaches—including surgical resection, chemotherapy, radiotherapy, or additional immunotherapies—may be required to achieve more meaningful clinical outcomes [267].

6. Considerations in Clinical Trials

Personalized vaccines for cancer have been explored in two primary clinical contexts: (1) as adjunct therapy for early-stage, operable tumors and (2) as maintenance therapy for advanced or metastatic disease. In the adjuvant setting, vaccines are typically administered following surgical tumor removal. They are often combined with chemotherapy or immune checkpoint blockade to target any remaining cancer cells and prevent micrometastases from spreading. The main outcome measured in these clinical trials is usually recurrence-free survival (RFS). Early-stage trials commonly have larger patient populations but require longer follow-up periods, leading to higher overall costs and delaying outcomes. In contrast, when used for metastatic cancers, the focus is on stabilizing disease progression, with endpoints commonly including progression-free survival (PFS). Recruitment can typically be performed more quickly and yield results in a shorter time frame but may show limited benefit in late-stage patients whose immune systems are already weakened, constraining the therapeutic impact of immune-based interventions.

The encouraging outcomes observed in trials involving resectable cancers may be attributed to the ability of T cells to destroy residual cancer cells before the establishment of a highly immunosuppressive tumor microenvironment. In contrast, patients with late-stage malignancies often exhibit weakened immune responses, which can limit the effectiveness of therapeutic vaccination. As such, the interval between tumor biopsy and the actual administration of a personalized vaccine—commonly referred to as needle-to-needle time—is a critical factor in treating advanced cancers. One potential approach to bridge this gap is to begin treatment with a ready-made vaccine targeting shared tumor-associated or tumor-specific antigens (TAA/TSA), particularly for patients who express common HLA types. This allows for an immediate immune response while the patient-specific vaccine is still being manufactured, enabling a timely transition to personalized immunotherapy. Looking ahead, the administration of cancer vaccines in individuals with early-stage disease or pre-cancerous conditions could pave the way for a preventative strategy in high-risk groups. Such a prophylactic approach would involve the use of frequently observed neoantigens, identified through large-scale data mining across cohorts or public repositories including The Genotype-Tissue Expression (GTEx) project and The Cancer Genome Atlas (TCGA).

7. Conclusions

Multiple factors influence the efficacy of personalized DNA vaccines, such as the characteristics of selected neoantigens, the type of vaccine delivery system, the hurdles in vaccination, and whether the patient has an immunocompetent or immunocompromised immune system. The ideal neoantigens should be highly specific to tumor cells, largely clonal across cancer cell populations, and capable of triggering strong immune responses. While accurately predicting TCR binding and immunogenicity remains difficult, ongoing improvements in data quality and computational modeling continue to enhance prediction accuracy. Innovations in vaccine technologies have also contributed to progress in the field. However, it is important to recognize that different vaccine modalities may elicit distinct immune profiles, potentially favoring CD4+ or CD8+ T cell responses to varying degrees [270]. Additional challenges to address in future studies include overcoming the immune-suppressive tumor microenvironment, reversing T cell dysfunction, and managing the complexities posed by tumor burden and metastasis. Critically, a fully functional immune system is essential for translating vaccine-induced immune responses into therapeutic outcomes. Beyond activating T cells, vaccines must also promote the development of memory cells to maintain long-term tumor surveillance. To this end, many clinical trials are exploring DNA cancer vaccines in combination with checkpoint blockade therapies, conventional chemotherapy, or as adjuvant treatments following tumor resection in early-stage disease [271]. The latest advancements in vaccine platforms and bioinformatic tools have produced encouraging clinical results. As these technologies continue to evolve, DNA cancer vaccines are expected to become a key component of future immunotherapy strategies.

Author Contributions: Conceptualization: A.A.W., T.W. and C.-F.H.; writing of manuscript: A.A.W., K.P., M.V., M.Z., Y.L., A.B., T.W. and C.-F.H.; reviewing of manuscript: All authors; study supervision: A.A.W., T.W. and C.-F.H. All authors have read and agreed to the published version of the manuscript.

Funding: This study was supported by the National Institutes of Health, National Cancer Institute Specialized Program of Research Excellence (SPORE) in Cervical Cancer grant (NIH/NCI P50CA098252 and R01CA295696).

Institutional Review Board Statement: Not applicable.

Informed Consent Statement: Not applicable.

Data Availability Statement: All data relevant to this review are included in the article. Data and materials are available upon reasonable request.

Acknowledgments: We thank everyone involved for their writing contributions and critical review of this manuscript. All figures are created with BioRender.com.

Conflicts of Interest: T.C.W. reports other from Papivax LLC and Papivax Biotech Inc. outside the submitted work. He is one of the cofounders of, and have an equity ownership interest in, Papivax LLC. In addition, T.C.W. owns Papivax Biotech Inc. stock and is a member of Papivax Biotech Inc.'s

Scientific Advisory Board. No disclosures were reported by the other authors. The companies have no roles in the design, execution, interpretation, or writing of the study.

Abbreviations

APC	Antigen-presenting cells
COVID-19	Coronavirus disease-2019
CPTAC	Clinical Proteomic Tumor Analysis Consortium
CTA	Cancer-testis antigen
CTL	Cytotoxic lymphocytes
DC	Dendritic cells
DNA	Deoxyribonucleic acid
EBV	Epstein–Barr virus
EGFR	Epidermal growth factor receptor
ELISpot	Enzyme-linked immunosorbent spot assay
FDA	Food and Drug Administration
FFPE	Formalin-fixed and paraffin-embedded
GM-CSF	Granulocyte macrophage-colony stimulating factor
GTEx	Genotype-Tissue Expression project
HBV	Hepatitis B virus
HCC	Hepatocellular carcinoma
HER	Human epidermal growth factor receptor
HLA	Human leukocyte antigen
HPV	Human papillomavirus
hTERT	Human telomerase reverse transcriptase
ICI	Immune checkpoint inhibitors
IDO	Indoleamine 2,3-dioxygenase
IFN-γ	Interferon gamma
IGFBP2	Insulin-like growth factor binding protein 2
IL	Interleukin
KRAS	Kirsten rat sarcoma virus
LNP	Lipid nanoparticles
MAGE	Melanoma antigen gene
MHC class I	Major histocompatibility complex class I
MHC class II	Major histocompatibility complex class II
mRNA	Messenger ribonucleic acid
NGS	Next-generation sequencing
NY-ESO-1	New York esophageal squamous cell carcinoma 1
PBMC	Peripheral blood mononuclear cells
PD-L1	Programmed death-ligand 1
PDAC	Pancreatic ductal adenocarcinoma
pMHC	peptide-MHC complex
PSA	Prostate-specific antigen
PSMA	Prostate-specific membrane antigen
RFS	Recurrence-free survival
RiboSeq	Ribosome profiling
RNA-seq	RNA sequencing
SNV	Single nucleotide variations
STING	Stimulator of interferon genes
TAA	Tumor-associated antigen
TCGA	The Cancer Genome Atlas
TCR	T cell receptor
TIL	Tumor infiltrating lymphocytes
TLR	Toll-like receptor

TMB	Tumor mutational burden
TNF	Tumor necrosis factor
TP53	Tumor protein p53
TSA	Tumor-specific antigen
WES	Whole exome sequencing
WGS	Whole genome sequencing
WT1	Wilms tumor 1

References

1. Ottensmeier, C.H.H.; Delord, J.P.; Lalanne, A.; Lantz, O.; Jamet, C.; Tavernaro, A.; Brandely-Talbot, M.; Grellier, B.; Bastien, B.; Makhloufi, H.; et al. Safety and immunogenicity of TG4050: A personalized cancer vaccine in head and neck carcinoma. *J. Clin. Oncol.* **2023**, *41*, 6082. [CrossRef]
2. Aggarwal, C.; Ben-Shachar, R.; Gao, Y.; Hyun, S.W.; Rivers, Z.; Epstein, C.; Kaneva, K.; Sangli, C.; Nimeiri, H.; Patel, J. Assessment of Tumor Mutational Burden and Outcomes in Patients with Diverse Advanced Cancers Treated with Immunotherapy. *JAMA Netw. Open* **2023**, *6*, e2311181. [CrossRef]
3. Quintanilha, J.C.F.; Storandt, M.H.; Graf, R.P.; Li, G.; Keller, R.; Lin, D.I.; Ross, J.S.; Huang, R.S.P.; Schrock, A.B.; Oxnard, G.R.; et al. Tumor Mutational Burden in Real-World Patients with Pancreatic Cancer: Genomic Alterations and Predictive Value for Immune Checkpoint Inhibitor Effectiveness. *JCO Precis Oncol.* **2023**, *7*, e2300092. [CrossRef]
4. Zhang, X.; Goedegebuure, S.P.; Chen, M.Y.; Mishra, R.; Zhang, F.; Yu, Y.Y.; Singhal, K.; Li, L.; Gao, F.; Myers, N.B.; et al. Neoantigen DNA vaccines are safe, feasible, and induce neoantigen-specific immune responses in triple-negative breast cancer patients. *Genome Med.* **2024**, *16*, 131. [CrossRef]
5. Yarchoan, M.; Gane, E.J.; Marron, T.U.; Perales-Linares, R.; Yan, J.; Cooch, N.; Shu, D.H.; Fertig, E.J.; Kagohara, L.T.; Bartha, G.; et al. Personalized neoantigen vaccine and pembrolizumab in advanced hepatocellular carcinoma: A phase 1/2 trial. *Nat. Med.* **2024**, *30*, 1044–1053. [CrossRef] [PubMed]
6. Kiyotani, K.; Toyoshima, Y.; Nakamura, Y. Personalized immunotherapy in cancer precision medicine. *Cancer Biol. Med.* **2021**, *18*, 955–965. [CrossRef] [PubMed]
7. Jou, J.; Harrington, K.J.; Zocca, M.B.; Ehrnrooth, E.; Cohen, E.E.W. The Changing Landscape of Therapeutic Cancer Vaccines-Novel Platforms and Neoantigen Identification. *Clin. Cancer Res.* **2021**, *27*, 689–703. [CrossRef] [PubMed]
8. Fan, T.; Zhang, M.; Yang, J.; Zhu, Z.; Cao, W.; Dong, C. Therapeutic cancer vaccines: Advancements, challenges, and prospects. *Signal Transduct. Target. Ther.* **2023**, *8*, 450. [CrossRef]
9. Hollingsworth, R.E.; Jansen, K. Turning the corner on therapeutic cancer vaccines. *npj Vaccines* **2019**, *4*, 7. [CrossRef]
10. Thomas, R.; Al-Khadairi, G.; Roelands, J.; Hendrickx, W.; Dermime, S.; Bedognetti, D.; Decock, J. NY-ESO-1 Based Immunotherapy of Cancer: Current Perspectives. *Front. Immunol.* **2018**, *9*, 947. [CrossRef]
11. Sahin, U.; Oehm, P.; Derhovanessian, E.; Jabulowsky, R.A.; Vormehr, M.; Gold, M.; Maurus, D.; Schwarck-Kokarakis, D.; Kuhn, A.N.; Omokoko, T.; et al. An RNA vaccine drives immunity in checkpoint-inhibitor-treated melanoma. *Nature* **2020**, *585*, 107–112. [CrossRef] [PubMed]
12. Papachristofilou, A.; Hipp, M.M.; Klinkhardt, U.; Früh, M.; Sebastian, M.; Weiss, C.; Pless, M.; Cathomas, R.; Hilbe, W.; Pall, G.; et al. Phase Ib evaluation of a self-adjuvanted protamine formulated mRNA-based active cancer immunotherapy, BI1361849 (CV9202), combined with local radiation treatment in patients with stage IV non-small cell lung cancer. *J. Immunother. Cancer* **2019**, *7*, 38. [CrossRef]
13. Gnjatic, S.; Altorki, N.K.; Tang, D.N.; Tu, S.M.; Kundra, V.; Ritter, G.; Old, L.J.; Logothetis, C.J.; Sharma, P. NY-ESO-1 DNA vaccine induces T-cell responses that are suppressed by regulatory T cells. *Clin. Cancer Res.* **2009**, *15*, 2130–2139. [CrossRef]
14. Xue, W.; Metheringham, R.L.; Brentville, V.A.; Gunn, B.; Symonds, P.; Yagita, H.; Ramage, J.M.; Durrant, L.G. SCIB2, an antibody DNA vaccine encoding NY-ESO-1 epitopes, induces potent antitumor immunity which is further enhanced by checkpoint blockade. *Oncoimmunology* **2016**, *5*, e1169353. [CrossRef] [PubMed]
15. van der Bruggen, P.; Traversari, C.; Chomez, P.; Lurquin, C.; De Plaen, E.; Van den Eynde, B.; Knuth, A.; Boon, T. A gene encoding an antigen recognized by cytolytic T lymphocytes on a human melanoma. *Science* **1991**, *254*, 1643–1647. [CrossRef]
16. Hannen, R.; Bartsch, J.W. Essential roles of telomerase reverse transcriptase hTERT in cancer stemness and metastasis. *FEBS Lett.* **2018**, *592*, 2023–2031. [CrossRef]
17. Teixeira, L.; Medioni, J.; Garibal, J.; Adotevi, O.; Doucet, L.; Durey, M.D.; Ghrieb, Z.; Kiladjian, J.J.; Brizard, M.; Laheurte, C.; et al. A First-in-Human Phase I Study of INVAC-1, an Optimized Human Telomerase DNA Vaccine in Patients with Advanced Solid Tumors. *Clin. Cancer Res.* **2020**, *26*, 588–597. [CrossRef]

18. Jo, J.H.; Kim, Y.T.; Choi, H.S.; Kim, H.G.; Lee, H.S.; Choi, Y.W.; Kim, D.U.; Lee, K.H.; Kim, E.J.; Han, J.H.; et al. Efficacy of GV1001 with gemcitabine/capecitabine in previously untreated patients with advanced pancreatic ductal adenocarcinoma having high serum eotaxin levels (KG4/2015): An open-label, randomised, Phase 3 trial. *Br. J. Cancer* **2024**, *130*, 43–52. [CrossRef]
19. Middleton, G.; Silcocks, P.; Cox, T.; Valle, J.; Wadsley, J.; Propper, D.; Coxon, F.; Ross, P.; Madhusudan, S.; Roques, T.; et al. Gemcitabine and capecitabine with or without telomerase peptide vaccine GV1001 in patients with locally advanced or metastatic pancreatic cancer (TeloVac): An open-label, randomised, phase 3 trial. *Lancet Oncol.* **2014**, *15*, 829–840. [CrossRef]
20. Vonderheide, R.H.; Kraynyak, K.A.; Shields, A.F.; McRee, A.J.; Johnson, J.M.; Sun, W.; Chintakuntlawar, A.V.; Pawlicki, J.; Sylvester, A.J.; McMullan, T.; et al. Phase 1 study of safety, tolerability and immunogenicity of the human telomerase (hTERT)-encoded DNA plasmids INO-1400 and INO-1401 with or without IL-12 DNA plasmid INO-9012 in adult patients with solid tumors. *J. Immunother. Cancer* **2021**, *9*, e003019. [CrossRef] [PubMed]
21. Reardon, D.A.; Brem, S.; Desai, A.S.; Bagley, S.J.; Kurz, S.C.; De La Fuente, M.I.; Nagpal, S.; Welch, M.R.; Hormigo, A.; Forsyth, P.A.J.; et al. Intramuscular (IM) INO-5401+INO-9012 with electroporation (EP) in combination with cemiplimab (REGN2810) in newly diagnosed glioblastoma. *J. Clin. Oncol.* **2022**, *40*, 2004. [CrossRef]
22. Madan, R.A.; Arlen, P.M.; Mohebtash, M.; Hodge, J.W.; Gulley, J.L. Prostvac-VF: A vector-based vaccine targeting PSA in prostate cancer. *Expert Opin. Investig. Drugs* **2009**, *18*, 1001–1011. [CrossRef] [PubMed]
23. Gulley, J.L.; Borre, M.; Vogelzang, N.J.; Ng, S.; Agarwal, N.; Parker, C.C.; Pook, D.W.; Rathenborg, P.; Flaig, T.W.; Carles, J.; et al. Phase III Trial of PROSTVAC in Asymptomatic or Minimally Symptomatic Metastatic Castration-Resistant Prostate Cancer. *J. Clin. Oncol.* **2019**, *37*, 1051–1061. [CrossRef]
24. Linch, M.; Papai, Z.; Takacs, I.; Imedio, E.R.; Kühnle, M.-C.; Derhovanessian, E.; Vogler, I.; Renken, S.; Graham, P.; Sahin, U.; et al. 421 A first-in-human (FIH) phase I/IIa clinical trial assessing a ribonucleic acid lipoplex (RNA-LPX) encoding shared tumor antigens for immunotherapy of prostate cancer; preliminary analysis of PRO-MERIT. *J. Immunother. Cancer* **2021**, *9*, A451. [CrossRef]
25. Patel, P.H.; Kockler, D.R. Sipuleucel-T: A vaccine for metastatic, asymptomatic, androgen-independent prostate cancer. *Ann. Pharmacother.* **2008**, *42*, 91–98. [CrossRef]
26. Small, E.J.; Schellhammer, P.F.; Higano, C.S.; Redfern, C.H.; Nemunaitis, J.J.; Valone, F.H.; Verjee, S.S.; Jones, L.A.; Hershberg, R.M. Placebo-controlled phase III trial of immunologic therapy with sipuleucel-T (APC8015) in patients with metastatic, asymptomatic hormone refractory prostate cancer. *J. Clin. Oncol.* **2006**, *24*, 3089–3094. [CrossRef]
27. Higano, C.S.; Schellhammer, P.F.; Small, E.J.; Burch, P.A.; Nemunaitis, J.; Yuh, L.; Provost, N.; Frohlich, M.W. Integrated data from 2 randomized, double-blind, placebo-controlled, phase 3 trials of active cellular immunotherapy with sipuleucel-T in advanced prostate cancer. *Cancer* **2009**, *115*, 3670–3679. [CrossRef] [PubMed]
28. Kantoff, P.W.; Higano, C.S.; Shore, N.D.; Berger, E.R.; Small, E.J.; Penson, D.F.; Redfern, C.H.; Ferrari, A.C.; Dreicer, R.; Sims, R.B.; et al. Sipuleucel-T immunotherapy for castration-resistant prostate cancer. *N. Engl. J. Med.* **2010**, *363*, 411–422. [CrossRef]
29. Crosby, E.J.; Gwin, W.; Blackwell, K.; Marcom, P.K.; Chang, S.; Maecker, H.T.; Broadwater, G.; Hyslop, T.; Kim, S.; Rogatko, A.; et al. Vaccine-Induced Memory $CD8^+$ T Cells Provide Clinical Benefit in HER2 Expressing Breast Cancer: A Mouse to Human Translational Study. *Clin. Cancer Res.* **2019**, *25*, 2725–2736. [CrossRef]
30. Kang, J.; Park, H.-H.; Choi, J.H.; Lim, J.; Jang, S.-Y.; Kim, M.-A.; Park, M.-K.; Park, Y.-H.; Lim, S.; Chung, C.-W.; et al. 897 AST-301, a pDNA-based cancer vaccine encoding HER2-ICD, enhances anti-tumor effect of HER2-ADC in a HER2-expressed gastric cancer xenograft model. *J. Immunother. Cancer* **2023**, *11*, A999. [CrossRef]
31. Lim, J.; Park, H.-H.; Choi, J.K.; Choi, J.H.; Kang, J.; Jang, S.-Y.; Kim, M.-A.; Park, M.-K.; Disis, M.L.; Joung, E.; et al. 817 AST-201 (pUMVC3-hIGFBP2 N-terminus) demonstrates anti-tumor effect in an ovarian cancer mouse model. *J. Immunother. Cancer* **2023**, *11*, A915. [CrossRef]
32. Han, H.S.; Wesolowski, R.; Fisher, C.; Gandhi, S.; Gwin, W.R.; Kowzun, M.J.; Gogineni, K.; Liu, H.; Costa, R.L.; Guerrero, J.; et al. A multicenter phase II study of vaccines to prevent recurrence in patients with HER-2-positive breast cancer. *J. Clin. Oncol.* **2023**, *41*, 532. [CrossRef]
33. Gwin, W.R.; Kuano, K.; Childs, J.; Symonds, L.K.; Coveler, A.L.; Liao, J.B.; Vinayak, S.; Disis, M.L. A phase II study of concurrent WOKVAC vaccination with neoadjuvant chemotherapy and HER2-targeted monoclonal antibody therapy. *J. Clin. Oncol.* **2023**, *41*, TPS636. [CrossRef]
34. Pan, R.Y.; Chung, W.H.; Chu, M.T.; Chen, S.J.; Chen, H.C.; Zheng, L.; Hung, S.I. Recent Development and Clinical Application of Cancer Vaccine: Targeting Neoantigens. *J. Immunol. Res.* **2018**, *2018*, 4325874. [CrossRef]
35. Romero, P.; Banchereau, J.; Bhardwaj, N.; Cockett, M.; Disis, M.L.; Dranoff, G.; Gilboa, E.; Hammond, S.A.; Hershberg, R.; Korman, A.J.; et al. The Human Vaccines Project: A roadmap for cancer vaccine development. *Sci. Transl. Med.* **2016**, *8*, 334ps9. [CrossRef] [PubMed]
36. de Martel, C.; Georges, D.; Bray, F.; Ferlay, J.; Clifford, G.M. Global burden of cancer attributable to infections in 2018: A worldwide incidence analysis. *Lancet Glob. Health* **2020**, *8*, e180–e190. [CrossRef] [PubMed]

37. Korzeniewski, N.; Treat, B.; Duensing, S. The HPV-16 E7 oncoprotein induces centriole multiplication through deregulation of Polo-like kinase 4 expression. *Mol. Cancer* **2011**, *10*, 61. [CrossRef] [PubMed]
38. Albert, E.; Laimins, L. Regulation of the Human Papillomavirus Life Cycle by DNA Damage Repair Pathways and Epigenetic Factors. *Viruses* **2020**, *12*, 744. [CrossRef] [PubMed]
39. Sofiani, V.H.; Veisi, P.; Rukerd, M.R.Z.; Ghazi, R.; Nakhaie, M. The complexity of human papilloma virus in cancers: A narrative review. *Infect. Agent Cancer* **2023**, *18*, 13. [CrossRef]
40. Klinghammer, K.; Saba, N.F.; Castelluci, E.; Colevas, A.D.; Rutkowski, T.; Greil, R.; Thurner, D.; Müller-Richter, U.; Di Giacomo, A.M.; Grewal, J.; et al. 155P BNT113 + pembrolizumab as first-line treatment in patients with unresectable recurrent/metastatic HNSCC: Preliminary safety data from AHEAD-MERIT. *Immuno. Oncol. Technol.* **2022**, *16*, 100267. [CrossRef]
41. Youn, J.W.; Hur, S.Y.; Woo, J.W.; Kim, Y.M.; Lim, M.C.; Park, S.Y.; Seo, S.S.; No, J.H.; Kim, B.G.; Lee, J.K.; et al. Pembrolizumab plus GX-188E therapeutic DNA vaccine in patients with HPV-16-positive or HPV-18-positive advanced cervical cancer: Interim results of a single-arm, phase 2 trial. *Lancet Oncol.* **2020**, *21*, 1653–1660. [CrossRef]
42. Gibson, M.K.; Savvides, P.; Worden, F.; Heimann-Nichols, E.; Wu, T.; Roden, R.; Chang, Y.-N. 677 Phase II trial assessing safety, efficacy and immune correlates of heterologous prime-boost with pBI-11 (IM) and TA-HPV (IM) plus pembrolizumab for advanced, PD-L1 CPS≥1, hrHPV+ Oropharyngeal cancer. *J. Immunother. Cancer* **2023**, *11*, A768. [CrossRef]
43. Peng, S.; Qiu, J.; Yang, A.; Yang, B.; Jeang, J.; Wang, J.W.; Chang, Y.N.; Brayton, C.; Roden, R.B.S.; Hung, C.F.; et al. Optimization of heterologous DNA-prime, protein boost regimens and site of vaccination to enhance therapeutic immunity against human papillomavirus-associated disease. *Cell Biosci.* **2016**, *6*, 16. [CrossRef] [PubMed]
44. Einstein, M.H.; Roden, R.B.S.; Ferrall, L.; Akin, M.; Blomer, A.; Wu, T.C.; Chang, Y.N. Safety Run-in of Intramuscular pNGVL4a-Sig/E7(detox)/HSP70 DNA and TA-CIN Protein Vaccination as Treatment for HPV16+ ASC-US, ASC-H, or LSIL/CIN1. *Cancer Prev. Res. (Phila)* **2023**, *16*, 219–227. [CrossRef] [PubMed]
45. Hillemanns, P.; Denecke, A.; Woelber, L.; Böhmer, G.; Jentschke, M.; Schjetne, K.W.; Bruins Slot, K.M.H.; Fredriksen, A.B. A Therapeutic Antigen-Presenting Cell-Targeting DNA Vaccine VB10.16 in HPV16-Positive High-Grade Cervical Intraepithelial Neoplasia: Results from a Phase I/IIa Trial. *Clin. Cancer Res.* **2022**, *28*, 4885–4892. [CrossRef]
46. Bhuyan, P.K.; Dallas, M.; Kraynyak, K.; Herring, T.; Morrow, M.; Boyer, J.; Duff, S.; Kim, J.; Weiner, D.B. Durability of response to VGX-3100 treatment of HPV16/18 positive cervical HSIL. *Hum. Vaccin. Immunother.* **2021**, *17*, 1288–1293. [CrossRef]
47. Huang, L.; Guo, Z.; Wang, F.; Fu, L. KRAS mutation: From undruggable to druggable in cancer. *Signal Transduct. Target Ther.* **2021**, *6*, 386. [CrossRef]
48. Gupta, R.G.; Li, F.; Roszik, J.; Lizée, G. Exploiting Tumor Neoantigens to Target Cancer Evolution: Current Challenges and Promising Therapeutic Approaches. *Cancer Discov.* **2021**, *11*, 1024–1039. [CrossRef] [PubMed]
49. Xia, H.; McMichael, J.; Becker-Hapak, M.; Onyeador, O.C.; Buchli, R.; McClain, E.; Pence, P.; Supabphol, S.; Richters, M.M.; Basu, A.; et al. Computational prediction of MHC anchor locations guides neoantigen identification and prioritization. *Sci. Immunol.* **2023**, *8*, eabg2200. [CrossRef]
50. Vilimas, T. Measuring Tumor Mutational Burden Using Whole-Exome Sequencing. *Methods Mol. Biol.* **2020**, *2055*, 63–91. [CrossRef]
51. Rizvi, N.A.; Hellmann, M.D.; Snyder, A.; Kvistborg, P.; Makarov, V.; Havel, J.J.; Lee, W.; Yuan, J.; Wong, P.; Ho, T.S.; et al. Cancer immunology. Mutational landscape determines sensitivity to PD-1 blockade in non-small cell lung cancer. *Science* **2015**, *348*, 124–128. [CrossRef] [PubMed]
52. Samstein, R.M.; Lee, C.H.; Shoushtari, A.N.; Hellmann, M.D.; Shen, R.; Janjigian, Y.Y.; Barron, D.A.; Zehir, A.; Jordan, E.J.; Omuro, A.; et al. Tumor mutational load predicts survival after immunotherapy across multiple cancer types. *Nat. Genet.* **2019**, *51*, 202–206. [CrossRef] [PubMed]
53. Charoentong, P.; Finotello, F.; Angelova, M.; Mayer, C.; Efremova, M.; Rieder, D.; Hackl, H.; Trajanoski, Z. Pan-cancer Immunogenomic Analyses Reveal Genotype-Immunophenotype Relationships and Predictors of Response to Checkpoint Blockade. *Cell Rep.* **2017**, *18*, 248–262. [CrossRef]
54. De Mattos-Arruda, L.; Vazquez, M.; Finotello, F.; Lepore, R.; Porta, E.; Hundal, J.; Amengual-Rigo, P.; Ng, C.K.Y.; Valencia, A.; Carrillo, J.; et al. Neoantigen prediction and computational perspectives towards clinical benefit: Recommendations from the ESMO Precision Medicine Working Group. *Ann. Oncol.* **2020**, *31*, 978–990. [CrossRef]
55. Shi, Y.; Jing, B.; Xi, R. Comprehensive analysis of neoantigens derived from structural variation across whole genomes from 2528 tumors. *Genome Biol.* **2023**, *24*, 169. [CrossRef]
56. Yewdell, J.W.; Antón, L.C.; Bennink, J.R. Defective ribosomal products (DRiPs): A major source of antigenic peptides for MHC class I molecules? *J. Immunol.* **1996**, *157*, 1823–1826. [CrossRef] [PubMed]
57. Turajlic, S.; Litchfield, K.; Xu, H.; Rosenthal, R.; McGranahan, N.; Reading, J.L.; Wong, Y.N.S.; Rowan, A.; Kanu, N.; Al Bakir, M.; et al. Insertion-and-deletion-derived tumour-specific neoantigens and the immunogenic phenotype: A pan-cancer analysis. *Lancet Oncol.* **2017**, *18*, 1009–1021. [CrossRef]

58. Hansen, U.K.; Ramskov, S.; Bjerregaard, A.M.; Borch, A.; Andersen, R.; Draghi, A.; Donia, M.; Bentzen, A.K.; Marquard, A.M.; Szallasi, Z.; et al. Tumor-Infiltrating T Cells From Clear Cell Renal Cell Carcinoma Patients Recognize Neoepitopes Derived From Point and Frameshift Mutations. *Front. Immunol.* **2020**, *11*, 373. [CrossRef]
59. Yang, W.; Lee, K.W.; Srivastava, R.M.; Kuo, F.; Krishna, C.; Chowell, D.; Makarov, V.; Hoen, D.; Dalin, M.G.; Wexler, L.; et al. Immunogenic neoantigens derived from gene fusions stimulate T cell responses. *Nat. Med.* **2019**, *25*, 767–775. [CrossRef]
60. Wei, Z.; Zhou, C.; Zhang, Z.; Guan, M.; Zhang, C.; Liu, Z.; Liu, Q. The Landscape of Tumor Fusion Neoantigens: A Pan-Cancer Analysis. *iScience* **2019**, *21*, 249–260. [CrossRef]
61. Romanish, M.T.; Cohen, C.J.; Mager, D.L. Potential mechanisms of endogenous retroviral-mediated genomic instability in human cancer. *Semin. Cancer Biol.* **2010**, *20*, 246–253. [CrossRef]
62. Schliehe, C.; Bitzer, A.; van den Broek, M.; Groettrup, M. Stable antigen is most effective for eliciting CD8+ T-cell responses after DNA vaccination and infection with recombinant vaccinia virus in vivo. *J. Virol.* **2012**, *86*, 9782–9793. [CrossRef]
63. Westcott, P.M.K.; Sacks, N.J.; Schenkel, J.M.; Ely, Z.A.; Smith, O.; Hauck, H.; Jaeger, A.M.; Zhang, D.; Backlund, C.M.; Beytagh, M.C.; et al. Low neoantigen expression and poor T-cell priming underlie early immune escape in colorectal cancer. *Nat. Cancer* **2021**, *2*, 1071–1085. [CrossRef]
64. Castro, A.; Zanetti, M.; Carter, H. Neoantigen Controversies. *Annu. Rev. Biomed. Data Sci.* **2021**, *4*, 227–253. [CrossRef]
65. Black, J.R.M.; McGranahan, N. Genetic and non-genetic clonal diversity in cancer evolution. *Nat. Rev. Cancer* **2021**, *21*, 379–392. [CrossRef] [PubMed]
66. Wright, B.W.; Yi, Z.; Weissman, J.S.; Chen, J. The dark proteome: Translation from noncanonical open reading frames. *Trends Cell Biol.* **2022**, *32*, 243–258. [CrossRef] [PubMed]
67. Starck, S.R.; Shastri, N. Nowhere to hide: Unconventional translation yields cryptic peptides for immune surveillance. *Immunol. Rev.* **2016**, *272*, 8–16. [CrossRef] [PubMed]
68. Kahles, A.; Lehmann, K.V.; Toussaint, N.C.; Hüser, M.; Stark, S.G.; Sachsenberg, T.; Stegle, O.; Kohlbacher, O.; Sander, C.; Rätsch, G. Comprehensive Analysis of Alternative Splicing Across Tumors from 8,705 Patients. *Cancer Cell* **2018**, *34*, 211–224.e216. [CrossRef]
69. Malarkannan, S.; Horng, T.; Shih, P.P.; Schwab, S.; Shastri, N. Presentation of out-of-frame peptide/MHC class I complexes by a novel translation initiation mechanism. *Immunity* **1999**, *10*, 681–690. [CrossRef]
70. Schwab, S.R.; Shugart, J.A.; Horng, T.; Malarkannan, S.; Shastri, N. Unanticipated antigens: Translation initiation at CUG with leucine. *PLoS Biol.* **2004**, *2*, e366. [CrossRef]
71. Jackson, R.; Kroehling, L.; Khitun, A.; Bailis, W.; Jarret, A.; York, A.G.; Khan, O.M.; Brewer, J.R.; Skadow, M.H.; Duizer, C.; et al. The translation of non-canonical open reading frames controls mucosal immunity. *Nature* **2018**, *564*, 434–438. [CrossRef]
72. Chong, C.; Coukos, G.; Bassani-Sternberg, M. Identification of tumor antigens with immunopeptidomics. *Nat. Biotechnol.* **2022**, *40*, 175–188. [CrossRef]
73. Ouspenskaia, T.; Law, T.; Clauser, K.R.; Klaeger, S.; Sarkizova, S.; Aguet, F.; Li, B.; Christian, E.; Knisbacher, B.A.; Le, P.M.; et al. Unannotated proteins expand the MHC-I-restricted immunopeptidome in cancer. *Nat. Biotechnol.* **2022**, *40*, 209–217. [CrossRef] [PubMed]
74. Ingolia, N.T.; Brar, G.A.; Stern-Ginossar, N.; Harris, M.S.; Talhouarne, G.J.; Jackson, S.E.; Wills, M.R.; Weissman, J.S. Ribosome profiling reveals pervasive translation outside of annotated protein-coding genes. *Cell Rep.* **2014**, *8*, 1365–1379. [CrossRef] [PubMed]
75. Goodenough, E.; Robinson, T.M.; Zook, M.B.; Flanigan, K.M.; Atkins, J.F.; Howard, M.T.; Eisenlohr, L.C. Cryptic MHC class I-binding peptides are revealed by aminoglycoside-induced stop codon read-through into the 3′ UTR. *Proc. Natl. Acad. Sci. USA* **2014**, *111*, 5670–5675. [CrossRef] [PubMed]
76. Bullock, T.N.; Eisenlohr, L.C. Ribosomal scanning past the primary initiation codon as a mechanism for expression of CTL epitopes encoded in alternative reading frames. *J. Exp. Med.* **1996**, *184*, 1319–1329. [CrossRef] [PubMed]
77. Saulquin, X.; Scotet, E.; Trautmann, L.; Peyrat, M.A.; Halary, F.; Bonneville, M.; Houssaint, E. +1 Frameshifting as a novel mechanism to generate a cryptic cytotoxic T lymphocyte epitope derived from human interleukin 10. *J. Exp. Med.* **2002**, *195*, 353–358. [CrossRef]
78. Malaker, S.A.; Penny, S.A.; Steadman, L.G.; Myers, P.T.; Loke, J.C.; Raghavan, M.; Bai, D.L.; Shabanowitz, J.; Hunt, D.F.; Cobbold, M. Identification of Glycopeptides as Posttranslationally Modified Neoantigens in Leukemia. *Cancer Immunol. Res.* **2017**, *5*, 376–384. [CrossRef]
79. Vigneron, N.; Stroobant, V.; Ferrari, V.; Abi Habib, J.; Van den Eynde, B.J. Production of spliced peptides by the proteasome. *Mol. Immunol.* **2019**, *113*, 93–102. [CrossRef]
80. Liepe, J.; Ovaa, H.; Mishto, M. Why do proteases mess up with antigen presentation by re-shuffling antigen sequences? *Curr. Opin. Immunol.* **2018**, *52*, 81–86. [CrossRef]

81. Ruiz Cuevas, M.V.; Hardy, M.P.; Hollý, J.; Bonneil, É.; Durette, C.; Courcelles, M.; Lanoix, J.; Côté, C.; Staudt, L.M.; Lemieux, S.; et al. Most non-canonical proteins uniquely populate the proteome or immunopeptidome. *Cell Rep.* **2021**, *34*, 108815. [CrossRef] [PubMed]
82. Sadeghi Najafabadi, S.A.; Bolhassani, A.; Aghasadeghi, M.R. Tumor cell-based vaccine: An effective strategy for eradication of cancer cells. *Immunotherapy* **2022**, *14*, 639–654. [CrossRef] [PubMed]
83. Berd, D. M-Vax: An autologous, hapten-modified vaccine for human cancer. *Expert Opin. Biol. Ther.* **2002**, *2*, 335–342. [CrossRef]
84. Sosman, J.A.; Sondak, V.K. Melacine: An allogeneic melanoma tumor cell lysate vaccine. *Expert Rev. Vaccines* **2003**, *2*, 353–368. [CrossRef]
85. Ogi, C.; Aruga, A. Clinical evaluation of therapeutic cancer vaccines. *Hum. Vaccin. Immunother.* **2013**, *9*, 1049–1057. [CrossRef]
86. Richters, M.M.; Xia, H.; Campbell, K.M.; Gillanders, W.E.; Griffith, O.L.; Griffith, M. Best practices for bioinformatic characterization of neoantigens for clinical utility. *Genome Med.* **2019**, *11*, 56. [CrossRef]
87. Ang, K.K.; Harris, J.; Wheeler, R.; Weber, R.; Rosenthal, D.I.; Nguyen-Tân, P.F.; Westra, W.H.; Chung, C.H.; Jordan, R.C.; Lu, C.; et al. Human papillomavirus and survival of patients with oropharyngeal cancer. *N. Engl. J. Med.* **2010**, *363*, 24–35. [CrossRef] [PubMed]
88. Roudko, V.; Greenbaum, B.; Bhardwaj, N. Computational Prediction and Validation of Tumor-Associated Neoantigens. *Front. Immunol.* **2020**, *11*, 27. [CrossRef]
89. Bohnert, R.; Vivas, S.; Jansen, G. Comprehensive benchmarking of SNV callers for highly admixed tumor data. *PLoS ONE* **2017**, *12*, e0186175. [CrossRef]
90. Pei, S.; Liu, T.; Ren, X.; Li, W.; Chen, C.; Xie, Z. Benchmarking variant callers in next-generation and third-generation sequencing analysis. *Brief. Bioinform.* **2021**, *22*, bbaa148. [CrossRef]
91. Sarwal, V.; Niehus, S.; Ayyala, R.; Kim, M.; Sarkar, A.; Chang, S.; Lu, A.; Rajkumar, N.; Darfci-Maher, N.; Littman, R.; et al. A comprehensive benchmarking of WGS-based deletion structural variant callers. *Brief. Bioinform.* **2022**, *23*, bbac221. [CrossRef] [PubMed]
92. Gallegos Ruiz, M.I.; Floor, K.; Rijmen, F.; Grünberg, K.; Rodriguez, J.A.; Giaccone, G. EGFR and K-ras mutation analysis in non-small cell lung cancer: Comparison of paraffin embedded versus frozen specimens. *Cell Oncol.* **2007**, *29*, 257–264. [CrossRef]
93. Cazzato, G.; Caporusso, C.; Arezzo, F.; Cimmino, A.; Colagrande, A.; Loizzi, V.; Cormio, G.; Lettini, T.; Maiorano, E.; Scarcella, V.S.; et al. Formalin-Fixed and Paraffin-Embedded Samples for Next Generation Sequencing: Problems and Solutions. *Genes* **2021**, *12*, 1472. [CrossRef]
94. Dodani, D.D.; Nguyen, M.H.; Morin, R.D.; Marra, M.A.; Corbett, R.D. Combinatorial and Machine Learning Approaches for Improved Somatic Variant Calling From Formalin-Fixed Paraffin-Embedded Genome Sequence Data. *Front. Genet.* **2022**, *13*, 834764. [CrossRef]
95. Trevarton, A.J.; Chang, J.T.; Symmans, W.F. Simple combination of multiple somatic variant callers to increase accuracy. *Sci. Rep.* **2023**, *13*, 8463. [CrossRef]
96. Junjun, R.; Zhengqian, Z.; Ying, W.; Jialiang, W.; Yongzhuang, L. A comprehensive review of deep learning-based variant calling methods. *Brief. Funct. Genom.* **2024**, *23*, 303–313. [CrossRef] [PubMed]
97. Quinn, E.M.; Cormican, P.; Kenny, E.M.; Hill, M.; Anney, R.; Gill, M.; Corvin, A.P.; Morris, D.W. Development of strategies for SNP detection in RNA-seq data: Application to lymphoblastoid cell lines and evaluation using 1000 Genomes data. *PLoS ONE* **2013**, *8*, e58815. [CrossRef]
98. Zhao, Y.; Wang, K.; Wang, W.L.; Yin, T.T.; Dong, W.Q.; Xu, C.J. A high-throughput SNP discovery strategy for RNA-seq data. *BMC Genom.* **2019**, *20*, 160. [CrossRef] [PubMed]
99. Liu, F.; Zhang, Y.; Zhang, L.; Li, Z.; Fang, Q.; Gao, R.; Zhang, Z. Systematic comparative analysis of single-nucleotide variant detection methods from single-cell RNA sequencing data. *Genome Biol.* **2019**, *20*, 242. [CrossRef]
100. CPTAC. Pan-Cancer Analysis Page. National Cancer Institute Proteomic Data Commons. Available online: https://pdc.cancer.gov/pdc/ (accessed on 27 August 2025).
101. Erhard, F.; Halenius, A.; Zimmermann, C.; L'Hernault, A.; Kowalewski, D.J.; Weekes, M.P.; Stevanovic, S.; Zimmer, R.; Dölken, L. Improved Ribo-seq enables identification of cryptic translation events. *Nat. Methods* **2018**, *15*, 363–366. [CrossRef]
102. Fedorova, A.D.; Tierney, J.A.S.; Michel, A.M.; Baranov, P.V. RiboGalaxy: A Galaxy-based Web Platform for Ribosome Profiling Data Processing—2023 Update. *J. Mol. Biol.* **2023**, *435*, 168043. [CrossRef] [PubMed]
103. Vizcaíno, J.A.; Kubiniok, P.; Kovalchik, K.A.; Ma, Q.; Duquette, J.D.; Mongrain, I.; Deutsch, E.W.; Peters, B.; Sette, A.; Sirois, I.; et al. The Human Immunopeptidome Project: A Roadmap to Predict and Treat Immune Diseases. *Mol. Cell Proteom.* **2020**, *19*, 31–49. [CrossRef]

104. Di Marco, M.; Schuster, H.; Backert, L.; Ghosh, M.; Rammensee, H.G.; Stevanović, S. Unveiling the Peptide Motifs of HLA-C and HLA-G from Naturally Presented Peptides and Generation of Binding Prediction Matrices. *J. Immunol.* **2017**, *199*, 2639–2651. [CrossRef]
105. Szolek, A.; Schubert, B.; Mohr, C.; Sturm, M.; Feldhahn, M.; Kohlbacher, O. OptiType: Precision HLA typing from next-generation sequencing data. *Bioinformatics* **2014**, *30*, 3310–3316. [CrossRef]
106. Kiyotani, K.; Mai, T.H.; Nakamura, Y. Comparison of exome-based HLA class I genotyping tools: Identification of platform-specific genotyping errors. *J. Hum. Genet.* **2017**, *62*, 397–405. [CrossRef]
107. Orenbuch, R.; Filip, I.; Comito, D.; Shaman, J.; Pe'er, I.; Rabadan, R. arcasHLA: High-resolution HLA typing from RNAseq. *Bioinformatics* **2020**, *36*, 33–40. [CrossRef]
108. Liu, C.; Yang, X.; Duffy, B.; Mohanakumar, T.; Mitra, R.D.; Zody, M.C.; Pfeifer, J.D. ATHLATES: Accurate typing of human leukocyte antigen through exome sequencing. *Nucleic Acids Res.* **2013**, *41*, e142. [CrossRef]
109. Boegel, S.; Löwer, M.; Schäfer, M.; Bukur, T.; de Graaf, J.; Boisguérin, V.; Türeci, O.; Diken, M.; Castle, J.C.; Sahin, U. HLA typing from RNA-Seq sequence reads. *Genome Med.* **2012**, *4*, 102. [CrossRef]
110. Profaizer, T.; Lázár-Molnár, E.; Close, D.W.; Delgado, J.C.; Kumánovics, A. HLA genotyping in the clinical laboratory: Comparison of next-generation sequencing methods. *Hla* **2016**, *88*, 14–24. [CrossRef] [PubMed]
111. Andreatta, M.; Nielsen, M. Gapped sequence alignment using artificial neural networks: Application to the MHC class I system. *Bioinformatics* **2016**, *32*, 511–517. [CrossRef] [PubMed]
112. Nielsen, M.; Lundegaard, C.; Blicher, T.; Lamberth, K.; Harndahl, M.; Justesen, S.; Røder, G.; Peters, B.; Sette, A.; Lund, O.; et al. NetMHCpan, a method for quantitative predictions of peptide binding to any HLA-A and -B locus protein of known sequence. *PLoS ONE* **2007**, *2*, e796. [CrossRef]
113. Jurtz, V.; Paul, S.; Andreatta, M.; Marcatili, P.; Peters, B.; Nielsen, M. NetMHCpan-4.0: Improved Peptide-MHC Class I Interaction Predictions Integrating Eluted Ligand and Peptide Binding Affinity Data. *J. Immunol.* **2017**, *199*, 3360–3368. [CrossRef]
114. Wieczorek, M.; Abualrous, E.T.; Sticht, J.; Álvaro-Benito, M.; Stolzenberg, S.; Noé, F.; Freund, C. Major Histocompatibility Complex (MHC) Class I and MHC Class II Proteins: Conformational Plasticity in Antigen Presentation. *Front. Immunol.* **2017**, *8*, 292. [CrossRef]
115. Rock, K.L.; Reits, E.; Neefjes, J. Present Yourself! By MHC Class I and MHC Class II Molecules. *Trends Immunol.* **2016**, *37*, 724–737. [CrossRef] [PubMed]
116. Andreatta, M.; Karosiene, E.; Rasmussen, M.; Stryhn, A.; Buus, S.; Nielsen, M. Accurate pan-specific prediction of peptide-MHC class II binding affinity with improved binding core identification. *Immunogenetics* **2015**, *67*, 641–650. [CrossRef]
117. Gfeller, D.; Bassani-Sternberg, M. Predicting Antigen Presentation-What Could We Learn From a Million Peptides? *Front. Immunol.* **2018**, *9*, 1716. [CrossRef]
118. IEDB Analysis Resource. Epitope Prediction and Analysis Tools. Available online: http://tools.iedb.org/main/ (accessed on 25 August 2025).
119. Yang, Y.; Wei, Z.; Cia, G.; Song, X.; Pucci, F.; Rooman, M.; Xue, F.; Hou, Q. MHCII-peptide presentation: An assessment of the state-of-the-art prediction methods. *Front. Immunol.* **2024**, *15*, 1293706. [CrossRef]
120. Bulik-Sullivan, B.; Busby, J.; Palmer, C.D.; Davis, M.J.; Murphy, T.; Clark, A.; Busby, M.; Duke, F.; Yang, A.; Young, L.; et al. Deep learning using tumor HLA peptide mass spectrometry datasets improves neoantigen identification. *Nat. Biotechnol.* **2018**, *37*, 55–63. [CrossRef] [PubMed]
121. Albert, B.A.; Yang, Y.; Shao, X.M.; Singh, D.; Smit, K.N.; Anagnostou, V.; Karchin, R. Deep neural networks predict class I major histocompatibility complex epitope presentation and transfer learn neoepitope immunogenicity. *Nat. Mach. Intell.* **2023**, *5*, 861–872. [CrossRef] [PubMed]
122. Shugay, M.; Bagaev, D.V.; Zvyagin, I.V.; Vroomans, R.M.; Crawford, J.C.; Dolton, G.; Komech, E.A.; Sycheva, A.L.; Koneva, A.E.; Egorov, E.S.; et al. VDJdb: A curated database of T-cell receptor sequences with known antigen specificity. *Nucleic Acids Res.* **2018**, *46*, D419–D427. [CrossRef] [PubMed]
123. Tickotsky, N.; Sagiv, T.; Prilusky, J.; Shifrut, E.; Friedman, N. McPAS-TCR: A manually curated catalogue of pathology-associated T cell receptor sequences. *Bioinformatics* **2017**, *33*, 2924–2929. [CrossRef]
124. Vita, R.; Mahajan, S.; Overton, J.A.; Dhanda, S.K.; Martini, S.; Cantrell, J.R.; Wheeler, D.K.; Sette, A.; Peters, B. The Immune Epitope Database (IEDB): 2018 update. *Nucleic Acids Res.* **2019**, *47*, D339–D343. [CrossRef] [PubMed]
125. Zhang, W.; Wang, L.; Liu, K.; Wei, X.; Yang, K.; Du, W.; Wang, S.; Guo, N.; Ma, C.; Luo, L.; et al. PIRD: Pan Immune Repertoire Database. *Bioinformatics* **2020**, *36*, 897–903. [CrossRef]
126. Nolan, S.; Vignali, M.; Klinger, M.; Dines, J.N.; Kaplan, I.M.; Svejnoha, E.; Craft, T.; Boland, K.; Pesesky, M.; Gittelman, R.M.; et al. A large-scale database of T-cell receptor beta (TCRβ) sequences and binding associations from natural and synthetic exposure to SARS-CoV-2. *Res. Sq.* **2020**, *16*, 1488851. [CrossRef]

127. 10× Genomics. Chromium Single Cell Immune Profiling. Available online: https://www.10xgenomics.com/products/single-cell-immune-profiling (accessed on 8 August 2025).
128. Fischer, D.S.; Wu, Y.; Schubert, B.; Theis, F.J. Predicting antigen specificity of single T cells based on TCR CDR3 regions. *Mol. Syst. Biol.* **2020**, *16*, e9416. [CrossRef]
129. Overall, S.A.; Toor, J.S.; Hao, S.; Yarmarkovich, M.; Sara, M.O.R.; Morozov, G.I.; Nguyen, S.; Japp, A.S.; Gonzalez, N.; Moschidi, D.; et al. High throughput pMHC-I tetramer library production using chaperone-mediated peptide exchange. *Nat. Commun.* **2020**, *11*, 1909. [CrossRef]
130. Meysman, P.; Barton, J.; Bravi, B.; Cohen-Lavi, L.; Karnaukhov, V.; Lilleskov, E.; Montemurro, A.; Nielsen, M.; Mora, T.; Pereira, P.; et al. Benchmarking solutions to the T-cell receptor epitope prediction problem: IMMREP22 workshop report. *ImmunoInformatics* **2023**, *9*, 100024. [CrossRef]
131. Grazioli, F.; Mösch, A.; Machart, P.; Li, K.; Alqassem, I.; O'Donnell, T.J.; Min, M.R. On TCR binding predictors failing to generalize to unseen peptides. *Front. Immunol.* **2022**, *13*, 1014256. [CrossRef]
132. Croce, G.; Bobisse, S.; Moreno, D.L.; Schmidt, J.; Guillame, P.; Harari, A.; Gfeller, D. Deep learning predictions of TCR-epitope interactions reveal epitope-specific chains in dual alpha T cells. *Nat. Commun.* **2024**, *15*, 3211. [CrossRef]
133. Habern, O. 2021 A Sequencing Approach to T-Cell Receptor-Antigen Recognition. 10× Genomics. Available online: https://www.10xgenomics.com/blog/a-sequencing-approach-to-t-cell-receptor-antigen-recognition (accessed on 18 July 2025).
134. McGranahan, N.; Furness, A.J.; Rosenthal, R.; Ramskov, S.; Lyngaa, R.; Saini, S.K.; Jamal-Hanjani, M.; Wilson, G.A.; Birkbak, N.J.; Hiley, C.T.; et al. Clonal neoantigens elicit T cell immunoreactivity and sensitivity to immune checkpoint blockade. *Science* **2016**, *351*, 1463–1469. [CrossRef] [PubMed]
135. Lang, F.; Schrörs, B.; Löwer, M.; Türeci, Ö.; Sahin, U. Identification of neoantigens for individualized therapeutic cancer vaccines. *Nat. Rev. Drug Discov.* **2022**, *21*, 261–282. [CrossRef]
136. Ragone, C.; Cavalluzzo, B.; Mauriello, A.; Tagliamonte, M.; Buonaguro, L. Lack of shared neoantigens in prevalent mutations in cancer. *J. Transl. Med.* **2024**, *22*, 344. [CrossRef]
137. Weller, M.; Butowski, N.; Tran, D.D.; Recht, L.D.; Lim, M.; Hirte, H.; Ashby, L.; Mechtler, L.; Goldlust, S.A.; Iwamoto, F.; et al. Rindopepimut with temozolomide for patients with newly diagnosed, EGFRvIII-expressing glioblastoma (ACT IV): A randomised, double-blind, international phase 3 trial. *Lancet Oncol.* **2017**, *18*, 1373–1385. [CrossRef]
138. Bagley, S.J.; Binder, Z.A.; Lamrani, L.; Marinari, E.; Desai, A.S.; Nasrallah, M.P.; Maloney, E.; Brem, S.; Lustig, R.A.; Kurtz, G.; et al. Repeated peripheral infusions of anti-EGFRvIII CAR T cells in combination with pembrolizumab show no efficacy in glioblastoma: A phase 1 trial. *Nat. Cancer* **2024**, *5*, 517–531. [CrossRef]
139. Laganà, A. Computational Approaches for the Investigation of Intra-tumor Heterogeneity and Clonal Evolution from Bulk Sequencing Data in Precision Oncology Applications. *Adv. Exp. Med. Biol.* **2022**, *1361*, 101–118. [CrossRef]
140. Xiao, Y.; Wang, X.; Zhang, H.; Ulintz, P.J.; Li, H.; Guan, Y. FastClone is a probabilistic tool for deconvoluting tumor heterogeneity in bulk-sequencing samples. *Nat. Commun.* **2020**, *11*, 4469. [CrossRef] [PubMed]
141. Roth, A.; Khattra, J.; Yap, D.; Wan, A.; Laks, E.; Biele, J.; Ha, G.; Aparicio, S.; Bouchard-Côté, A.; Shah, S.P. PyClone: Statistical inference of clonal population structure in cancer. *Nat. Methods* **2014**, *11*, 396–398. [CrossRef]
142. Miller, C.A.; White, B.S.; Dees, N.D.; Griffith, M.; Welch, J.S.; Griffith, O.L.; Vij, R.; Tomasson, M.H.; Graubert, T.A.; Walter, M.J.; et al. SciClone: Inferring clonal architecture and tracking the spatial and temporal patterns of tumor evolution. *PLoS Comput. Biol.* **2014**, *10*, e1003665. [CrossRef] [PubMed]
143. Hundal, J.; Kiwala, S.; McMichael, J.; Miller, C.A.; Xia, H.; Wollam, A.T.; Liu, C.J.; Zhao, S.; Feng, Y.Y.; Graubert, A.P.; et al. pVACtools: A Computational Toolkit to Identify and Visualize Cancer Neoantigens. *Cancer Immunol. Res.* **2020**, *8*, 409–420. [CrossRef] [PubMed]
144. Kodysh, J.; Rubinsteyn, A. OpenVax: An Open-Source Computational Pipeline for Cancer Neoantigen Prediction. *Methods Mol. Biol.* **2020**, *2120*, 147–160. [CrossRef]
145. Li, B.; Jing, P.; Zheng, G.; Pi, C.; Zhang, L.; Yin, Z.; Xu, L.; Qiu, J.; Gu, H.; Qiu, T.; et al. Neo-intline: Integrated pipeline enables neoantigen design through the in-silico presentation of T-cell epitope. *Signal. Transduct. Target. Ther.* **2023**, *8*, 397. [CrossRef]
146. Rubinsteyn, A.; Kodysh, J.; Hodes, I.; Mondet, S.; Aksoy, B.A.; Finnigan, J.P.; Bhardwaj, N.; Hammerbacher, J. Computational Pipeline for the PGV-001 Neoantigen Vaccine Trial. *Front. Immunol.* **2017**, *8*, 1807. [CrossRef]
147. Schmittel, A.; Keilholz, U.; Scheibenbogen, C. Evaluation of the interferon-gamma ELISPOT-assay for quantification of peptide specific T lymphocytes from peripheral blood. *J. Immunol. Methods* **1997**, *210*, 167–174. [CrossRef] [PubMed]
148. Godard, B.; Gazagne, A.; Gey, A.; Baptiste, M.; Vingert, B.; Pegaz-Fiornet, B.; Strompf, L.; Fridman, W.H.; Glotz, D.; Tartour, E. Optimization of an elispot assay to detect cytomegalovirus-specific CD8+ T lymphocytes. *Hum. Immunol.* **2004**, *65*, 1307–1318. [CrossRef] [PubMed]
149. Czerkinsky, C.C.; Nilsson, L.A.; Nygren, H.; Ouchterlony, O.; Tarkowski, A. A solid-phase enzyme-linked immunospot (ELISPOT) assay for enumeration of specific antibody-secreting cells. *J. Immunol. Methods* **1983**, *65*, 109–121. [CrossRef]

150. Slota, M.; Lim, J.B.; Dang, Y.; Disis, M.L. ELISpot for measuring human immune responses to vaccines. *Expert Rev. Vaccines* **2011**, *10*, 299–306. [CrossRef]
151. Korzeniewski, C.; Callewaert, D.M. An enzyme-release assay for natural cytotoxicity. *J. Immunol. Methods* **1983**, *64*, 313–320. [CrossRef]
152. Weigelin, B.; den Boer, A.T.; Wagena, E.; Broen, K.; Dolstra, H.; de Boer, R.J.; Figdor, C.G.; Textor, J.; Friedl, P. Cytotoxic T cells are able to efficiently eliminate cancer cells by additive cytotoxicity. *Nat. Commun.* **2021**, *12*, 5217. [CrossRef]
153. Gao, S.; Wu, Z.; Arnold, B.; Diamond, C.; Batchu, S.; Giudice, V.; Alemu, L.; Raffo, D.Q.; Feng, X.; Kajigaya, S.; et al. Single-cell RNA sequencing coupled to TCR profiling of large granular lymphocyte leukemia T cells. *Nat. Commun.* **2022**, *13*, 1982. [CrossRef] [PubMed]
154. Frank, M.L.; Lu, K.; Erdogan, C.; Han, Y.; Hu, J.; Wang, T.; Heymach, J.V.; Zhang, J.; Reuben, A. T-Cell Receptor Repertoire Sequencing in the Era of Cancer Immunotherapy. *Clin. Cancer Res.* **2023**, *29*, 994–1008. [CrossRef]
155. Kato, T.; Matsuda, T.; Ikeda, Y.; Park, J.H.; Leisegang, M.; Yoshimura, S.; Hikichi, T.; Harada, M.; Zewde, M.; Sato, S.; et al. Effective screening of T cells recognizing neoantigens and construction of T-cell receptor-engineered T cells. *Oncotarget* **2018**, *9*, 11009–11019. [CrossRef] [PubMed]
156. Zong, S.; Mi, T.; Flores, L.G., 2nd; Alpert, A.; Olivares, S.; Patel, K.; Maiti, S.; McNamara, G.; Cooper, L.J.N.; Torikai, H. Very rapid cloning, expression and identifying specificity of T-cell receptors for T-cell engineering. *PLoS ONE* **2020**, *15*, e0228112. [CrossRef] [PubMed]
157. Danilova, L.; Anagnostou, V.; Caushi, J.X.; Sidhom, J.W.; Guo, H.; Chan, H.Y.; Suri, P.; Tam, A.; Zhang, J.; Asmar, M.E.; et al. The Mutation-Associated Neoantigen Functional Expansion of Specific T Cells (MANAFEST) Assay: A Sensitive Platform for Monitoring Antitumor Immunity. *Cancer Immunol. Res.* **2018**, *6*, 888–899. [CrossRef]
158. Guil-Luna, S.; Sedlik, C.; Piaggio, E. Humanized Mouse Models to Evaluate Cancer Immunotherapeutics. *Annu. Rev. Cancer Biol.* **2021**, *5*, 119–136. [CrossRef]
159. Zhang, X.; Kim, S.; Hundal, J.; Herndon, J.M.; Li, S.; Petti, A.A.; Soysal, S.D.; Li, L.; McLellan, M.D.; Hoog, J.; et al. Breast Cancer Neoantigens Can Induce $CD8^+$ T-Cell Responses and Antitumor Immunity. *Cancer Immunol. Res.* **2017**, *5*, 516–523. [CrossRef]
160. Vijh, S.; Pilip, I.M.; Pamer, E.G. Effect of antigen-processing efficiency on in vivo T cell response magnitudes. *J. Immunol.* **1998**, *160*, 3971–3977. [CrossRef]
161. Lopez, J.S.; Camidge, R.; Iafolla, M.; Rottey, S.; Schuler, M.; Hellmann, M.; Balmanoukian, A.; Dirix, L.; Gordon, M.; Sullivan, R.; et al. A phase Ib study to evaluate RO7198457, an individualized Neoantigen Specific immunoTherapy (iNeST), in combination with atezolizumab in patients with locally advanced or metastatic solid tumors. *Cancer Res.* **2020**, *80*, CT301. [CrossRef]
162. Van Pul, K.M.; Fransen, M.F.; van de Ven, R.; de Gruijl, T.D. Immunotherapy Goes Local: The Central Role of Lymph Nodes in Driving Tumor Infiltration and Efficacy. *Front. Immunol.* **2021**, *12*, 643291. [CrossRef] [PubMed]
163. Cochran, A.J.; Huang, R.R.; Lee, J.; Itakura, E.; Leong, S.P.; Essner, R. Tumour-induced immune modulation of sentinel lymph nodes. *Nat. Rev. Immunol.* **2006**, *6*, 659–670. [CrossRef]
164. Norbury, C.C.; Basta, S.; Donohue, K.B.; Tscharke, D.C.; Princiotta, M.F.; Berglund, P.; Gibbs, J.; Bennink, J.R.; Yewdell, J.W. CD8+ T cell cross-priming via transfer of proteasome substrates. *Science* **2004**, *304*, 1318–1321. [CrossRef]
165. Ho, N.I.; Huis In't Veld, L.G.M.; Raaijmakers, T.K.; Adema, G.J. Adjuvants Enhancing Cross-Presentation by Dendritic Cells: The Key to More Effective Vaccines? *Front. Immunol.* **2018**, *9*, 2874. [CrossRef]
166. Wiethoff, C.M.; Middaugh, C.R. Barriers to nonviral gene delivery. *J. Pharm. Sci.* **2003**, *92*, 203–217. [CrossRef] [PubMed]
167. Hobernik, D.; Bros, M. DNA Vaccines-How Far From Clinical Use? *Int. J. Mol. Sci.* **2018**, *19*, 3605. [CrossRef] [PubMed]
168. Disis, M.L.N.; Guthrie, K.A.; Liu, Y.; Coveler, A.L.; Higgins, D.M.; Childs, J.S.; Dang, Y.; Salazar, L.G. Safety and Outcomes of a Plasmid DNA Vaccine Encoding the ERBB2 Intracellular Domain in Patients with Advanced-Stage ERBB2-Positive Breast Cancer: A Phase 1 Nonrandomized Clinical Trial. *JAMA Oncol.* **2023**, *9*, 71–78. [CrossRef]
169. Schalk, J.A.; Mooi, F.R.; Berbers, G.A.; van Aerts, L.A.; Ovelgönne, H.; Kimman, T.G. Preclinical and clinical safety studies on DNA vaccines. *Hum. Vaccin.* **2006**, *2*, 45–53. [CrossRef]
170. Fioretti, D.; Iurescia, S.; Rinaldi, M. Recent advances in design of immunogenic and effective naked DNA vaccines against cancer. *Recent. Pat. Anticancer. Drug Discov.* **2014**, *9*, 66–82. [CrossRef]
171. Faurez, F.; Dory, D.; Le Moigne, V.; Gravier, R.; Jestin, A. Biosafety of DNA vaccines: New generation of DNA vectors and current knowledge on the fate of plasmids after injection. *Vaccine* **2010**, *28*, 3888–3895. [CrossRef] [PubMed]
172. Khobragade, A.; Bhate, S.; Ramaiah, V.; Deshpande, S.; Giri, K.; Phophle, H.; Supe, P.; Godara, I.; Revanna, R.; Nagarkar, R.; et al. Efficacy, safety, and immunogenicity of the DNA SARS-CoV-2 vaccine (ZyCoV-D): The interim efficacy results of a phase 3, randomised, double-blind, placebo-controlled study in India. *Lancet* **2022**, *399*, 1313–1321. [CrossRef]
173. Ndeupen, S.; Qin, Z.; Jacobsen, S.; Bouteau, A.; Estanbouli, H.; Igyártó, B.Z. The mRNA-LNP platform's lipid nanoparticle component used in preclinical vaccine studies is highly inflammatory. *iScience* **2021**, *24*, 103479. [CrossRef]

174. Baden, L.R.; El Sahly, H.M.; Essink, B.; Kotloff, K.; Frey, S.; Novak, R.; Diemert, D.; Spector, S.A.; Rouphael, N.; Creech, C.B.; et al. Efficacy and Safety of the mRNA-1273 SARS-CoV-2 Vaccine. *N. Engl. J. Med.* **2021**, *384*, 403–416. [CrossRef]
175. Liu, M.A. A Comparison of Plasmid DNA and mRNA as Vaccine Technologies. *Vaccines* **2019**, *7*, 37. [CrossRef]
176. Ledwith, B.J.; Manam, S.; Troilo, P.J.; Barnum, A.B.; Pauley, C.J.; Griffiths, T.G., 2nd; Harper, L.B.; Beare, C.M.; Bagdon, W.J.; Nichols, W.W. Plasmid DNA vaccines: Investigation of integration into host cellular DNA following intramuscular injection in mice. *Intervirology* **2000**, *43*, 258–272. [CrossRef]
177. Li, Y.D.; Chi, W.Y.; Su, J.H.; Ferrall, L.; Hung, C.F.; Wu, T.C. Coronavirus vaccine development: From SARS and MERS to COVID-19. *J. Biomed. Sci.* **2020**, *27*, 104. [CrossRef] [PubMed]
178. Soltani, S.; Farahani, A.; Dastranj, M.; Momenifar, N.; Mohajeri, P.; Emamie, A.D. Dna Vaccine: Methods and Mechanisms. *Adv. Hum. Biol.* **2018**, *8*, 132–139. [CrossRef]
179. Jorritsma, S.H.T.; Gowans, E.J.; Grubor-Bauk, B.; Wijesundara, D.K. Delivery methods to increase cellular uptake and immunogenicity of DNA vaccines. *Vaccine* **2016**, *34*, 5488–5494. [CrossRef]
180. Hauser, H.; Chen, S.Y. Augmentation of DNA vaccine potency through secretory heat shock protein-mediated antigen targeting. *Methods* **2003**, *31*, 225–231. [CrossRef] [PubMed]
181. Trimble, C.L.; Peng, S.; Kos, F.; Gravitt, P.; Viscidi, R.; Sugar, E.; Pardoll, D.; Wu, T.C. A phase I trial of a human papillomavirus DNA vaccine for HPV16+ cervical intraepithelial neoplasia 2/3. *Clin. Cancer Res.* **2009**, *15*, 361–367. [CrossRef]
182. Hung, C.F.; Hsu, K.F.; Cheng, W.F.; Chai, C.Y.; He, L.; Ling, M.; Wu, T.C. Enhancement of DNA vaccine potency by linkage of antigen gene to a gene encoding the extracellular domain of Fms-like tyrosine kinase 3-ligand. *Cancer Res.* **2001**, *61*, 1080–1088.
183. Choi, Y.J.; Hur, S.Y.; Kim, T.J.; Hong, S.R.; Lee, J.K.; Cho, C.H.; Park, K.S.; Woo, J.W.; Sung, Y.C.; Suh, Y.S.; et al. A Phase II, Prospective, Randomized, Multicenter, Open-Label Study of GX-188E, an HPV DNA Vaccine, in Patients with Cervical Intraepithelial Neoplasia 3. *Clin. Cancer Res.* **2020**, *26*, 1616–1623. [CrossRef]
184. Cheng, W.F.; Hung, C.F.; Chai, C.Y.; Hsu, K.F.; He, L.; Ling, M.; Wu, T.C. Tumor-specific immunity and antiangiogenesis generated by a DNA vaccine encoding calreticulin linked to a tumor antigen. *J. Clin. Investig.* **2001**, *108*, 669–678. [CrossRef]
185. Garcia, F.; Petry, K.U.; Muderspach, L.; Gold, M.A.; Braly, P.; Crum, C.P.; Magill, M.; Silverman, M.; Urban, R.G.; Hedley, M.L.; et al. ZYC101a for treatment of high-grade cervical intraepithelial neoplasia: A randomized controlled trial. *Obstet. Gynecol.* **2004**, *103*, 317–326. [CrossRef]
186. Matijevic, M.; Hedley, M.L.; Urban, R.G.; Chicz, R.M.; Lajoie, C.; Luby, T.M. Immunization with a poly (lactide co-glycolide) encapsulated plasmid DNA expressing antigenic regions of HPV 16 and 18 results in an increase in the precursor frequency of T cells that respond to epitopes from HPV 16, 18, 6 and 11. *Cell Immunol.* **2011**, *270*, 62–69. [CrossRef]
187. Kabachinski, G.; Schwartz, T.U. The nuclear pore complex--structure and function at a glance. *J. Cell Sci.* **2015**, *128*, 423–429. [CrossRef]
188. Dean, D.A. Cell-specific targeting strategies for electroporation-mediated gene delivery in cells and animals. *J. Membr. Biol.* **2013**, *246*, 737–744. [CrossRef]
189. Cervia, L.D.; Yuan, F. Current Progress in Electrotransfection as a Nonviral Method for Gene Delivery. *Mol. Pharm.* **2018**, *15*, 3617–3624. [CrossRef]
190. Dietz, W.M.; Skinner, N.E.; Hamilton, S.E.; Jund, M.D.; Heitfeld, S.M.; Litterman, A.J.; Hwu, P.; Chen, Z.Y.; Salazar, A.M.; Ohlfest, J.R.; et al. Minicircle DNA is superior to plasmid DNA in eliciting antigen-specific CD8+ T-cell responses. *Mol. Ther.* **2013**, *21*, 1526–1535. [CrossRef]
191. Chen, Z.Y.; He, C.Y.; Ehrhardt, A.; Kay, M.A. Minicircle DNA vectors devoid of bacterial DNA result in persistent and high-level transgene expression in vivo. *Mol. Ther.* **2003**, *8*, 495–500. [CrossRef] [PubMed]
192. Boye, C.; Arpag, S.; Francis, M.; DeClemente, S.; West, A.; Heller, R.; Bulysheva, A. Reduction of plasmid vector backbone length enhances reporter gene expression. *Bioelectrochemistry* **2022**, *144*, 107981. [CrossRef] [PubMed]
193. Darquet, A.M.; Cameron, B.; Wils, P.; Scherman, D.; Crouzet, J. A new DNA vehicle for nonviral gene delivery: Supercoiled minicircle. *Gene Ther.* **1997**, *4*, 1341–1349. [CrossRef]
194. Bigger, B.W.; Tolmachov, O.; Collombet, J.M.; Fragkos, M.; Palaszewski, I.; Coutelle, C. An araC-controlled bacterial cre expression system to produce DNA minicircle vectors for nuclear and mitochondrial gene therapy. *J. Biol. Chem.* **2001**, *276*, 23018–23027. [CrossRef] [PubMed]
195. Mayrhofer, P.; Blaesen, M.; Schleef, M.; Jechlinger, W. Minicircle-DNA production by site specific recombination and protein-DNA interaction chromatography. *J. Gene Med.* **2008**, *10*, 1253–1269. [CrossRef]
196. Williams, J.A.; Luke, J.; Johnson, L.; Hodgson, C. pDNAVACCultra vector family: High throughput intracellular targeting DNA vaccine plasmids. *Vaccine* **2006**, *24*, 4671–4676. [CrossRef]
197. Luke, J.; Carnes, A.E.; Hodgson, C.P.; Williams, J.A. Improved antibiotic-free DNA vaccine vectors utilizing a novel RNA based plasmid selection system. *Vaccine* **2009**, *27*, 6454–6459. [CrossRef]
198. Williams, J.A.; Paez, P.A. Improving cell and gene therapy safety and performance using next-generation Nanoplasmid vectors. *Mol. Ther. Nucleic Acids* **2023**, *32*, 494–503. [CrossRef]

199. Adie, T.; Orefo, I.; Kysh, D.; Kondas, K.; Thapa, S.; Extance, J.; Duncan, T.; Rothwell, P.J. dbDNA™: An advanced platform for genetic medicines. *Drug Discov. Today* **2022**, *27*, 374–377. [CrossRef]
200. Chalmers, Z.R.; Connelly, C.F.; Fabrizio, D.; Gay, L.; Ali, S.M.; Ennis, R.; Schrock, A.; Campbell, B.; Shlien, A.; Chmielecki, J.; et al. Analysis of 100,000 human cancer genomes reveals the landscape of tumor mutational burden. *Genome Med.* **2017**, *9*, 34. [CrossRef] [PubMed]
201. Zehir, A.; Benayed, R.; Shah, R.H.; Syed, A.; Middha, S.; Kim, H.R.; Srinivasan, P.; Gao, J.; Chakravarty, D.; Devlin, S.M.; et al. Mutational landscape of metastatic cancer revealed from prospective clinical sequencing of 10,000 patients. *Nat. Med.* **2017**, *23*, 703–713. [CrossRef] [PubMed]
202. Alexandrov, L.B.; Nik-Zainal, S.; Wedge, D.C.; Aparicio, S.A.; Behjati, S.; Biankin, A.V.; Bignell, G.R.; Bolli, N.; Borg, A.; Børresen-Dale, A.L.; et al. Signatures of mutational processes in human cancer. *Nature* **2013**, *500*, 415–421. [CrossRef] [PubMed]
203. Cullinan, D.; McLellan, M.; Zhang, X.; Vickery, T.; Myers, N.; Sturmoski, M.; Ruzinova, M.; Hundal, J.; Miller, C.; Griffith, M.; et al. Preliminary Results Of A Phase Ib Clinical Trial Of A Neoantigen Dna Vaccine For Pancreatic Cancer. *HPB* **2020**, *22*, S12–S13. [CrossRef]
204. Ochsenreither, S.; Anguera, G.; Dieter, S.; Trikalinos, N.; Fu, S.; Fernández, B.C.; Ferrándiz, A.C.; Kim, S.Y.; Rodriguez, L.M.; Berg, K.C.G.; et al. Induction of neoantigen-specific immune responses by VB10.NEO in combination with atezolizumab in heavily pretreated patients with advanced solid tumors: Final analysis of the phase 1b VB N-02 trial. *J. Clin. Oncol.* **2025**, *43*, 2639. [CrossRef]
205. Shah, K.; Ganapathy, A.; Borkowski, A.; Shah, N.; Bansal, D.; Beck, R.; Knoche, E.M.; Picus, J.; Reimers, M.A.; Roth, B.J.; et al. A pilot trial of neoantigen DNA vaccine in combination with nivolumab/ipilimumab and prostvac in metastatic hormone-sensitive prostate cancer (mHSPC). *J. Clin. Oncol.* **2022**, *40*, 5068. [CrossRef]
206. Johanns, T.M.; Garfinkle, E.A.R.; Miller, K.E.; Livingstone, A.J.; Roberts, K.F.; Rao Venkata, L.P.; Dowling, J.L.; Chicoine, M.R.; Dacey, R.G.; Zipfel, G.J.; et al. Integrating Multisector Molecular Characterization into Personalized Peptide Vaccine Design for Patients with Newly Diagnosed Glioblastoma. *Clin. Cancer Res.* **2024**, *30*, 2729–2742. [CrossRef]
207. ClinicalTrials.gov. Neoantigen-based Personalized DNA Vaccine with Retifanlimab PD-1 Blockade Therapy in Patients with Newly Diagnosed, Unmethylated Glioblastoma. (NCT05743595). Identifier: NCT05743595. Available online: https://clinicaltrials.gov/study/NCT05743595 (accessed on 27 August 2025).
208. ClinicalTrials.gov. Neoepitope_based Personalized DNA Vaccine Approach in Pediatric Patients with Recurrent Brain Tumors. (NCT03988283). Identifier: NCT03988283. Available online: https://clinicaltrials.gov/study/NCT03988283 (accessed on 27 August 2025).
209. ClinicalTrials.gov. PolyImmune {Durvalumad (MEDI4736) and Tremelimumab} & Vaccine Ochaestrated Treatment for Patients with Advanced/Metastatic Renal Cell Carcinoma (PIVOT-RCC). (NCT03598816). Identifier: NCT03598816. Available online: https://clinicaltrials.gov/study/NCT03598816 (accessed on 27 August 2025).
210. ClinicalTrials.gov. Personalized Neoantigen Vaccine in Combination with Durvalumab (MEDI4736) in Extensive Stage Small Cell Lung Cancer. (NCT04397003) Identifier: NCT04397003. Available online: https://clinicaltrials.gov/study/NCT04397003 (accessed on 27 August 2025).
211. Daniela, K.-K.; Nadia, V.; Michail, A.P.; Mads, L.; Thomas, T.; Nikolas, H.T.; Christian, G.; Anders, J.; Thomas, S.J.; Britt, W.L.; et al. 623 AI-designed personalized neoantigen vaccine, EVX-02, induces robust T-cell responses in melanoma patients. *J. Immunother. Cancer* **2023**, *11*, 623. [CrossRef]
212. Thomas, S.K.; Cha, S.C.; Smith, D.L.; Kim, K.H.; Parshottam, S.R.; Rao, S.; Popescu, M.; Lee, V.Y.; Neelapu, S.S.; Kwak, L.W. Phase I study of an active immunotherapy for asymptomatic phase Lymphoplasmacytic lymphoma with DNA vaccines encoding antigen-chemokine fusion: Study protocol. *BMC Cancer* **2018**, *18*, 187. [CrossRef] [PubMed]
213. Szymura, S.J.; Wang, L.; Zhang, T.; Cha, S.C.; Song, J.; Dong, Z.; Anderson, A.; Oh, E.; Lee, V.; Wang, Z.; et al. Personalized neoantigen vaccines as early intervention in untreated patients with lymphoplasmacytic lymphoma: A non-randomized phase 1 trial. *Nat. Commun.* **2024**, *15*, 6874. [CrossRef] [PubMed]
214. King, D.A.; Smith, A.R.; Pineda, G.; Nakano, M.; Michelini, F.; Goedegebuure, S.P.; Thyparambil, S.; Liao, W.-L.; McCormick, A.; Ju, J.; et al. Complete Remission of Widely Metastatic Human Epidermal Growth Factor Receptor 2–Amplified Pancreatic Adenocarcinoma After Precision Immune and Targeted Therapy with Description of Sequencing and Organoid Correlates. *JCO Precis. Oncol.* **2023**, *7*, e2100489. [CrossRef]
215. Garfinkle, E.A.; Miller, K.E.; Livingstone, A.J.; Perales-Linares, R.; Cooch, N.; Perales-Puchalt, A.; Rochestie, S.; Peters, J.; Sardesai, N.Y.; Gillanders, W.E.; et al. Abstract 1174: Incorporation of multisector analysis into the design of personalized DNA vaccines for patients with newly diagnosed glioblastoma. *Cancer Res.* **2024**, *84*, 1174. [CrossRef]
216. Pandya, A.; Shah, Y.; Kothari, N.; Postwala, H.; Shah, A.; Parekh, P.; Chorawala, M.R. The future of cancer immunotherapy: DNA vaccines leading the way. *Med. Oncol.* **2023**, *40*, 200. [CrossRef]

217. Xia, Q.; Zhang, F.F.; Geng, F.; Liu, C.L.; Wang, Y.Q.; Xu, P.; Lu, Z.Z.; Xie, Y.; Wu, H.; Chen, Y.; et al. Improvement of anti-tumor immunity of fibroblast activation protein α based vaccines by combination with cyclophosphamide in a murine model of breast cancer. *Cell Immunol.* **2016**, *310*, 89–98. [CrossRef] [PubMed]
218. Jagodinsky, J.C.; Harari, P.M.; Morris, Z.S. The Promise of Combining Radiation Therapy with Immunotherapy. *Int. J. Radiat. Oncol. Biol. Phys.* **2020**, *108*, 6–16. [CrossRef]
219. Rupp, T.; Genest, L.; Babin, D.; Legrand, C.; Hunault, M.; Froget, G.; Castagné, V. Anti-CTLA-4 and anti-PD-1 immunotherapies repress tumor progression in preclinical breast and colon model with independent regulatory T cells response. *Transl. Oncol.* **2022**, *20*, 101405. [CrossRef]
220. Zappasodi, R.; Serganova, I.; Cohen, I.J.; Maeda, M.; Shindo, M.; Senbabaoglu, Y.; Watson, M.J.; Leftin, A.; Maniyar, R.; Verma, S.; et al. CTLA-4 blockade drives loss of T(reg) stability in glycolysis-low tumours. *Nature* **2021**, *591*, 652–658. [CrossRef]
221. Soong, R.S.; Trieu, J.; Lee, S.Y.; He, L.; Tsai, Y.C.; Wu, T.C.; Hung, C.F. Xenogeneic human p53 DNA vaccination by electroporation breaks immune tolerance to control murine tumors expressing mouse p53. *PLoS ONE* **2013**, *8*, e56912. [CrossRef]
222. Yang, B.; Jeang, J.; Yang, A.; Wu, T.C.; Hung, C.F. DNA vaccine for cancer immunotherapy. *Hum. Vaccin. Immunother.* **2014**, *10*, 3153–3164. [CrossRef] [PubMed]
223. Dhatchinamoorthy, K.; Colbert, J.D.; Rock, K.L. Cancer Immune Evasion Through Loss of MHC Class I Antigen Presentation. *Front. Immunol.* **2021**, *12*, 636568. [CrossRef] [PubMed]
224. Cheever, M.A.; Allison, J.P.; Ferris, A.S.; Finn, O.J.; Hastings, B.M.; Hecht, T.T.; Mellman, I.; Prindiville, S.A.; Viner, J.L.; Weiner, L.M.; et al. The prioritization of cancer antigens: A national cancer institute pilot project for the acceleration of translational research. *Clin. Cancer Res.* **2009**, *15*, 5323–5337. [CrossRef] [PubMed]
225. Cornel, A.M.; Mimpen, I.L.; Nierkens, S. MHC Class I Downregulation in Cancer: Underlying Mechanisms and Potential Targets for Cancer Immunotherapy. *Cancers* **2020**, *12*, 1760. [CrossRef]
226. Propper, D.J.; Chao, D.; Braybrooke, J.P.; Bahl, P.; Thavasu, P.; Balkwill, F.; Turley, H.; Dobbs, N.; Gatter, K.; Talbot, D.C.; et al. Low-dose IFN-gamma induces tumor MHC expression in metastatic malignant melanoma. *Clin. Cancer Res.* **2003**, *9*, 84–92.
227. Parikh, F.; Duluc, D.; Imai, N.; Clark, A.; Misiukiewicz, K.; Bonomi, M.; Gupta, V.; Patsias, A.; Parides, M.; Demicco, E.G.; et al. Chemoradiotherapy-induced upregulation of PD-1 antagonizes immunity to HPV-related oropharyngeal cancer. *Cancer Res.* **2014**, *74*, 7205–7216. [CrossRef]
228. Barker, H.E.; Paget, J.T.; Khan, A.A.; Harrington, K.J. The tumour microenvironment after radiotherapy: Mechanisms of resistance and recurrence. *Nat. Rev. Cancer* **2015**, *15*, 409–425. [CrossRef]
229. van Meir, H.; Nout, R.A.; Welters, M.J.; Loof, N.M.; de Kam, M.L.; van Ham, J.J.; Samuels, S.; Kenter, G.G.; Cohen, A.F.; Melief, C.J.; et al. Impact of (chemo)radiotherapy on immune cell composition and function in cervical cancer patients. *Oncoimmunology* **2017**, *6*, e1267095. [CrossRef] [PubMed]
230. Dersh, D.; Phelan, J.D.; Gumina, M.E.; Wang, B.; Arbuckle, J.H.; Holly, J.; Kishton, R.J.; Markowitz, T.E.; Seedhom, M.O.; Fridlyand, N.; et al. Genome-wide Screens Identify Lineage- and Tumor-Specific Genes Modulating MHC-I- and MHC-II-Restricted Immunosurveillance of Human Lymphomas. *Immunity* **2021**, *54*, 116–131.e110. [CrossRef] [PubMed]
231. Bailey, C.; Pich, O.; Thol, K.; Watkins, T.B.K.; Luebeck, J.; Rowan, A.; Stavrou, G.; Weiser, N.E.; Dameracharla, B.; Bentham, R.; et al. Origins and impact of extrachromosomal DNA. *Nature* **2024**, *635*, 193–200. [CrossRef] [PubMed]
232. Pecorino, L.T.; Verhaak, R.G.W.; Henssen, A.; Mischel, P.S. Extrachromosomal DNA (ecDNA): An origin of tumor heterogeneity, genomic remodeling, and drug resistance. *Biochem. Soc. Trans.* **2022**, *50*, 1911–1920. [CrossRef]
233. Bafna, V.; Mischel, P.S. Extrachromosomal DNA in Cancer. *Annu. Rev. Genom. Hum. Genet.* **2022**, *23*, 29–52. [CrossRef]
234. Melief, C.J.; van der Burg, S.H. Immunotherapy of established (pre)malignant disease by synthetic long peptide vaccines. *Nat. Rev. Cancer* **2008**, *8*, 351–360. [CrossRef]
235. Shen, L.; Zhang, J.; Lee, H.; Batista, M.T.; Johnston, S.A. RNA Transcription and Splicing Errors as a Source of Cancer Frameshift Neoantigens for Vaccines. *Sci. Rep.* **2019**, *9*, 14184. [CrossRef]
236. Lange, J.T.; Rose, J.C.; Chen, C.Y.; Pichugin, Y.; Xie, L.; Tang, J.; Hung, K.L.; Yost, K.E.; Shi, Q.; Erb, M.L.; et al. The evolutionary dynamics of extrachromosomal DNA in human cancers. *Nat. Genet.* **2022**, *54*, 1527–1533. [CrossRef]
237. Wu, A.A.; Drake, V.; Huang, H.-S.; Chiu, S.; Zheng, L. Reprogramming the tumor microenvironment: Tumor-induced immunosuppressive factors paralyze T cells. *OncoImmunology* **2015**, *4*, e1016700. [CrossRef]
238. Maley, C.C.; Aktipis, A.; Graham, T.A.; Sottoriva, A.; Boddy, A.M.; Janiszewska, M.; Silva, A.S.; Gerlinger, M.; Yuan, Y.; Pienta, K.J.; et al. Classifying the evolutionary and ecological features of neoplasms. *Nat. Rev. Cancer* **2017**, *17*, 605–619. [CrossRef] [PubMed]
239. Merlo, L.M.; Pepper, J.W.; Reid, B.J.; Maley, C.C. Cancer as an evolutionary and ecological process. *Nat. Rev. Cancer* **2006**, *6*, 924–935. [CrossRef]
240. Thomas, D.; Radhakrishnan, P. Tumor-stromal crosstalk in pancreatic cancer and tissue fibrosis. *Mol. Cancer* **2019**, *18*, 14. [CrossRef] [PubMed]

241. Yamamoto, K.; Iwadate, D.; Kato, H.; Nakai, Y.; Tateishi, K.; Fujishiro, M. Targeting the Metabolic Rewiring in Pancreatic Cancer and Its Tumor Microenvironment. *Cancers* **2022**, *14*, 4351. [CrossRef]
242. Dey, A.; Varelas, X.; Guan, K.L. Targeting the Hippo pathway in cancer, fibrosis, wound healing and regenerative medicine. *Nat. Rev. Drug Discov.* **2020**, *19*, 480–494. [CrossRef]
243. Lee, J.H.; Massagué, J. TGF-β in developmental and fibrogenic EMTs. *Semin. Cancer Biol.* **2022**, *86*, 136–145. [CrossRef]
244. Gonzalez, D.M.; Medici, D. Signaling mechanisms of the epithelial-mesenchymal transition. *Sci. Signal* **2014**, *7*, re8. [CrossRef]
245. Minchinton, A.I.; Tannock, I.F. Drug penetration in solid tumours. *Nat. Rev. Cancer* **2006**, *6*, 583–592. [CrossRef] [PubMed]
246. Kohli, K.; Pillarisetty, V.G.; Kim, T.S. Key chemokines direct migration of immune cells in solid tumors. *Cancer Gene Ther.* **2022**, *29*, 10–21. [CrossRef] [PubMed]
247. Furumoto, K.; Soares, L.; Engleman, E.G.; Merad, M. Induction of potent antitumor immunity by in situ targeting of intratumoral DCs. *J. Clin. Investig.* **2004**, *113*, 774–783. [CrossRef]
248. Olive, K.P.; Jacobetz, M.A.; Davidson, C.J.; Gopinathan, A.; McIntyre, D.; Honess, D.; Madhu, B.; Goldgraben, M.A.; Caldwell, M.E.; Allard, D.; et al. Inhibition of Hedgehog signaling enhances delivery of chemotherapy in a mouse model of pancreatic cancer. *Science* **2009**, *324*, 1457–1461. [CrossRef]
249. Finn, O.J. The dawn of vaccines for cancer prevention. *Nat. Rev. Immunol.* **2018**, *18*, 183–194. [CrossRef]
250. Sahin, U.; Türeci, Ö. Personalized vaccines for cancer immunotherapy. *Science* **2018**, *359*, 1355–1360. [CrossRef]
251. Melief, C.J. Cancer immunotherapy by dendritic cells. *Immunity* **2008**, *29*, 372–383. [CrossRef] [PubMed]
252. Ott, P.A.; Hu, Z.; Keskin, D.B.; Shukla, S.A.; Sun, J.; Bozym, D.J.; Zhang, W.; Luoma, A.; Giobbie-Hurder, A.; Peter, L.; et al. An immunogenic personal neoantigen vaccine for patients with melanoma. *Nature* **2017**, *547*, 217–221. [CrossRef] [PubMed]
253. Sahin, U.; Derhovanessian, E.; Miller, M.; Kloke, B.P.; Simon, P.; Löwer, M.; Bukur, V.; Tadmor, A.D.; Luxemburger, U.; Schrörs, B.; et al. Personalized RNA mutanome vaccines mobilize poly-specific therapeutic immunity against cancer. *Nature* **2017**, *547*, 222–226. [CrossRef]
254. Labani-Motlagh, A.; Ashja-Mahdavi, M.; Loskog, A. The Tumor Microenvironment: A Milieu Hindering and Obstructing Antitumor Immune Responses. *Front. Immunol.* **2020**, *11*, 940. [CrossRef]
255. Gabai, Y.; Assouline, B.; Ben-Porath, I. Senescent stromal cells: Roles in the tumor microenvironment. *Trends Cancer* **2023**, *9*, 28–41. [CrossRef]
256. Topalian, S.L.; Taube, J.M.; Anders, R.A.; Pardoll, D.M. Mechanism-driven biomarkers to guide immune checkpoint blockade in cancer therapy. *Nat. Rev. Cancer* **2016**, *16*, 275–287. [CrossRef] [PubMed]
257. Dong, H.; Strome, S.E.; Salomao, D.R.; Tamura, H.; Hirano, F.; Flies, D.B.; Roche, P.C.; Lu, J.; Zhu, G.; Tamada, K.; et al. Tumor-associated B7-H1 promotes T-cell apoptosis: A potential mechanism of immune evasion. *Nat. Med.* **2002**, *8*, 793–800. [CrossRef]
258. Derynck, R.; Turley, S.J.; Akhurst, R.J. TGFβ biology in cancer progression and immunotherapy. *Nat. Rev. Clin. Oncol.* **2021**, *18*, 9–34. [CrossRef]
259. Munn, D.H.; Mellor, A.L. Indoleamine 2,3-dioxygenase and tumor-induced tolerance. *J. Clin. Investig.* **2007**, *117*, 1147–1154. [CrossRef]
260. Saraiva, M.; Vieira, P.; O'Garra, A. Biology and therapeutic potential of interleukin-10. *J. Exp. Med.* **2020**, *217*, e20190418. [CrossRef]
261. Farmer, E.; Cheng, M.A.; Hung, C.F.; Wu, T.C. Vaccination Strategies for the Control and Treatment of HPV Infection and HPV-Associated Cancer. *Recent Results Cancer Res.* **2021**, *217*, 157–195. [CrossRef]
262. Hauge, A.; Rofstad, E.K. Antifibrotic therapy to normalize the tumor microenvironment. *J. Transl. Med.* **2020**, *18*, 207. [CrossRef]
263. Cha, J.H.; Chan, L.C.; Li, C.W.; Hsu, J.L.; Hung, M.C. Mechanisms Controlling PD-L1 Expression in Cancer. *Mol. Cell* **2019**, *76*, 359–370. [CrossRef]
264. Lee, N.Y.; Sherman, E.J.; Schöder, H.; Wray, R.; Boyle, J.O.; Singh, B.; Grkovski, M.; Paudyal, R.; Cunningham, L.; Zhang, Z.; et al. Hypoxia-Directed Treatment of Human Papillomavirus-Related Oropharyngeal Carcinoma. *J. Clin. Oncol.* **2024**, *42*, 940–950. [CrossRef] [PubMed]
265. Leone, R.D.; Powell, J.D. Fueling the Revolution: Targeting Metabolism to Enhance Immunotherapy. *Cancer Immunol. Res.* **2021**, *9*, 255–260. [CrossRef]
266. McLane, L.M.; Abdel-Hakeem, M.S.; Wherry, E.J. CD8 T Cell Exhaustion During Chronic Viral Infection and Cancer. *Annu. Rev. Immunol.* **2019**, *37*, 457–495. [CrossRef] [PubMed]
267. Cafri, G.; Gartner, J.J.; Zaks, T.; Hopson, K.; Levin, N.; Paria, B.C.; Parkhurst, M.R.; Yossef, R.; Lowery, F.J.; Jafferji, M.S.; et al. mRNA vaccine-induced neoantigen-specific T cell immunity in patients with gastrointestinal cancer. *J. Clin. Investig.* **2020**, *130*, 5976–5988. [CrossRef]
268. Zhang, Z.; Liu, S.; Zhang, B.; Qiao, L.; Zhang, Y.; Zhang, Y. T Cell Dysfunction and Exhaustion in Cancer. *Front. Cell Dev. Biol.* **2020**, *8*, 17. [CrossRef] [PubMed]

269. De Visser, K.E.; Joyce, J.A. The evolving tumor microenvironment: From cancer initiation to metastatic outgrowth. *Cancer Cell* **2023**, *41*, 374–403. [CrossRef] [PubMed]
270. Koup, R.A.; Douek, D.C. Vaccine design for CD8 T lymphocyte responses. *Cold Spring Harb. Perspect. Med.* **2011**, *1*, a007252. [CrossRef] [PubMed]
271. Riaz, N.; Havel, J.J.; Makarov, V.; Desrichard, A.; Urba, W.J.; Sims, J.S.; Hodi, F.S.; Martín-Algarra, S.; Mandal, R.; Sharfman, W.H.; et al. Tumor and Microenvironment Evolution during Immunotherapy with Nivolumab. *Cell* **2017**, *171*, 934–949.e916. [CrossRef] [PubMed]

Journal of *Personalized Medicine*

MDPI

Communication

The Role of Stereotactic Body Radiotherapy (SBRT) in Oligoprogressive Renal Cell Carcinoma (RCC) Treated with ICIs–TKIs: A Retrospective Multicentric Study

Maria La Vecchia [1], Manuela Federico [1,*], Dario Aiello [1], Valentina Zagardo [2], Antonella Mazzonello [1], Lorella Testa [1], Leonarda La Paglia [1], Tiziana Bruno [1] and Ivan Fazio [1]

1 Unità Operativa di Radioterapia Oncologica, Casa di Cura Macchiarella, 90138 Palermo, Italy; lavecchiamaria8@gmail.com (M.L.V.); dario_aiello@msn.com (D.A.); antonellamazzonella@alice.it (A.M.); lorellatesta@tiscali.it (L.T.); dina.lapaglia@gmail.com (L.L.P.); brtiziana@libero.it (T.B.); ivanfazio27@gmail.com (I.F.)

2 Unità Operativa di Radioterapia Oncologica, Rem Radioterapia srl, 95029 Viagrande, Italy; valentina.zagardo@gmail.com

* Correspondence: manuela.fed@gmail.com

Abstract: Background: This multicentric, retrospective study investigated the use of stereotactic body radiotherapy (SBRT) in patients (pts) with metastatic renal cell carcinoma (mRCC) who experienced oligoprogression during a combination therapy with an immune checkpoint inhibitor (ICI) and a tyrosine–kinase inhibitor (TKI). Methods: We retrospectively evaluated 34 pts affected by oligoprogressive RCC treated with an ICI–TKI combination between January 2020 and December 2023. SBRT was delivered to each site of oligoprogressive metastatic disease. After SBRT, pts were given follow-up clinical evaluations. 6–12–18-month local control (LC) rates and median next-line treatment-free survival (NEST-FS) were the primary endpoints. The secondary endpoints were overall response rate (ORR), clinical benefits and safety. Results: After a median follow-up of 24 months, 6–12–18-month LC rates were 100%, 71% and 43%, respectively, and the median NEST-FS was 20 months. ORR was 90%, while clinical benefit was 100%. No > G2 adverse events related to SBRT were recorded. Conclusions: In our study, SBRT for oligoprogressive mRCC turned out to be a safe and useful treatment which was able to preserve current treatment. Further prospective studies are necessary to explore the effects of the ICIs–TKIs combination and SBRT upon oligoprogressive sites in mRCC.

Keywords: renal cell carcinoma; immunotherapy; stereotactic body radiotherapy

1. Introduction

Renal cell carcinoma (RCC) represents about 2.4% of all cancers in adults, with more than 400,000 new cases diagnosed worldwide per year [1].

The 5-year survival rate for kidney cancer for all patients (pts) is approximately 71%.

Survival rates strongly depend on disease stage, declining to 67% when locoregional disease (stage III) is detected and 12% in pts with distant metastases [2,3].

About 25–30% of pts with locally advanced disease present synchronous metastases and a proportion between 15 and 25% will develop metastases after nephrectomy [4,5].

The standard of care for pts with metastatic RCC (mRCC) is systemic therapy [3].

At present, therapeutic options for first-line systemic treatment of mRCC include the following:

- combination therapies with an immune checkpoint inhibitor (ICI) and a tyrosine–kinase inhibitor (TKI);
- combination therapy with two ICIs;
- monotherapy with a TKI.

Combination therapies using ICIs–TKIs and ICI–ICI were shown to be more effective than monotherapy with a TKI in intermediate and poor-risk (according to IMDC criteria) mRCC.

Particularly, KEYNOTE426, Checkmate 9ER and Clear trials explored the use of axitinib–pembrolizumab, cabozantinib–nivolumab and lenvatinib–pembrolizumab combinations, respectively, showing they are more effective than monotherapy with sunitinib [6,7].

The Checkmate214 trial, instead, compared a ipilimumab–nivolumab combination to monotherapy with sunitinib, showing longer median progression-free survival (PFS) and overall survival (OS) for the ICI–ICI combination [7].

Unfortunately, even during these very effective systemic treatments, resistances to drugs are developed [8].

Resistance to systemic therapy manifests as generalized or oligometastatic (OM) disease progression. The OM state is an intermediate state that may benefit from local treatments, such as surgery or radiotherapy (RT) [9].

Through the use of stereotactic body radiotherapy technique (SBRT), which delivers high doses in small volumes, the radioresistance of RCC has been overcome. Moreover, SBRT may activate the immune system against tumor cells, improving the effect of immunotherapy and delaying the change of systemic treatment [10,11].

Evidence has shown that SBRT used to treat OM disease guarantees a good local control (LC) with a tolerable toxicity in the management of many tumors [12] and in the treatment of associated tumor symptoms; for example, in the case of a tumor thrombus in the inferior vena cava, it can shrink edema and improve pts' quality of life [13].

SABR-COMET is the first phase II randomized trial that assessed the impact of SBRT in patients with oligometastases belonging to multiple histologies. According to lesion location, which is the main cause of significant differences in LC rates, the overall long-term LC was better in patients who underwent SBRT [14].

Moreover, a long-term analysis of SABR-COMET showed improvements in OS with a median benefit of 22 months after a 5-year follow-up [14].

Therefore, even in mRCC, by using this strategy and combining RT with ICIs-based systemic treatments, LC may increase [9]. This study explores the role of SBRT in oligoprogressive mRCC treated with a first-line ICIs–TKIs combination.

2. Materials and Methods

We retrospectively evaluated 34 oligoprogressive mRCC pts and 56 metastases treated with ablative SBRT at the Department of Radiation Oncology of the Casa di Cura Macchiarella (Palermo, Italy) and at REM Department of IOM (Viagrande, Italy) between January 2020 and December 2023.

All pts signed an informed consent form before undergoing SBRT.

The indication for SBRT was given according to the following criteria: (1) Performance Status 0–2, (2) histologically proven primary RCC, (3) oligoprogressive lesion(s) during an ICIs–TKIs combination (<5 metastases), (4) oligoprogression detected after at least 6 months from the beginning of ICIs–TKIs treatment, and (5) almost 6 months follow-up. Pts receiving conventional fractionated radiation therapy, with the number of lesions at >5, without histologically proven primary RCC, were excluded. Patients with brain mts were excluded. Enrolled pts undergoing SBRT were treated with a dose of at least 6 Gy per fraction to a biologically effective dose (BED) of at least 90 Gy, using an α/β ratio of 3 Gy. Pts underwent computed tomography (CT)-based SBRT planning with a 3–5 mm slice thickness. Suitable immobilization devices were used, according to the site of the lesion. Diagnostic CT and MRI were co-registered with the planning CT to more accurately identify the target. Gross tumor volume (GTV), defined by means of morphologic and/or metabolic diagnostic instruments, was equivalent to the clinical target volume (CTV). The planning target volume (PTV) was defined by adding an isotropic 3–5 mm margin to the CTV. Organs at risk were delineated depending on the tumor site. The dose prescription depended on the volume and localization of oligometastases (OM). SBRT was delivered by

Linac-based external beam radiation with daily Image-Guided Radiotherapy (IGRT). Before each treatment, image guidance with kilovoltage (kV) cone beam CT scans were acquired and appropriate adjustments were made to correlate bony anatomy. In lung treatment, breath control was performed with lung protocols cone beam CT and respiratory gating. During SBRT, TKIs were interrupted. All pts underwent consecutive daily sessions from Monday to Friday, and no discontinuity of treatment was observed.

After SBRT, pts were radiologically evaluated with CTCT or magnetic resonance imaging (MRI), depending on baseline imaging. The LC of each lesion was assessed according to Response Evaluation Criteria from the Solid Tumors RECIST criteria. Disease progression at >5 metastatic sites led to a change of systemic treatment. If further oligoprogression occurred, a new course of SBRT was proposed if less than 5 new metastases were diagnosed. SBRT retreatment was not allowed.

Statistical Analysis

The primary endpoints were 6–12–18-month LC rates, defined as complete response (CR) and partial response (PR) of any duration or stable disease (SD) for at least 6 months from the start of RT in oligoprogressive sites. As coprimary endpoint, we chose next-line treatment-free survival (NEST-FS), defined as the time from the beginning of first-line systemic treatment to the change of systemic treatment. NEST-FS was first investigated and used as an endpoint in clinical trials exploring the use of metastases-directed therapies in other tumors, like prostate cancer, but has never been used in kidney cancer. However, it seems to be the most suitable endpoint to evaluate the role of metastases-directed therapies in oligoprogressive tumor disease. The secondary endpoints were overall response rate (ORR), defined as CR or PR of any duration after the start of RT, clinical benefits and safety.

3. Results

3.1. Patients Characteristics

A total of 34 pts with 56 oligoprogressive lesions receiving SBRT were retrospectively analyzed. The median age was 61 years (range 44–82). We evaluated 4 females and 30 males; 20, 10 and 4 pts had an ECOG PS of 0, 1 and 2, respectively. Pts'clinical characteristics are listed in Table 1. For mRCC, all pts received a first-line ICIs–TKIs combination. Particularly, 20 pts received a combination of axitinib–pembrolizumab, while 14 pts received cabozantinib–nivolumab. The best response to an ICIs–TKIs combination before SBRT was CR in 7, PR in 12 and SD in 15 pts. Imaging techniques used to detect oligoprogressive sites and evaluate responses to MDT were CT in 30 pts and MRI in 14 pts.

Table 1. Patients characteristics.

Variable	n	%
Age		
≤61	22	65
>61	12	35
Sex		
Male	30	88
Female	4	12
Performance status		
0	20	59
1	10	29
2	4	12
Metastatic sites undergone SBRT (56 metastases)		

Table 1. *Cont.*

Variable	n	%
bone	14	41
lung	20	58
lymph node	16	47
liver	2	6
adrenal	4	11
Imaging techniques		
CT	30	88
MRI	14	41
Systemic Therapy		
axitinib-pembrolizumab	20	59
cabozantinib-nivolumab	14	40
SBRT dose per fraction		
30 in 6 Gy per fractions	30	54
37.5 Gy in 7.5 Gy per fractions	22	38
50 Gy in 10 Gy per fractions	3	4
40 Gy in 8 Gy per fractions	1	2

SBRT was delivered to 14 bone, 16 nodal, 20 lung, 2 liver and 4 adrenal metastases. The median SBRT fraction and total dose were 6 Gy (6–10) and 30 Gy (30–50), respectively. The median number of fractions was 5 (3–5).

3.2. Treatment Outcomes

Treatment outcomes are summarized in Table 2.

Table 2. Treatment outcomes.

OUTCOMES	
6 months-LC	100%
12 months-LC	70%
24 months-LC	41%
Median NEST	20 months
SBRT RESPONSE RATE	
CR	53%
PR	35%
SD	20%
ORR	88%
Clinical Benefits	100%

The median follow-up was 24 months (range 6–42); 6–12–18-month LC rates were 100%, 70% and 41% respectively.

The median NEST-FS was 20 months (12–not reached). All pts had performed imaging control after a single course of SBRT: 53% experienced a CR, 35% a PR and 20% SD. No progressive disease was recorded. The ORR was 88% while the clinical benefit was 100%.

No > G2 adverse events related to SBRT were recorded.

4. Discussion

In mRCC progressing under first-line systemic treatment, the historical standard of care was based on the interruption of the current therapy and switching to a new line of treatment [14]. Historically, RCC has been considered a radioresistant tumor and RT was used only as palliative treatment, especially for brain and painful bone metastases. [15] In the last few years, with the employment of SBRT as a curative treatment to control oligoprogressive sites, radioresistance can be overcome and current therapy can be preserved [15,16].

In fact, according to the literature, it seems that SBRT overcomes the paradigm of the exclusively palliative role of RT in mRCC in favor of an active and safe treatment option that can be integrated into a multidisciplinary strategy to improve patients' clinical outcomes.

To date, the results of the Delphi consensus on the use of SBRT in oligometastatic and oligoprogressive RCC divided expert opinion. However, 71% of panelists would recommend SABR as a valid option for delaying the change of systemic therapy in oligoprogressive disease in selected cases, and they suggest a minimum acceptable time of 6 months from the start of systemic therapy to SABR to avoid systemic treatment change [17]. Several studies showed that the addition of RT to systemic treatment with ICIs and TKIs induced cell death through the release of molecules known as damage-associated molecular patterns (DAMPs). Moreover, evidence also demonstrated that tumor cell populations with a significant survival advantage are not confined within the boundaries of an organ site but can successfully spread to and reseed other sites [17–19]. DAMPs make cancer cells more susceptible to a cytotoxic immune response, preventing metastasis-to-metastasis seeding [20–22]. Furthermore, the current literature has shown that SBRT on RCC metastases provides fair LC with acceptable toxicity [23,24].

Altoos et al. [23], after a 2-year follow-up, reported a LC rate of 93.4% with SBRT (vs. 35.27% with conventional RT) regarding 53 lesions in pts with extracranial disease. In this study, no pts reported severe adverse events. In a study conducted by Stinauer R.et al. [24], the univariate analysis showed a correlation between higher doses per fraction and LC in patients with mRCC. To our knowledge, all the retrospective studies in the literature investigated the role of SBRT in a heterogeneous series of pts who underwent different systemic therapies (chemotherapy, target therapy or immunotherapy).

Our study, instead, assessed the role of SBRT in patients treated with an ICIs–TKIs combination exclusively.

Our results showed that SBRT improved LC in pts treated with an ICIs–TKIs combination and the results seem to be similar to previous studies, although conducted on pts undergoing different types of therapies and without any significant toxicity.

As a coprimary endpoint, we chose NEST-FS. NEST-FS is an endpoint used to explore the activity and efficacy of SBRT in oligoprogressive disease to prolong current treatments and delay the change of systemic therapies. It was used especially in metastatic oligoprogressive prostate cancer.

To our knowledge, this endpoint has never been used in oligoprogressive mRCC.

Hannan et al., in a phase II clinical trial, showed that sequential SBRT to oligoprogressive mRCC metastases prolonged the duration of ongoing systemic therapy by >6 mo in at least 40% of patients [25].

Cheung et al., instead, showed that the use of SBRT, in oligoprogressive mRCC patients who had previous stability or response after 3 months of TKI therapy, guarantees a LC rate of 93% (95% CI 71–98%) at 1 year, with a median time to change in systemic therapy of 12.6 months [26].

Although our study included a very heterogeneous cohort of nodal, spine and visceral metastases, our results confirm that SBRT may provide good LC, with a 20-month median NEST-FS. Moreover, no severe acute and late toxicities were reported.

Nevertheless, the retrospective nature of these studies does not claim to obtain a strong level of evidence.

Therefore, further prospective studies are warranted to select patients who may benefit from SBRT in oligoprogressive mRCC and establish the optimal schedule of treatment to guarantee the best clinical oncological outcomes as possible.

5. Conclusions

SBRT upon oligoprogressive sites in mRCC treated with an ICIs–TKIs combination is an effective and feasible therapeutic strategy to overcome resistance to systemic treatment with a good local control and without significant toxicities. Further investigations are needed to obtain a strong level of evidence.

Author Contributions: Methodology, M.F.; Resources, M.L.V., V.Z., A.M., L.T., L.L.P. and T.B.; Writing—review & editing, I.F.; Project administration, D.A. All authors have read and agreed to the published version of the manuscript.

Funding: This research received no external funding.

Institutional Review Board Statement: The study was conducted in accordance with the Declaration of Helsinki. Ethical approval was waived due to the retrospective nature of the study.

Informed Consent Statement: Not applicable.

Data Availability Statement: No new data were created or analyzed in this study. Data sharing is not applicable to this paper.

Conflicts of Interest: The authors declare no conflicts of interest.

References

1. Tomoyuki, M.; Suguru, K. Epidemiology and Prevention of Renal Cell Carcinoma. *Cancers* **2022**, *14*, 4059. [CrossRef] [PubMed]
2. Motzer, R.J.; Hutson, T.E. Overall survival and updated results for sunitinib compared with interferon alfa in patients with metastatic renal cell carcinoma. *J. Clin. Oncol.* **2009**, *27*, 3584–3590. [CrossRef] [PubMed]
3. LINEE GUIDA AIOM 2021.
4. Rabinovitch, R.A.; Zelefsky, M.J. Patterns of failure following surgical resection of renal cell carcinoma: Implications for adjuvant local and systemic therapy. *J. Clin. Oncol.* **1994**, *12*, 206–212. [CrossRef]
5. Kim, S.P.; Weight, C.J. Outcomes and clinico pathologic variables associated with late recurrence after nephrectomy for localized renal cell carcinoma. *Urology* **2011**, *78*, 1101–1106. [CrossRef]
6. Powles, T.; Plimack, E.R.; Soulières, D.; Waddell, T.; Stus, V.; Gafanov, R.; Nosov, D.; Pouliot, F.; Melichar, B.; Vynnychenko, I.; et al. Pembrolizumab plus axitinib versus sunitinib monotherapy as first-line treatment of advanced renal cell carcinoma (KEYNOTE-426): Extended follow-up from a randomised, open-label, phase 3 trial. *N. Engl. J. Med.* **2019**, *380*, 1116–1127. [CrossRef]
7. Choueiri, T.K.; Powles, T.; Burotto, M.; Escudier, B.; Bourlon, M.T.; Zurawski, B.; Oyervides Juárez, V.M.; Hsieh, J.J.; Basso, U.; Shah, A.Y.; et al. Nivolumab plus Cabozantinib versus Sunitinib for Advanced Renal-Cell Carcinoma. *N. Engl. J. Med.* **2021**, *384*, 829–841. [CrossRef] [PubMed]
8. Motzer, R.J.; Tannir, N.M. Nivolumab plus ipilimumab versus sunitinib in advanced renal cell carcinoma. *N. Engl. J. Med.* **2018**, *378*, 1277–1290. [CrossRef]
9. Choueiri, T.K.; Motzer, R.J. Systemic therapy for metastatic renal-cell carcinoma. *N. Engl. J. Med.* **2017**, *376*, 354–366. [CrossRef]
10. Hellman, S.; Weichselbaum, R.R. Oligometastases. *J. Clin. Oncol.* **1995**, *13*, 8–10. [CrossRef]
11. Zagardo, V.; Harikar, M.; Ferini, G. Is an immune-oriented use of radiation therapy possible? An increasingly open question under the spotlight of immunotherapy. *Oncologie* **2024**, *26*, 487–491.
12. Sun, X.; Gan, L.; Na, A.; Ge, L.; Chen, B.; Liu, J. Combination with Stereotactic Body Radiotherapy Offers a Promising Strategy to Overcome Resistance to Immunotherapy in Advanced Renal Cell Cancer. *J. Oncol.* **2019**, *2019*, 1483406. [CrossRef]
13. Zagardo, V.; Cuccia, F.; Piras, A.; Parisi, S.; Sciacca, M.; Ferrantelli, G.; Latteri, F.; Ferini, G. Radiotherapy directed to inferior vena cava tumor thrombus among patients with renal cell carcinoma: An illustrative case and review of the literature. *Oncologie* **2024**. [CrossRef]
14. Palma, D.A.; Olson, R.; Harrow, S.; Gaede, S.; Louie, A.V.; Haasbeek, C.; Mulroy, L.; Lock, M.; Rodrigues, G.B.; Yaremko, B.P.; et al. Stereotactic Ablative Radiotherapy for the Comprehensive Treatment of Oligometastatic Cancers: Long-Term Results of the SABR-COMET Phase II Randomized Trial. *J. Clin. Oncol.* **2020**, *38*, 2830–2838. [CrossRef] [PubMed]
15. Alt, A.L.; Boorjian, S.A. Survival after complete surgical resection of multiple metastases from renal cell carcinoma. *Cancer* **2011**, *117*, 2873–2882. [CrossRef] [PubMed]
16. Victor, C.T.-S.; Rech, A.J. Radiation and dual checkpoint blockade activate non-redundant immune mechanisms in cancer. *Nature* **2015**, *520*, 373–377. [CrossRef] [PubMed]
17. Marvaso, G.; Jereczek-Fossa, B.A.; Zaffaroni, M.; Vincini, M.G.; Corrao, G.; Andratschke, N.; Balagamwala, E.H.; Bedke, J.; Blanck, O.; Capitanio, U.; et al. Delphi consensus on stereotactic ablative radiotherapy for oligometastatic and oligoprogressive renal cell carcinoma—A European Society for Radiotherapy and Oncology study endorsed by the European Association of Urology. *Lancet Oncol.* **2024**, *25*, e193–e204. [CrossRef] [PubMed]

18. Escudier, B.; Porta, C. Renal cell carcinoma: ESMO clinical practice guidelines for diagnosis, treatment and follow-up. *Ann. Oncol.* **2019**, *30*, 706–720. [CrossRef]
19. Zhang, Y.; Schoenhals, J. Stereotactic ablative radiation therapy (SAbR) used to defer systemic therapy in oligometastatic renal cell cancer. *Int. J. Radiat. Oncol. Biol. Phys.* **2019**, *105*, 367–375. [CrossRef]
20. Sharabi, A.B.; Nirschl, C.J. Stereotactic radiation therapy augments antigen-specific PD-1-mediated antitumor immune responses via cross-presentation of tumor antigen. *Cancer Immunol. Res.* **2015**, *3*, 345–355. [CrossRef]
21. Ahmed, M.M.; Hodge, J.W. Harnessing the potential of radiation-induced immune modulation for cancer therapy. *Cancer Immunol. Res.* **2013**, *1*, 280–284. [CrossRef]
22. Formenti, S.C.; Demaria, S. Radiation therapy to convert the tumor into an in situ vaccine. *Int. J. Radiat. Oncol. Biol. Phys.* **2012**, *84*, 879–880. [CrossRef]
23. Altoos, B.; Amini, A. Local control rates of metastatic renal cell carcinoma (RCC) to thoracic, abdominal, and soft tissue lesions using stereotactic body radiotherapy (SBRT). *Radiat. Oncol.* **2015**, *10*, 218. [CrossRef] [PubMed]
24. Stinauer, M.A.; Kavanagh, B.D.; Schefter, T.E.; Gonzalez, R.; Flaig, T.; Lewis, K.; Robinson, W.; Chidel, M.; Glode, M.; Raben, D. Stereotactic body radiation therapy for melanoma and renal cell carcinoma: Impact of single fraction equivalent dose on local control. *Radiat. Oncol.* **2011**, *6*, 34. [CrossRef] [PubMed]
25. Hannan, R.; Christensen, M.; Hammers, H.; Christie, A.; Paulman, B.; Lin, D.; Garant, A.; Arafat, W.; Courtney, K.; Bowman, I.; et al. Phase II trial of stereotactic ablative radiation for oligoprogressive metastatic kidney cancer. *Eur. Urol. Oncol.* **2022**, *5*, 216–224. [CrossRef] [PubMed]
26. Cheung, P.; Patel, S. Stereotactic Radiotherapy for Oligoprogression in Metastatic Renal Cell Cancer Patients Receiving Tyrosine Kinase Inhibitor Therapy: A Phase 2 Prospective Multicenter Study. *Eur. Urol.* **2021**, *80*, 693–700. [CrossRef]

Journal of
Personalized Medicine

MDPI

Article

The Immunomodulatory Potential of Concurrent High-Dose Radiotherapy and Immune Checkpoint Inhibitor Cemiplimab in Advanced Cutaneous Squamous Cell Carcinoma: Initial Results

Maria Chiara Lo Greco [1,*], Giorgia Marano [1], Roberto Milazzotto [2], Rocco Luca Emanuele Liardo [2], Irene Finocchiaro [1], Madalina La Rocca [1], Antonio Basile [3,4], Pietro Valerio Foti [3,4], Stefano Palmucci [3,4], Emanuele David [3,4], Stefano Pergolizzi [1] and Corrado Spatola [2,4]

1 Radiation Oncology Unit, Department of Biomedical, Dental and Morphological and Functional Imaging Sciences, University of Messina, 98122 Messina, Italy; giorgiamarano@gmail.com (G.M.); irene.finocchiaro.com@gmail.com (I.F.); madalina.larocca@gmail.com (M.L.R.); stefano.pergolizzi@unime.it (S.P.)
2 Radiation Oncology Unit, University Hospital Policlinico "G. Rodolico-San Marco", 95123 Catania, Italy; r.milazzotto@policlinico.unict.it (R.M.); lucaliardo@hotmail.com (R.L.E.L.); cor_spatola@hotmail.com (C.S.)
3 Radiology I Unit, University Hospital Policlinico "G. Rodolico-San Marco", 95123 Catania, Italy; basile.antonello73@gmail.com (A.B.); pietrofoti@hotmail.com (P.V.F.); spalmucci@unict.it (S.P.); david.emanuele@yahoo.it (E.D.)
4 Department of Medical Surgical Sciences and Advanced Technologies "G.F. Ingrassia", University of Catania, 95123 Catania, Italy
* Correspondence: mariachiaralg@gmail.com

Abstract: In this retrospective case series, we investigate the synergistic effect and the immunomodulatory potential of combination radiotherapy and immunotherapy on 11 patients affected by locally advanced or metastatic cutaneous squamous cell carcinoma (CSCC), treated at our institution between 2020 and 2023. The primary endpoints of this study are objective tumor response, assessed by Immunotherapy Response Evaluation Criteria in Solid Tumors (iRECIST), and time to treatment failure (disease progression). In all patients, surgery was deemed not amenable, due to its potential functional and aesthetic impact. Therefore, upon multidisciplinary agreement, radiotherapy and immunotherapy with cemiplimab were alternatively administered. After 6 months, an early objective tumor response was observed in 9/11 patients, with 17/20 cutaneous lesions (85%) presenting either a complete or partial response. Only 2/11 patients, with a total of 3/20 cutaneous lesions (15%), had stable disease. These benefits persisted at a longer follow-up (21.4 ± 9.7 months), with no patients presenting disease progression. Despite the retrospective nature of this study and small sample size, our experience highlights the ability of concomitant radiotherapy and cemiplimab to promote an early objective response in patients with advanced CSCC. Moreover, in our population, the clinical benefits were also related to a longer progression-free survival, without any safety alert reported.

Keywords: squamous cell cancer; high-dose radiotherapy; abscopal effect; cemiplimab

1. Introduction

Cutaneous squamous cell carcinoma (CSCC) is the second most prevalent form of non-melanoma skin cancer (NMSC), accounting for 25% of cases and nearly 75% of NMSC-related deaths [1].

CSCC typically originates from epidermal keratinocytes and manifests as a spectrum of progressively advanced malignancies, ranging from precursor actinic keratosis to in situ carcinoma, followed by invasive and finally metastatic CSCC [2]. Because of this spectrum of conditions, the therapeutic approaches available for this malignancy also vary according to the severity of the stage.

The first-line treatment option for most CSCCs is surgery with adequate margins. However, in cases of inoperable disease or high post-operative risk, radiation therapy can be performed, offering satisfactory cosmetic and functional outcomes [3].

Radiation treatment can be performed with beams of electrons, photons, surface brachytherapy, or protons, as experimented in our center, for squamous cell carcinomas of the conjunctiva or porocarcinomas [4–6].

In locally advanced or metastatic CSCC, several systemic agents have been shown to have clinical benefits, including chemotherapy, epidermal growth factor receptor (EGFR)-targeted therapy, and immunotherapy with programmed cell death-1 (PD-1) inhibitors [7]. Nevertheless, the optimal approach in this setting remains unclear, with no established consensus on first-line systemic treatment.

Given the promising results of combining radiotherapy and immunotherapy for several malignancies such as advanced melanoma, head and neck district CSCC, and non-small-cell lung cancer [8–11], we performed a retrospective case series study, investigating the synergistic effect and immunomodulatory potential of this combination on 11 patients with locally advanced CSCC, treated at our institution between 2020 and 2023. The primary endpoints of this study are objective tumor response, assessed by Immunotherapy Response Evaluation Criteria in Solid Tumors (iRECIST), and time to treatment failure (disease progression). The feasibility of the combined treatment was evaluated using the Common Terminology Criteria for Adverse Events (CTCAE v4.0).

2. Materials and Methods

For this retrospective case series, 11 patients with locally advanced or metastatic CSCC treated at the University of Catania between 2020 and 2023 have been selected. The inclusion criteria were age > 18 years, single or multiple cutaneous lesions with a histological diagnosis of CSCC, clinical and radiological diagnosis of locally advanced or metastatic disease, radiotherapy treatment, and immunotherapy with cemiplimab. The patients' characteristics are summarized in Table 1.

Table 1. Patients' characteristics.

Patients' Characteristics		%
Sex	Male	63.6%
	Female	36.6%
Age	<65	18.1%
	65–75	36.6%
	>75	45.4%
PS ECOG	0	45.4%
	1	36.6%
	2	9%
	3	0%
Stage	Locally advanced	63.3%
	Metastatic	36.3%
N. of lesions	Single (1)	36.3%
	Multiple (2)	45.5%
	Multiple (≥3)	18.1%
Lesion's location	High-risk areas	40%
	Medium-risk areas	40%
	Low-risk areas	20%

At baseline, all patients presented one or more ulcerated, patchy, papulonodular, papillomatous, or exophytic lesions, specifically in sun-exposed skin areas (the face, the scalp, and the backs of the hands) and other non-exposed areas (i.e., trunk, feet).

Biopsy and histological examination were performed to obtain diagnosis confirmation of CSCC. In detail, a total of 20 skin lesions were identified in a population of 11 patients.

Following this, additional imaging techniques such as contrast-enhanced Computed Tomography (CT) or Magnetic Resonance Imaging (MRI) were performed to assess the depth of invasion. Assessment of in-transit regional lymph node metastases was made with an accurate physical examination, ultrasonography, and PET-CT when needed. Tumor staging was established according to the TNM (tumor, node, and metastasis) American Joint Committee on Cancer (AJCC) criteria, with all patients being affected by either locally advanced or metastatic SCC.

Surgery was deemed not amenable due to its potential functional and aesthetic impact; therefore, radiotherapy and immunotherapy with cemiplimab were offered to the patients, upon multidisciplinary agreement.

To design a unique and tailored radiotherapy treatment, each patient underwent a simulation process through a CT scan (3–5 mm slice spacing) without contrast enhancement. Since the patient's position must be the same for both initial simulation and subsequent treatment, different immobilization devices (based on tumor locations) were used to obtain an optimal setup.

After CT image acquisition, the treatment planning software Raystation® (Ray Search Laboratories) version 12, was used for target volume definition and dose solutions. During the contour delineation phase, the gross tumor volume (GTV) was outlined, including the primary tumor and positive nodes (when present). The clinical target volume (CTV) was then delineated and successively expanded to obtain a planning target volume (PTV). After the delineation phase, a personalized plan was built up by the medical physicist, in synergy with the radiation oncologist, respecting the dose limits of any organ at risk (OAR) to minimize the side effects of the treatment. All patients received a 0.5 cm thick water bolus that had increased PTV coverage.

External-beam radiation therapy was delivered through an Elekta VERSA HD® linear accelerator, using electron beams or photon beams through either a 3D-conformal technique (3D-CRT) or a static step-and-shot intensity-modulated technique (IMRT), based on the conformation of the target. During the entire course of radiotherapy treatment, patients were set up daily by using one sagittal and two lateral tattoos and lasers. A kilovoltage cone-beam computer tomography image-guided radiotherapy (KV CBCT IGRT) system was used two times a week to check patients' setups. All treatments were performed on a HexaPod® (ELEKTA) carbon fiber robotic treatment table capable of performing corrections in all 6 degrees of freedom. Patients with face or scalp lesions were monitored through daily optical surface-guided imaging (VisionRT–AlignRT®).

Different fractionation schedules were used, including conventionally fractionated radiation therapy (CFRT) or hypofractionated radiation therapy (HFRT). BED was calculated using an alpha/beta ratio of 10. Radiotherapy schedules are summarized in Table 2.

Table 2. Radiotherapy treatment schedules and BED.

Radiotherapy Schedules		BED (α/β = 10)	%
Conventionally fractionated radiotherapy	2–60 Gy	72	15%
	2–66 Gy	79.2	15%
Hypofractionated radiotherapy	4–40 Gy	56	20%
	5–40 Gy	60	40%
	5–50 Gy	75	10%

Cemiplimab 350 mg was administered intravenously over 30 min triweekly (Q3W) until disease progression or unmanageable toxicity.

The primary endpoints of this study are objective tumor response, assessed by iRECIST criteria, and time to treatment failure (disease progression). In this regard, patients were clinically and radiologically evaluated at baseline and quarterly after the end of the treatment. Diagnostic imaging included CT, MRI, and Positron Emission Tomography (PET)–CT scan.

To determine the feasibility and toxicity rates of the combined treatment, all patients were clinically and hematologically evaluated, once a week during the treatment course, and quarterly after the end of this. Toxicity data were collected according to CTCAE v4.0.

3. Results

From 2020 to 2023, a series of 11 patients with locally advanced or metastatic CSCC were treated at the University of Catania with radiotherapy, either to single or multiple cutaneous lesions, and immunotherapy with cemiplimab. In total, seven patients presented with locally advanced disease, while four patients presented with metastatic disease. Furthermore, four patients presented a single lesion, while five and two patients presented two or more lesions, respectively, up to a total of twenty lesions. Regarding tumor locations, eight (40%) lesions were located in high-risk areas (mask areas of the face, genitalia, hands, and feet), eight (40%) lesions were in medium-risk areas (cheeks, forehead, scalp, neck, and pretibial), and four (20%) lesions were in low-risk areas (trunk and extremities, excluding hands and feet), as reported in Table 1.

All lesions were treated with radiotherapy, accounting for a total of 20 lesions treated, with either CFRT or HFRT.

Regarding radiotherapy, doses and fractionation schedules were tailored based on patients' conditions and target volumes. In standard conditions, in patients with good performance status and large tumor size (>2 cm), the preferred schedule was CFRT, delivered using a daily dose of 2 Gy, five times a week, up to a total dose of 60 Gy. In the case of high-risk features, dose escalation was performed, up to 66 Gy.

On the contrary, in frail and old patients, those unable to perform daily sessions, or in the case of small lesions (<2 cm), the preferred schedule was HFRT, delivered using a fractional dose of 4–5 Gy, two times a week, up to a total dose of 40–50 Gy (Table 2).

Regarding systemic treatment, all patients received cemiplimab 350 mg, Q3W until disease progression or unmanageable toxicity.

All patients were clinically and hematologically evaluated, once a week during the treatment course and quarterly after the end of this. In terms of early toxicities, only five patients reported grade I–II toxicities, either related to immunotherapy (diarrhea, fatigue, nausea, and constipation) or radiotherapy (radiation dermatitis). No patient reported either early grade III toxicities or late toxicities.

To determine short-term efficacy, patients were clinically and radiologically examined at baseline and quarterly after the end of the treatment, and the response was evaluated according to the iRECIST criteria.

After 6 months, an early clinical and radiological response was observed in 9/11 patients, with 17/20 lesions (85%) presenting either a complete or partial response (Figures 1–3). Only 2/11 patients, with a total of 3/20 lesions (15%), had stable disease. The benefits in terms of early response persisted at longer follow-up (21.4 $\pm$ 9.7 months), with no patients presenting disease progression.

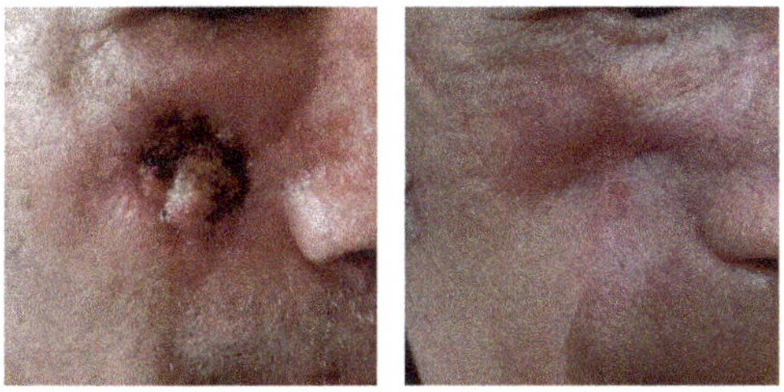

(a) (b)

Figure 1. Patient with locally advanced CSCC of the right cheek (area M) at baseline (**a**) and after treatment (**b**).

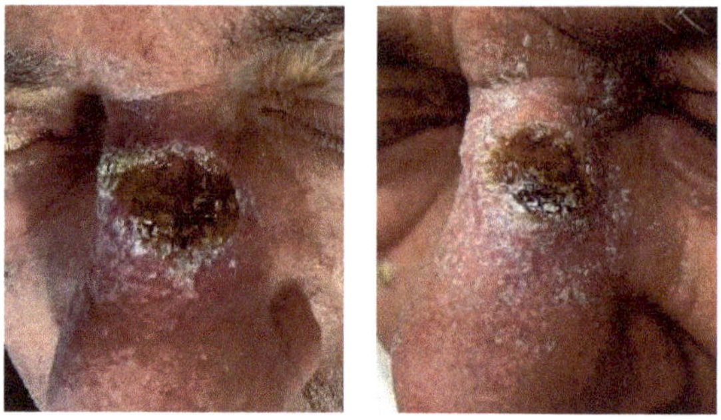

(a) (b)

Figure 2. Patient with locally advanced CSCC of the nose (area H) at baseline (**a**) and after treatment (**b**).

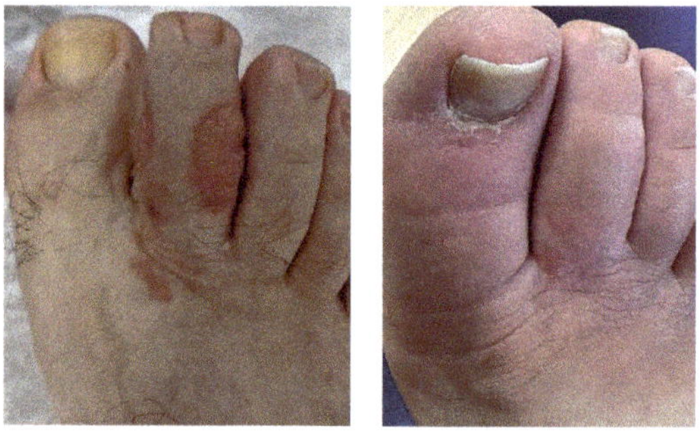

(a) (b)

Figure 3. Patient with locally advanced CSCC of the left foot (area H) at baseline (**a**) and after treatment (**b**).

4. Discussion

4.1. Theoretical and Practical Bases for Immunotherapy

Even though the incidence of advanced CSCC is increasing, an established consensus on the first-line treatment to administer to this population is still missing [12].

Regarding chemotherapy, even though no agent is currently specifically approved in this setting, cisplatin, either alone or in combination with 5-fluorouracil (5-FU), represents a therapeutic option for patients who require additional treatment beyond surgery and radiotherapy [13]. Regarding EGFR-target therapy, different tyrosine kinase inhibitors (erlotinib, gefitinib) and monoclonal antibodies (cetuximab or panitumumab) have been investigated in the recurrent and metastatic setting [14–17]. Nevertheless, evidence supporting this approach is still limited.

A major and practice-changing breakthrough in advanced CSCC happened when, in September 2018, the Food and Drug Administration (FDA) approved cemiplimab as an option for patients with metastatic or locally advanced cSCC who are not candidates for surgery or radiotherapy.

In detail, cemiplimab is a high-affinity, highly potent human immunoglobulin G4 (IgG4) anti-PD-1 receptor monoclonal antibody that has demonstrated efficacy in terms of overall response rate and long-term durable response, with a very effective disease control rate in patients with advanced and metastatic CSCC [18]. The mechanism of action is based on the inhibition of PD-1 receptor activity by cemiplimab. Indeed, this recombinant human IgG4 monoclonal antibody binds the receptor, blocking its interactions with programmed cell death ligand-1 and -2 (PD-L1 and PD-L2). The inhibition of the PD-1 pathway results in an immune checkpoint-enhancing T-cell-mediated response, leading to T-cell activation and proliferation against tumor cells [19].

The approval of cemiplimab was based on the results of two early-phase clinical trials that enrolled 163 patients with advanced CSCC in the United States, Australia, and Europe. The first trial was a phase 1 study (NCT02383212) evaluating cemiplimab in patients with advanced malignancies. The second trial was a pivotal phase 2 clinical trial (NCT02760498) specifically assessing cemiplimab in advanced CSCC. Response rates were consistent in both the phase 1 cohorts (50%) and the phase 2 cohort (47%). Additionally, the characteristics of tumor responses demonstrated the efficacy of cemiplimab for treating CSCC in immunocompetent patients. On the other hand, adverse events assessed by investigators were grade 1 or 2 events, with only 8% and 7% of patients in the phase 1 cohorts and the phase 2 cohort discontinuing treatment due to adverse events [18].

Along with cemiplimab, other anti-PD-1 agents are under evaluation in CSCC, such as Pembrolizumab in patients with recurrent/metastatic or locally advanced unresectable CSCC (NCT03284424) and in patients with locally advanced CSCC after surgery and radiation (NCT03833167), and nivolumab as monotherapy in patients with locally advanced/metastatic CSCC (NCT04204837, NCT03834233).

The theoretical bases for the administration of immunotherapy come from the evidence that CSCC has an elevated tumor mutation burden (TMB) and, consequently, is susceptible to higher responsiveness to immune checkpoint inhibitors. Indeed, although skin carcinogenesis is multifactorial, the primary risk factor is represented by prolonged exposure to ultraviolet (UV) radiation, which causes nearly 90% of non-melanoma skin cell cancers [18]. The cumulative exposure to ultraviolet radiation induces different categories of DNA damage in skin cells, such as cyclobutene pyrimidine dimers (CPD), 6-4 photoproducts (6-4 PP), DNA strand breaks, and crosslinks. When these damages cannot be repaired, they become genetic mutations, promoting skin carcinogenesis and increasing TMB load [20,21]. In turn, the accumulation of somatic modification induces the expression of neoantigens (fractions of nonsynonymous mutations that become exposed as epitopes), which can trigger an anticancer response by the immune system. Specifically, neoantigens can activate CD8+ cytotoxic T cells (CTLs) which recognize the peptide bound to major histocompatibility complex class I (MHC I) on tumor cells, and hence initiate tumor cell lysis. Finally, during tumor cell lysis, CTLs release cytotoxic molecules that lead to the destruction of the tumor cell [22].

Given the evidence in the literature that the most robust responses to PD-1/PD-L1 blockade have been seen in tumors with high TMB load, this biomarker and other TMB-derived measures (neoantigens, neoepitopes, and mutation clonality) are all currently under investigation to further stratify patients most likely to respond to immunotherapy.

4.2. *The Synergistic Effect of Radiotherapy*

Even though anti-PD-1 agents have been demonstrated to improve both disease control rate and overall response rate in patients with advanced and metastatic CSCC [18,23], research on how to further enhance SCC outcomes is currently ongoing. In this regard, radiotherapy represents a helpful resource [24,25].

In detail, radiotherapy can provide a synergistic benefit in combination with PD-1 inhibition for patients with CSCC, in terms of both local and distant tumor control, in a T-cell-dependent manner [26,27]. The theoretical basis supporting this combination can be explained through the abscopal effect.

The abscopal effect is a sporadic clinical event that happens when local therapy, typically radiotherapy, induces the shrinkage of a tumoral lesion at a distance from the irradiated site. One of the key components of the abscopal effect is Damage-Associated Molecular Patterns (DAMPs), which play a crucial role in the immune response during tissue damage. In detail, when ionizing radiation induces the death of a tumor cell, the latter induces the release of DAMPs, such as high-motility group box 1 (HMGB1), heat shock proteins (HSPs), calreticulin membrane exposure, and glucose-regulated protein

96 (GP96). In turn, DAMPs promote the activation of dendritic cells through the TLR4 pathway, while HMGB1 promotes dendritic cell maturation, thanks to the pro-inflammatory cytokines (TNF-a, IL-1, IL-6, and IL-8) produced by monocytes [28]. Another important key component is represented by DNA damage induced by ionizing radiation. In detail, DNA fragments that gain access to the cytosol of irradiated cells lead the expression of IFN genes. These genes, in turn, promote the activation of the STING pathway, which enhances anti-tumor CD8+ cells in tumor-draining lymph nodes (TLDNs). Once activated in the TLDNs, tumor-specific CD8 T cells start migrating, guided by inflammatory cytokines and chemokines, extravasating and infiltrating the tumor site. Radiation-induced upregulation of major histocompatibility class I antigens (MHC- I), NKG2D ligands, and death receptors on the cancer cells improves the recognition and killing of the cancer cells by cytotoxic CD8 T cells. In summary, the abscopal effect demonstrates the intricate interplay between local treatments, immune responses, and systemic anti-tumor effects, potentially leading to remarkable clinical outcomes in cancer patients [29].

Even if rare, this effect has been reported in the literature for various types of cancers, including both solid and liquid tumors. Regarding skin cancer, cases of Merkel cell carcinoma and melanoma have been reported in the literature. Regarding CSCC, studies have been investigating the potential immunogenic effect of radiotherapy to stimulate responses in distant nonirradiated sites.

A recently published work demonstrated the benefit of delivering concurrent radiotherapy with cemiplimab, in terms of local effect, but not in terms of distant effect [30]. In detail, this work was the first real-life retrospective study investigating concomitant radiotherapy to cemiplimab as a significant therapeutic strategy. The authors showed that the addition of radiotherapy to cemiplimab enables an earlier clinical–radiological response, with a median duration of 5.5 months in the cemiplimab group versus 3 months in the concomitant therapy group. The response to treatment was prolonged despite discontinuation of cemiplimab, with 91.6% and 83.3% patients in complete or partial remission at 6 months and 1 year after cessation of cemiplimab and no switch to another oncological treatment, respectively. Radiation therapy also provided a therapeutic effect in 83.3% of the patients in the concomitant group, without increasing the occurrence of adverse events [30].

Based on the above-mentioned literature data, we performed a retrospective case series study, investigating the synergistic effect and the immunomodulatory potential of concomitant radiotherapy and immunotherapy. The results of this study (despite its limitations) support the use of this combination to promote objective tumor response and slow disease progression.

Although further investigations are necessary, we can reasonably conclude that the theoretical foundations supporting the synergistic effect of radiotherapy and immunotherapy have the potential to translate into positive clinical outcomes.

5. Conclusions

In this retrospective case series, we investigate combination radiotherapy and immunotherapy in 11 patients affected by locally advanced or metastatic CSCC treated at our institution between 2020 and 2023. In total, seven patients presented with locally advanced disease, while four patients presented metastatic disease. Furthermore, four patients presented a single lesion, while three and two patients, respectively, presented two or more lesions, up to a total of twenty lesions. The primary endpoints of this study are objective tumor response, assessed by iRECIST criteria, and time to treatment failure (disease progression).

Despite the retrospective nature of this study, the small sample size, and the lack of a control group, our experience highlights the ability of concomitant radiotherapy and cemiplimab to promote an early clinical–radiological objective response in patients with advanced CSCC, durable with time. Indeed, after 6 months, 85% of CSCC lesions presented either a complete or partial response, while only 15% had stable disease. The benefits in terms of early response persisted at longer follow-up (21.4 ± 9.7 months), with no patients presenting disease progression. No patient reported either early grade III toxicities or late toxicities related to the treatment.

Since local therapy has been delivered to each lesion, it is not possible to conclude whether radiotherapy stimulated the abscopal effect or not. However, we can affirm that it has enhanced early clinical and radiological responses, positively impacting progression-free survival rates.

Even if it is not possible to make practice recommendations, we hope that the results of this study could serve as a basis for designing future larger, randomized, controlled trials, and improve the cooperation between dermatologists, medical oncologists, and radiation oncologists with the common objective of improving patients' outcomes.

Author Contributions: Data curation, I.F. and M.L.R.; investigation, R.M.; methodology, R.L.E.L., A.B., P.V.F., S.P. (Stefano Palmucci) and E.D.; supervision, S.P. (Stefano Pergolizzi) and C.S.; writing—original draft, M.C.L.G. and G.M.; writing—review and editing, M.C.L.G. and R.M. All authors have read and agreed to the published version of the manuscript.

Funding: This research received no external funding.

Institutional Review Board Statement: This study was conducted in accordance with the Declaration of Helsinki. Ethical review and approval were waived for this study due to its retrospective, non-interventional nature.

Informed Consent Statement: Informed consent was obtained from all subjects involved in this study.

Data Availability Statement: The data presented in this study are available on request from the corresponding author. The data are not publicly available due to privacy restrictions.

Conflicts of Interest: The authors declare no conflicts of interest.

References

1. Khayyati Kohnehshahri, M.; Sarkesh, A.; Mohamed Khosroshahi, L.; HajiEsmailPoor, Z.; Aghebati-Maleki, A.; Yousefi, M.; Aghebati-Maleki, L. Current status of skin cancers with a focus on immunology and immunotherapy. *Cancer Cell Int.* **2023**, *23*, 174. [CrossRef] [PubMed]
2. Ratushny, V.; Gober, M.D.; Hick, R.; Ridky, T.W.; Seykora, J.T. From keratinocyte to cancer: The pathogenesis and modeling of cutaneous squamous cell carcinoma. *J. Clin. Investig.* **2012**, *122*, 464–472. [CrossRef] [PubMed]
3. Muto, P.; Pastore, F. Radiotherapy in the adjuvant and advanced setting of CSCC. *Dermatol. Pract. Concept.* **2021**, *11*, e2021168S. [CrossRef]
4. Fionda, B.; Placidi, E.; Rosa, E.; Lancellotta, V.; Stimato, G.; De Angeli, M.; Ciardo, F.G.; Cornacchione, P.; Siebert, F.A.; Tagliaferri, L.; et al. Multilayer intensity modulated contact interventional radiotherapy (brachytherapy): Stretching the therapeutic window in skin cancer. *J. Contemp. Brachytherapy* **2023**, *15*, 220–223. [CrossRef] [PubMed]
5. Milazzotto, R.; Liardo RL, E.; Privitera, G.; Raffaele, L.; Salamone, V.; Arena, F.; Pergolizzi, S.; Cuttone, G.; Cirrone GA, P.; Russo, A.; et al. Proton beam radiotherapy of locally advanced or recurrent conjunctival squamous cell carcinoma: Experience of the CATANA Centre. *J. Radiother. Pract.* **2022**, *21*, 97–104. [CrossRef]
6. Tocco, A.; Privitera, G.; Raffaele, L.; Salamone, V.; Scoglio, C.; Milazzotto, R.; Marletta, D.; Cuttone, G.; Cirrone GA, P.; Russo, A.; et al. Porocarcinoma of the eyelid treated with proton beam radiotherapy: Case report and literature review. *Acta Medica Mediterr.* **2018**, *34*, 709–712. [CrossRef]
7. García-Foncillas, J.; Tejera-Vaquerizo, A.; Sanmartín, O.; Rojo, F.; Mestre, J.; Martín, S.; Azinovic, I.; Mesía, R. Update on Management Recommendations for Advanced Cutaneous Squamous Cell Carcinoma. *Cancers* **2022**, *14*, 629. [CrossRef] [PubMed]
8. Chicas-Sett, R.; Morales-Orue, I.; Rodriguez-Abreu, D.; Lara-Jimenez, P. Combining radiotherapy and ipilimumab induces clinically relevant radiation-induced abscopal effects in metastatic melanoma patients: A systematic review. *Clin. Transl. Radiat. Oncol.* **2018**, *9*, 5–11. [CrossRef] [PubMed]
9. Forner, D.; Horwich, P.; Trites, J.R.; Hollenhorst, H.; Bullock, M.; Lamond, N.W.D. The abscopal effect in head-and-neck squamous cell carcinoma treated with radiotherapy and nivolumab: A case report and literature review. *Curr. Oncol.* **2020**, *27*, 330–335. [CrossRef]
10. Koller, K.M.; Mackley, H.B.; Liu, J.; Wagner, H.; Talamo, G.; Schell, T.D.; Pameijer, C.; Neves, R.I.; Anderson, B.; Kokolus, K.M.; et al. Improved survival and complete response rates in patients with advanced melanoma treated with concurrent ipilimumab and radiotherapy versus ipilimumab alone. *Cancer Biol. Ther.* **2017**, *18*, 36–42. [CrossRef]
11. Theelen WS, M.E.; Chen, D.; Verma, V.; Hobbs, B.P.; Peulen HM, U.; Aerts JG, J.V.; Bahce, I.; Niemeijer AL, N.; Chang, J.Y.; de Groot, P.M.; et al. Pembrolizumab with or without radiotherapy for metastatic non-small-cell lung cancer: A pooled analysis of two randomised trials. *Lancet Respir. Med.* **2021**, *9*, 467–475. [CrossRef] [PubMed]

12. Fitzgerald, K.; Tsai, K.K. Systemic therapy for advanced cutaneous squamous cell carcinoma. *Semin. Cutan. Med. Surg.* **2019**, *38*, E67–E74. [CrossRef] [PubMed]
13. Schmults, C.D.; Blitzblau, R.; Aasi, S.Z.; Alam, M.; Andersen, J.S.; Baumann, B.C.; Bordeaux, J.; Chen, P.L.; Chin, R.; Contreras, C.M.; et al. Squamous Cell Skin Cancer, Version 1.2022 Featured Updates to the NCCN Guidelines. *JNCCN J. Natl. Compr. Cancer Netw.* **2021**, *19*, 1382–1394. [CrossRef] [PubMed]
14. Foote, M.C.; Mcgrath, M.; Guminski, A.; Hughes BG, M.; Meakin, J.; Thomson, D.; Zarate, D.; Simpson, F.; Porceddu, S.V. Phase II study of single agent panitumumab in patients with incurable cutaneous squamous cell carcinoma Downloaded from. *Ann. Oncol. Adv. Access* **2014**, *25*, 2047–2052. [CrossRef] [PubMed]
15. Gold, K.A.; Kies, M.S.; William, W.N.; Johnson, F.M.; Lee, J.J.; Glisson, B.S. Erlotinib in the treatment of recurrent or metastatic cutaneous squamous cell carcinoma: A single-arm phase 2 clinical trial. *Cancer* **2018**, *124*, 2169–2173. [CrossRef] [PubMed]
16. Maubec, E.; Petrow, P.; Scheer-Senyarich, I.; Duvillard, P.; Lacroix, L.; Gelly, J.; Certain, A.; Duval, X.; Crickx, B.; Buffard, V.; et al. Phase II study of cetuximab as first-line single-drug therapy in patients with unresectable squamous cell carcinoma of the skin. *J. Clin. Oncol.* **2011**, *29*, 3419–3426. [CrossRef]
17. William, W.N.; Feng, L.; Ferrarotto, R.; Ginsberg, L.; Kies, M.; Lippman, S.; Glisson, B.; Kim, E.S. Gefitinib for patients with incurable cutaneous squamous cell carcinoma: A single-arm phase II clinical trial. *J. Am. Acad. Dermatol.* **2017**, *77*, 1110–1113.e2. [CrossRef] [PubMed]
18. Migden, M.R.; Rischin, D.; Schmults, C.D.; Guminski, A.; Hauschild, A.; Lewis, K.D.; Chung, C.H.; Hernandez-Aya, L.; Lim, A.M.; Chang AL, S.; et al. PD-1 Blockade with Cemiplimab in Advanced Cutaneous Squamous-Cell Carcinoma. *N. Engl. J. Med.* **2018**, *379*, 341–351. [CrossRef]
19. Lee, A.; Duggan, S.; Deeks, E.D. Cemiplimab: A Review in Advanced Cutaneous Squamous Cell Carcinoma. *Drugs* **2020**, *80*, 813–819. [CrossRef]
20. Teng, Y.; Yu, Y.; Li, S.; Huang, Y.; Xu, D.; Tao, X.; Fan, Y. Ultraviolet Radiation and Basal Cell Carcinoma: An Environmental Perspective. *Front. Public Health* **2021**, *9*, 666528. [CrossRef]
21. Falchook, G.S.; Leidner, R.; Stankevich, E.; Piening, B.; Bifulco, C.; Lowy, I.; Fury, M.G. Responses of metastatic basal cell and cutaneous squamous cell carcinomas to anti-PD1 monoclonal antibody REGN2810. *J. Immunother. Cancer* **2016**, *4*, 70. [CrossRef] [PubMed]
22. Gubin, M.M.; Artyomov, M.N.; Mardis, E.R.; Schreiber, R.D. Tumor neoantigens: Building a framework for personalized cancer immunotherapy. *J. Clin. Investig.* **2015**, *125*, 3413–3421. [CrossRef] [PubMed]
23. Rischin, D.; Khushalani, N.I.; Schmults, C.D.; Guminski, A.; Chang AL, S.; Lewis, K.D.; Lim, A.M.; Hernandez-Aya, L.; Hughes BG, M.; Schadendorf, D.; et al. Integrated analysis of a phase 2 study of cemiplimab in advanced cutaneous squamous cell carcinoma: Extended follow-up of outcomes and quality of life analysis. *J. Immunother. Cancer* **2021**, *9*, e002757. [CrossRef] [PubMed]
24. Ferini, G.; Palmisciano, P.; Forte, S.; Viola, A.; Martorana, E.; Parisi, S.; Valenti, V.; Fichera, C.; Umana, G.E.; Pergolizzi, S. Advanced or Metastatic Cutaneous Squamous Cell Carcinoma: The Current and Future Role of Radiation Therapy in the Era of Immunotherapy. *Cancers* **2022**, *14*, 1871. [CrossRef] [PubMed]
25. Ferini, G.; Castorina, P.; Valenti, V.; Illari, S.I.; Sachpazidis, I.; Castorina, L.; Marrale, M.; Pergolizzi, S. A Novel Radiotherapeutic Approach to Treat Bulky Metastases Even from Cutaneous Squamous Cell Carcinoma: Its Rationale and a Look at the Reliability of the Linear-Quadratic Model to Explain Its Radiobiological Effects. *Front. Oncol.* **2022**, *12*, 809279. [CrossRef] [PubMed]
26. Dovedi, S.J.; Cheadle, E.J.; Popple, A.L.; Poon, E.; Morrow, M.; Stewart, R.; Yusko, E.C.; Sanders, C.M.; Vignali, M.; Emerson, R.O.; et al. Fractionated radiation therapy stimulates antitumor immunity mediated by both resident and infiltrating polyclonal T-cell populations when combined with PD-1 blockade. *Clin. Cancer Res.* **2017**, *23*, 5514–5526. [CrossRef] [PubMed]
27. Twyman-Saint Victor, C.; Rech, A.J.; Maity, A.; Rengan, R.; Pauken, K.E.; Stelekati, E.; Benci, J.L.; Xu, B.; Dada, H.; Odorizzi, P.M.; et al. Radiation and dual checkpoint blockade activate non-redundant immune mechanisms in cancer. *Nature* **2015**, *520*, 373–377. [CrossRef] [PubMed]
28. Janopaul-Naylor, J.R.; Shen, Y.; Qian, D.C.; Buchwald, Z.S. The abscopal effect: A review of pre-clinical and clinical advances. *Int. J. Mol. Sci.* **2021**, *22*, 11061. [CrossRef] [PubMed]
29. Reits, E.A.; Hodge, J.W.; Herberts, C.A.; Groothuis, T.A.; Chakraborty, M.; Wansley, E.K.; Camphausen, K.; Luiten, R.M.; De Ru, A.H.; Neijssen, J.; et al. Radiation modulates the peptide repertoire, enhances MHC class I expression, and induces successful antitumor immunotherapy. *J. Exp. Med.* **2006**, *203*, 1259–1271. [CrossRef]
30. Bailly-Caillé, B.; Kottler, D.; Morello, R.; Lecornu, M.; Kao, W.; Meyer, E.; Dompmartin, A.; L'Orphelin, J.M. Real-Life Study of the Benefit of Concomitant Radiotherapy with Cemiplimab in Advanced Cutaneous Squamous Cell Carcinoma (cSCC): A Retrospective Cohort Study. *Cancers* **2023**, *15*, 495. [CrossRef]

Journal of *Personalized Medicine*

MDPI

Case Report

Unexpected Transient Glioblastoma Regression in a Patient Previously Treated with Bacillus Calmette–Guérin Therapy: A Case Report and Immunomodulatory Effects Hypothesis

Gianluca Scalia [1,*], Gianluca Ferini [2], Salvatore Marrone [3], Maurizio Salvati [4], Vicky Yamamoto [5], Babak Kateb [6], Reinhard Schulte [7], Stefano Forte [8] and Giuseppe Emmanuele Umana [9]

1 Neurosurgery Unit, Department of Head and Neck Surgery, Garibaldi Hospital, 95123 Catania, Italy
2 Department of Radiation Oncology, Istituto Oncologico del Mediterraneo, 95029 Viagrande, Italy; gianluca.ferini@grupposamed.com
3 Neurosurgical Clinic, AOUP "Paolo Giaccone", Post Graduate Residency Program in Neurologic Surgery, Department of Biomedicine Neurosciences and Advanced Diagnostics, School of Medicine, University of Palermo, 90127 Palermo, Italy; salvo.mr89@gmail.com
4 Department of Neurosurgery, Policlinico "Tor Vergata", University of Rome "Tor Vergata", 00133 Rome, Italy; salvati.maurizio@libero.it
5 University of Southern California-Norris Comprehensive Cancer Center, Los Angeles, CA 90033, USA; vyamamot@usc.edu
6 Brain Mapping Foundation, Los Angeles, CA 90272, USA; babak.kateb@worldbrainmapping.org
7 School of Medicine, Loma Linda University, Loma Linda, CA 11085, USA; schulte@llu.edu
8 Genomics and Experimental Oncology Unit, Istituto Oncologico del Mediterraneo, 95029 Viagrande, Catania, Italy; stefano.forte@grupposamed.com
9 Department of Neurosurgery, Gamma Knife and Trauma Center, Cannizzaro Hospital, 95126 Catania, Italy; umana.nch@gmail.com
* Correspondence: gianluca.scalia@outlook.it

Abstract: (1) Background: Glioblastoma multiforme (GBM) is a highly aggressive brain tumor with limited treatment options and poor prognosis. Bacillus Calmette–Guérin (BCG), a live attenuated strain of Mycobacterium bovis, has been used as an immunotherapeutic agent in bladder cancer and has shown non-specific beneficial effects. This report presents a unique case of GBM regression following BCG therapy for bladder cancer, suggesting the potential systemic immunomodulatory effects of BCG on GBM. (2) Case Presentation: A 67-year-old male with a history of bladder cancer treated with BCG presented with neurological symptoms. Imaging revealed two GBM lesions, and surgery was performed to remove one. Subsequently, the patient experienced complete tumor regression after initial stability. (3) Conclusions: This case highlights the potential of BCG or other immunotherapies in GBM treatment and underscores the need for further research. Understanding the immunomodulatory effects of BCG on GBM could lead to innovative therapies for this devastating disease; although, overcoming the immune evasion mechanisms in the brain is a significant challenge. Further investigation is warranted to explore this promising avenue of research.

Keywords: glioblastoma; Bacillus Calmette–Guérin; bladder cancer; regression; immunomodulatory effects; case report

1. Introduction

Glioblastoma multiforme (GBM) stands as the most prevalent primary malignant brain tumor in adults, characterized by its aggressive growth pattern and resistance to treatment. Despite standardized treatment protocols involving maximal safe surgical removal, followed by radiotherapy and chemotherapy utilizing temozolomide, the median survival rate for patients remains disappointingly low. Consequently, there exists an urgent demand for more effective therapies targeting GBM. Bacillus Calmette–Guérin (BCG), a live attenuated strain of Mycobacterium bovis, has a long history of use as a vaccine for tuberculosis and as an immunotherapeutic agent in bladder cancer treatment. The BCG vaccine has shown non-specific beneficial effects, reducing morbidity and mortality from various types of infections and potentially some malignancies [1,2]. In bladder cancer, BCG therapy induces a potent local immune response leading to the destruction of cancer cells [3,4]. This report presents a unique case in which a patient, previously treated with BCG for bladder cancer, subsequently developed GBM, which then regressed completely. This occurrence raises the possibility of systemic immunomodulatory effects induced by BCG influencing the course of GBM.

2. Case Presentation

A 67-year-old male was referred to our emergency department due to the progressive deterioration of his consciousness. His previous medical history was positive for bladder cancer diagnosed 6 years earlier, and he had been treated for 5 years with topical bladder BCG instillations. The patient also had a history of arterial hypertension.

2.1. Clinical Examination and Findings

The clinical examination revealed a Glasgow Coma Scale (GCS) score of 10/15 and left-sided hemianopia. A detailed physical examination was impossible due to the poor neurological condition of the patient.

2.2. Imaging and Initial Diagnosis

A head CT scan showed two lesions: the largest located to the right, temporally and posteriorly, and a smaller one positioned medially and anteriorly to it. The midline shift was approximately 12 mm. The patient underwent an urgent brain MRI with Gadolinium to better characterize the two lesions, measuring 70 × 40 mm^2 and 17 × 18 mm^2, both associated with peritumoral edema and central necrosis (Figure 1).

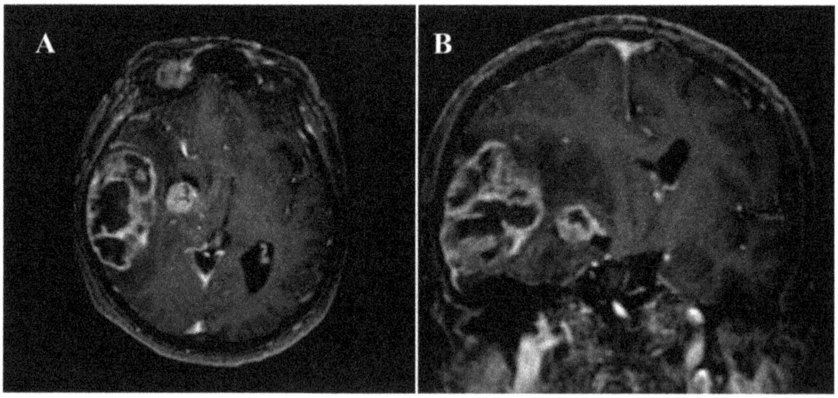

Figure 1. Preoperative T1-weighted brain MRI axial (**A**) and coronal (**B**) sequences with gadolinium reveal the presence of lesions with irregular margins, containing diffuse necrotic and hemorrhagic/hemosiderin-rich intralesional components. It exhibits pathological and heterogeneous contrast enhancement, localized in the right lateral temporal region. This lesion measures approximately 70 mm antero-posteriorly, 40 mm medio-laterally, and 56 mm cranio-caudally. It is associated with a substantial perifocal edema extending into the temporal, deep frontoparietal, and ipsilateral nucleus-capsule. Another smaller lesion of similar significance and characteristics, with a rounded morphology, is observed in the ipsilateral temporo-mesial region.

2.3. Further Diagnostic Tests

The patient also underwent a PET-FDG total body scan and a CT scan with contrast enhancement, which excluded systemic lesions.

2.4. Initial Surgical Intervention

An urgent right temporal craniotomy was performed to remove the larger lesion, but the procedure was quickly stopped due to intraoperative seizures, and the smaller lesion was left in place. The postoperative period was uneventful, and the patient progressively fully recovered. Postoperative imaging showed complete removal of the larger lesion and the stability of the smaller one (Figure 2).

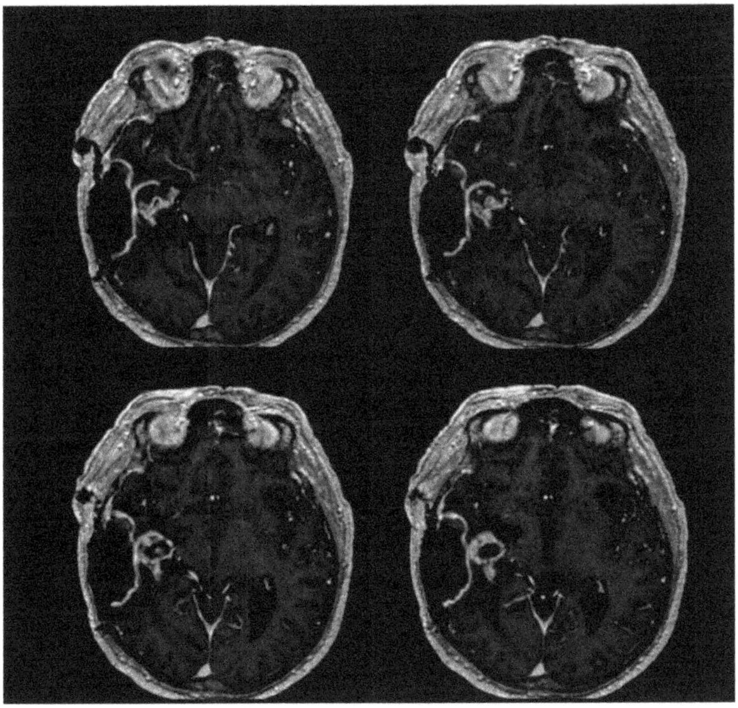

Figure 2. Postoperative T1-weighted brain MRI axial sequences with gadolinium demonstrate the complete removal of the larger lesion and the stability of the smaller temporo-mesial right lesion.

2.5. Histological Examination

Histological examination documented the lesion as a high-grade glial tumor, wildtype IDH, with extensive necrosis and microvascular proliferation consistent with glioblastoma (WHO grade IV). MGMT methylation was observed (32%).

2.6. Treatment and Follow-Up

Post-operatively, the patient was prescribed levetiracetam at a dosage of 500 mg twice daily for a duration of 4 weeks to manage the risk of seizures. Additionally, a course of Dexamethasone, initially administered at 4 mg twice daily for 15 days, was gradually tapered down to mitigate inflammation and cerebral edema caused by the surgery. The patient started the Stupp protocol and underwent serial MRI scans with Gadolinium every 3 months. During follow-up, tumor stability was observed for about 1 year. Afterward, MRI scans documented no recurrence in the operative field and complete tumor regression of the unresected lesion. Serial MRI scans with Gadolinium, spectroscopy, perfusion studies, and PET-met confirmed the regression of the glioma (Figure 3).

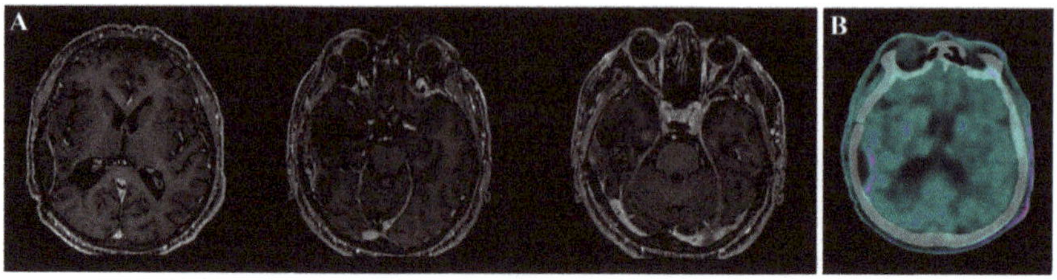

Figure 3. One-year follow-up postoperative T1-weighted brain MRI axial sequences with gadolinium reveal locoregional meningeal enhancement in the absence of neoangiogenesis signs on perfusion study. The previously observed right temporo-mesial lesion shows no enhancement and exhibits no signs of neoangiogenesis in the perfusion study (**A**). The 11C-methionine PET/CT brain examination documents a mild, heterogeneous tracer accumulation along the right temporo-parietal surgical cavity margin, with no additional abnormalities or asymmetries detected in the remaining brain areas. This is indicative of the absence of cerebral disease (**B**).

2.7. Disease Progression

The patient appeared to be tumor-free for almost 1 year, but 21 months after surgery he developed a recurrence of bladder cancer, and BCG therapy was administered. After 1 month, two new brain lesions appeared: one in the right paratrigonal area and another infiltrating the splenium of the corpus callosum on the left side; no recurrence of the original lesions on the right was detected (Figure 4).

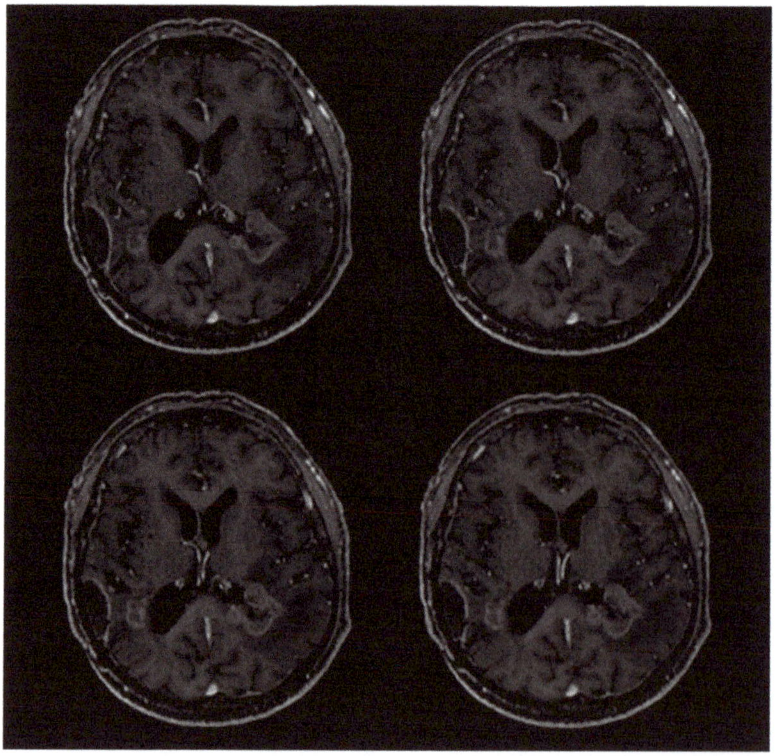

Figure 4. T1-weighted postoperative brain MRI sequences at more than one year of follow-up reveal two new brain lesions: one in the right para-trigonal area and another infiltrating the splenium of the corpus callosum on the left side. There is no evidence of recurrence of the previous lesions on the right.

2.8. End-of-Life Care

It was decided to withdraw the patient from any treatment due to the severity of the tumor spread. The patient died a few days later, 22 months after surgery.

3. Discussion

BCG, an attenuated microorganism derived from Mycobacterium bovis, becomes avirulent after undergoing several laboratory processes. Its capacity to stimulate an effective immune response makes it valuable in vaccinations against tuberculosis and leprosy in high-endemic areas. It is also utilized in neurology for the immunomodulation treatment of multiple sclerosis and in oncology [4].

In urology, it has been used towards non-muscle-invasive bladder cancer, resulting in reduced recurrence and progression. This is achieved by stimulating in situ innate and acquired immunity, thereby providing focused control of tumor expansion [1,2]. Additionally, BCG can directly induce tumor necrosis through free radical-mediated oxidative stress, boosting the immune response, or in certain cases, causing controlled cell death or apoptosis [3].

Recent studies have shown that neoplastic cells can phagocytize the bacillus through endocytosis, which, once internalized, activates intrinsic caspase-dependent pathways aimed at cellular death, facilitating a cytoreductive effect [4]. This internalization does not occur in healthy urothelium cells. Despite the stronger capacity in less differentiated neoplastic cells, there are evident cases of under-response or non-responsiveness to the bacillus [5]. This is likely due to the bacillus's paradoxical ability to inhibit other cytokine-mediated cytotoxic signals intended to ensure neoplastic cell death [6]. As a result, both the cytotoxic and immunomodulatory effects of BCG continue to be investigated through in vitro and in vivo experiments.

GBM is a neurosurgical disease with a poor prognosis. However, advancements in chemotherapy and radiotherapy, such as the Stupp protocol, have increased survival from six months to two years for patients with GBM IDH-mutant [7].

Rare cases of pathology regression have been reported, where off-label usage of drugs for vasogenic edema (such as dexamethasone) is hypothesized to inhibit inflammation mediators like metalloproteinase and adrenomedullin. These factors affect neo-angiogenesis underlying tumor proliferation and its expansion [8]. Corticosteroids, along with antiepileptic drugs (levetiracetam, valproate), are believed to increase neoplastic cells' chemotherapy sensitivity by interfering with the activity of specific D cyclins involved in stem cell transformation [9]. Indeed, a unique case of the regression of a glioblastoma following therapy with dexamethasone and levetiracetam has already been reported [10]. Levetiracetam has also been invoked as a trigger for unexpected, likely immune-related events in patients previously submitted to radiotherapy [11]. Several studies have proven that such an antiepileptic drug may act as a sensitizer of concurrent chemoradiotherapy in glioblastoma, enhancing its antitumor efficacy and, ultimately, prolonging patients' survival [12–15]. An almost complete regression of a recurrent anaplastic oligodendroglioma was reported in a patient treated with levetiracetam in addition to temozolomide and dexamethasone [16].

In the 1970s, Albright demonstrated a hypersensitivity reaction in GBM patients after BCG inoculation [17], and in 1985, Knerich et al. used BCG as immunotherapy in combination with chemotherapy for brain tumors (both primary and metastatic) [18]. Current research is focusing on testing vaccines capable of immunizing the body against specific molecular receptors on the membrane of neoplastic cells.

The use of bacterial microorganisms like Vibrio cholerae for pre-immunizing mice with anaplastic ependymoblastomas appears to stimulate an immune response that interferes with neoplastic proliferation and increases median survival [19].

Specific antibodies against tumor cells were extracted from Macaca Fascicularis primates' serum after being inoculated with BCG and human glioma cell cultures. This extraction confirmed the effectiveness and non-toxicity of the serum, as it stimulated a hyperimmune response without attacking the autologous tissues (encephalomyelitis) [20].

However, there are limited studies explaining the immunotherapeutic function of BCG in human glioma and its potential role in tumor regression. The development of hybrid vaccines, which combine the microbiological component BCG with autologous neoplastic cells that have lost their ability to divide due to radiation but can still be processed and recognized by the immune system, has made significant progress in research [21]. However, there are still many unanswered questions about the mechanism of action and efficacy of this approach in tumor immunobiology.

The mechanisms by which BCG achieves this involve both innate and adaptive immunity. BCG is known to stimulate toll-like receptor 2 (TLR2), leading to the activation of the NF-κB pathway and the subsequent release of pro-inflammatory cytokines such as TNF-α, IL-1, IL-6, and IL-12. Furthermore, BCG stimulates the maturation of dendritic cells, enhances the cytotoxicity of natural killer (NK) cells, and promotes the activation and proliferation of both CD4+ and CD8+ T cells [22].

The possibility of BCG having systemic immunomodulatory effects that could influence the course of other malignancies, including GBM, is intriguing. The regression of GBM in this case could be hypothesized to result from an enhanced systemic immune response induced by BCG, possibly involving the activation of NK cells or cytotoxic T cells against GBM cells, or the production of cytokines that inhibit tumor growth or promote apoptosis of cancer cells.

However, it is also possible that the observed regression of GBM in this case is coincidental and unrelated to BCG therapy. Besides the above-mentioned possible role of dexamethasone and levetiracetam, the components of STUPP protocol may also have been a determinant in achieving the observed tumor disappearance: the event of complete response to chemoradiotherapy or temozolomide alone occurred rarely [23,24]. Given the rarity of spontaneous regression in GBM, which was reported as transient (like in our case) in only two other patients [25,26], the temporal relationship to BCG therapy suggests a possible causal relationship, but this cannot be confirmed based on a single case. Furthermore, bladder cancer recurrence followed by the development of two new lesions described here might be related to each other. One hypothesis could be that the bladder recurrence was the expression of the BCG-related lack of immune coverage, leading to both recurrences. However, even surgery could be added to the list of the above determinant factors, lying as a further confounder behind the cause of the observed result. Indeed, surgical procedures (intended both as biopsy and resection of the primary tumor or metastases) may elicit immunologic surveillance through proinflammatory injuries leading up to complete regression of any residual macroscopic distant tumor [27]. This very rare phenomenon has been reported for a variety of tumor histologies, although not yet for gliomas [25,26,28–30].

A comprehensive theory would bring into play all the afore-mentioned factors: it is possible that the subtotal resection, functioning as an immune un-blocker thanks to its association with radiotherapy, temozolomide, levetiracetam, and dexamethasone, may have facilitated the host immune system to cross-react against the residual glioblastoma cells after a long-standing stimulation with BCG. The latter, once stopped for several months, might have been insufficient to imprint an effective immunological memory to prevent and contrast the subsequent bladder and brain recurrences. Further studies, including preclinical studies in animal models and clinical trials in patients, are needed to investigate whether BCG or other forms of immunotherapy could be effective in the treatment of GBM.

Despite the uncertainty, this case raises important questions about the potential role of immunotherapy in the treatment of GBM and provides a rationale for further research in this area.

It is hoped that such research will contribute to the development of more effective therapies for GBM. Given the significant challenge that this aggressive cancer presents, it is crucial to explore all potential therapeutic avenues, including those that might seem unexpected. The potential immunomodulatory effects of BCG, a treatment traditionally associated with bladder cancer and tuberculosis, certainly fall within this category.

The immune system has long been known to play a crucial role in cancer development and progression but harnessing it effectively for cancer therapy has been a significant challenge [27]. The success of immunotherapies such as checkpoint inhibitors in various cancers has underscored the potential of this approach, and the possibility that BCG might have similar effects in GBM is an exciting prospect that warrants further investigation [31].

However, it is worth noting that the complex immunological environment of the brain and the immunosuppressive nature of GBM present specific challenges for immunotherapy in this context. GBM has various mechanisms to evade and suppress the immune response, including the production of immunosuppressive cytokines, the recruitment of regulatory T cells, and the expression of immune checkpoint molecules [32–35]. Overcoming these mechanisms will be a key challenge in the development of effective immunotherapies for GBM.

4. Conclusions

The intriguing case showcasing transient GBM regression after Bacillus Calmette–Guérin (BCG) therapy for bladder cancer prompts a critical need for a meticulous investigation into its underlying mechanisms and therapeutic prospects. While the precise mechanisms remain enigmatic, the potential systemic immunomodulatory effects of BCG on GBM warrant in-depth scrutiny. This scenario prompts pivotal inquiries into the complex interplay between systemic immune responses and the intricate microenvironment within GBM. An extensive exploration into the prospective immunomodulatory roles of BCG or analogous immunotherapies in GBM therapy holds significant promise. However, GBM's innate immunosuppressive strategies, including cytokine secretion, regulatory T cell recruitment, and immune checkpoint expression, pose formidable challenges. The clinical implications are profound, suggesting a potential avenue for refining GBM treatment strategies by harnessing immune responses. Despite the success of analogous treatments in other cancers, overcoming GBM's intrinsic immunosuppression necessitates rigorous investigation and innovative approaches. Interdisciplinary collaboration is imperative to elucidate the intricate dynamics between immunotherapy and GBM. Thorough preclinical investigations and meticulously designed clinical trials are imperative to ascertain the potential efficacy of BCG or similar immunotherapeutic interventions in reshaping GBM treatment paradigms. While this case signifies the intriguing potential of BCG-induced immunomodulation in GBM, comprehensive research is imperative. Successful exploration could offer new avenues for combatting this formidable disease, offering renewed optimism for individuals grappling with GBM's challenges.

Author Contributions: Conceptualization, G.E.U., G.S. and S.M.; methodology, G.E.U., G.S. and G.F.; software, G.E.U. and G.S.; validation, G.E.U., M.S., V.Y., B.K., R.S., S.F. and G.F.; formal analysis, G.S. and G.F.; investigation, G.E.U., G.S., S.M. and M.S.; resources, G.S. and G.F.; data curation, G.E.U. and G.S.; writing—original draft preparation, G.E.U., G.S., S.M. and G.F.; writing—review and editing, G.E.U., G.F. and G.S.; visualization, M.S., V.Y., B.K., R.S., S.F. and G.S.; supervision, G.E.U. and G.S.; project administration, G.E.U. funding acquisition, G.F. All authors have read and agreed to the published version of the manuscript.

Funding: This research received no external funding.

Institutional Review Board Statement: Not applicable.

Informed Consent Statement: Written informed consent has been obtained from the patient's next of kin to publish this paper.

Data Availability Statement: No new data were created or analysed in this study.

Acknowledgments: We would like to extend our gratitude to all those who contributed to the successful completion of this medical research, including colleagues, mentors, and our supportive friends and families.

Conflicts of Interest: The authors declare no conflict of interest.

References

1. Sandes, E.; Lodillinsky, C.; Cwirenbaum, R.; Argüelles, C.; Casabé, A.; Eiján, A.M. Cathepsin B is involved in the apoptosis intrinsic pathway induced by Bacillus Calmette-Guérin in transitional cancer cell lines. *Int. J. Mol. Med.* **2007**, *20*, 823–828. [CrossRef]
2. Yu, D.S.; Wu, C.L.; Ping, S.Y.; Keng, C.; Shen, K.H. Bacille Calmette-Guerin can induce cellular apoptosis of urothelial cancer directly through toll-like receptor 7 activation. *Kaohsiung J. Med. Sci.* **2015**, *31*, 391–397. [CrossRef] [PubMed]
3. Choi, S.Y.; Kim, S.J.; Chi, B.H.; Kwon, J.K.; Chang, I.H. Modulating the internalization of bacille Calmette-Guérin by cathelicidin in bladder cancer cells. *Urology* **2015**, *85*, 964.e7–964.e12. [CrossRef] [PubMed]
4. Geckin, B.; Konstantin Föhse, F.; Domínguez-Andrés, J.; Netea, M.G. Trained immunity: Implications for vaccination. *Curr. Opin. Immunol.* **2022**, *77*, 102190. [CrossRef] [PubMed]
5. Holla, S.; Ghorpade, D.S.; Singh, V.; Bansal, K.; Balaji, K.N. Mycobacterium bovis BCG promotes tumor cell survival from tumor necrosis factor-α-induced apoptosis. *Mol. Cancer* **2014**, *13*, 210. [CrossRef] [PubMed]
6. Ryk, C.; Koskela, L.R.; Thiel, T.; Wiklund, N.P.; Steineck, G.; Schumacher, M.C.; de Verdier, P.J. Outcome after BCG treatment for urinary bladder cancer may be influenced by polymorphisms in the NOS_2 and NOS_3 genes. *Redox Biol.* **2015**, *6*, 272–277. [CrossRef] [PubMed]
7. Biau, J.; Chautard, E.; De Schlichting, E.; Dupic, G.; Pereira, B.; Fogli, A.; Müller-Barthélémy, M.; Dalloz, P.; Khalil, T.; Dillies, A.F.; et al. Radiotherapy plus temozolomide in elderly patients with GBM: A "real-life" report. *Radiat. Oncol.* **2017**, *12*, 197. [CrossRef] [PubMed]
8. Takahashi, K.; Udono-Fujimori, R.; Totsune, K.; Murakami, O.; Shibahara, S. Suppression of cytokine-induced expression of adrenomedullin and endothelin-1 by dexamethasone in T98G human GBM cells. *Peptides* **2003**, *24*, 1053–1062. [CrossRef]
9. Li, X.N.; Shu, Q.; Su, J.M.; Perlaky, L.; Blaney, S.M.; Lau, C.C. Valproic acid induces growth arrest, apoptosis, and senescence in medulloblastomas by increasing histone hyperacetylation and regulating expression of p21Cip1, CDK4, and CMYC. *Mol. Cancer Ther.* **2005**, *4*, 1912–1922. [CrossRef]
10. Peddi, P.; Ajit, N.E.; Burton, G.V.; El-Osta, H. Regression of a glioblastoma multiforme: Spontaneous versus a potential antineoplastic effect of dexamethasone and levetiracetam. *BMJ Case Rep.* **2016**, *2016*, bcr2016217393. [CrossRef]
11. Sindoni, A.; Severo, C.; Vadala', R.E.; Ferini, G.; Mazzei, M.M.; Vaccaro, M.; IatÌ, G.; Pontoriero, A.; Pergolizzi, S. Levetiracetam-induced radiation recall dermatitis in a patient undergoing stereotactic radiotherapy. *J. Dermatol.* **2016**, *43*, 1440–1441. [CrossRef]
12. Hwang, K.; Kim, J.; Kang, S.G.; Jung, T.Y.; Kim, J.H.; Kim, S.H.; Kang, S.H.; Hong, Y.K.; Kim, T.M.; Kim, Y.J.; et al. Levetiracetam as a sensitizer of concurrent chemoradiotherapy in newly diagnosed glioblastoma: An open-label phase 2 study. *Cancer Med.* **2022**, *11*, 371–379. [CrossRef]
13. Pallud, J.; Huberfeld, G.; Dezamis, E.; Peeters, S.; Moiraghi, A.; Gavaret, M.; Guinard, E.; Dhermain, F.; Varlet, P.; Oppenheim, C.; et al. Effect of Levetiracetam Use Duration on Overall Survival of Isocitrate Dehydrogenase Wild-Type Glioblastoma in Adults: An Observational Study. *Neurology* **2022**, *98*, e125–e140. [CrossRef]
14. Roh, T.H.; Moon, J.H.; Park, H.H.; Kim, E.H.; Hong, C.K.; Kim, S.H.; Kang, S.G.; Chang, J.H. Association between survival and levetiracetam use in glioblastoma patients treated with temozolomide chemoradiotherapy. *Sci. Rep.* **2020**, *10*, 10783. [CrossRef]
15. Kim, Y.H.; Kim, T.; Joo, J.D.; Han, J.H.; Kim, Y.J.; Kim, I.A.; Yun, C.H.; Kim, C.Y. Survival benefit of levetiracetam in patients treated with concomitant chemoradiotherapy and adjuvant chemotherapy with temozolomide for glioblastoma multiforme. *Cancer* **2015**, *121*, 2926–2932. [CrossRef]
16. Kumar, A.A.; Abraham Koshy, A. Regression of Recurrent High-Grade Glioma with Temozolomide, Dexamethasone, and Levetiracetam: Case Report and Review of the Literature. *World Neurosurg.* **2017**, *108*, 990.e11–990.e16. [CrossRef]
17. Albright, L.; Seab, J.A.; Ommaya, A.K. Intracerebral delayed hypersensitivity reactions in GBM multiforme patients. *Cancer* **1977**, *39*, 1331–1336. [CrossRef]
18. Knerich, R.; Robustelli della Cuna, G.; Butti, G.; Pavesi, L.; Adinolfi, D.; Preti, P.; Locatelli, D. Chemotherapy plus immunotherapy for patients with primary and metastatic brain tumors. *J. Neurosurg. Sci.* **1985**, *29*, 19–24.
19. Albright, L.; Madigan, J.C.; Gaston, M.R.; Houchens, D.P. Therapy in an intracerebral murine glioma model, using Bacillus Calmette-Guérin, neuraminidase-treated tumor cells, and 1-(2-chloroethyl)-3-cyclohexyl-1-nitrosourea. *Cancer Res.* **1975**, *35*, 658–665.
20. Wikstrand, C.J.; Bigner, D.D. Hyperimmunization of non-human primates with BCG-CW and cultured human glioma-derived cells. Production of reactive antisera and absence of EAE induction. *J. Neuroimmunol.* **1981**, *1*, 249–260. [CrossRef]
21. Holladay, F.P.; Heitz-Turner, T.; Bayer, W.L.; Wood, G.W. Autologous tumor cell vaccination combined with adoptive cellular immunotherapy in patients with grade III/IV astrocytoma. *J. Neurooncol.* **1996**, *27*, 179–189. [CrossRef] [PubMed]
22. van Puffelen, J.H.; Keating, S.T.; Oosterwijk, E.; van der Heijden, A.G.; Netea, M.G.; Joosten, L.A.B.; Vermeulen, S.H. Trained immunity as a molecular mechanism for BCG immunotherapy in bladder cancer. *Nat. Rev. Urol.* **2020**, *17*, 513–525. [CrossRef] [PubMed]
23. Parlato, C.; Barbarisi, M.; Moraci, M.; Moraci, A. Surgery, radiotherapy and temozolomide in treating high-grade gliomas. *Front. Biosci.* **2006**, *11*, 1280–1283. [CrossRef] [PubMed]
24. Laigle-Donadey, F.; Figarella-Branger, D.; Chinot, O.; Taillandier, L.; Cartalat-Carel, S.; Honnorat, J.; Kaloshi, G.; Delattre, J.Y.; Sanson, M. Up-front temozolomide in elderly patients with glioblastoma. *J. Neurooncol.* **2010**, *99*, 89–94. [CrossRef] [PubMed]

25. Yamasaki, F.; Takayasu, T.; Nosaka, R.; Haratake, D.; Arihiro, K.; Ueno, H.; Shimomura, R.; Akiyama, Y.; Sugiyama, K.; Matsumoto, M.; et al. Transient spontaneous regression of brainstem glioblastoma. *J. Neurosurg. Sci.* **2018**, *62*, 610–612. [CrossRef] [PubMed]
26. Gandhoke, C.S.; Ansari, M.T.; Syal, S.K.; Singh, D.; Saran, R.K. Spontaneous Regression of a Suspected Temporal lobe Glioblastoma Multiforme and its Re-appearance at a Different Site. *JCR* **2017**, *7*, 214–218. [CrossRef]
27. Zhang, Y.; Zhang, Z. The history and advances in cancer immunotherapy: Understanding the characteristics of tumor-infiltrating immune cells and their therapeutic implications. *Cell Mol. Immunol.* **2020**, *17*, 807–821. [CrossRef]
28. Žarković, N.; Jaganjac, M.; Žarković, K.; Gęgotek, A.; Skrzydlewska, E. Spontaneous Regression of Cancer: Revealing Granulocytes and Oxidative Stress as the Crucial Double-edge Sword. *Front. Biosci. (Landmark Ed.)* **2022**, *27*, 119. [CrossRef]
29. Pokhrel, B.; Chidharla, A.; Neupane, P. Spontaneous Regression of the Pulmonary Metastases in Adenoid Cystic Carcinoma of the Parotid Gland: A Case Report. *Cureus* **2022**, *14*, e30783. [CrossRef]
30. Roseman, J.M. Regression of locally recurrent squamous cell carcinoma of the skin following excision of a metastasis: With review of the literature. *J. Surg. Oncol.* **1988**, *39*, 213–214. [CrossRef]
31. Arrieta, V.A.; Dmello, C.; McGrail, D.J.; Brat, D.J.; Lee-Chang, C.; Heimberger, A.B.; Chand, D.; Stupp, R.; Sonabend, A.M. Immune checkpoint blockade in glioblastoma: From tumor heterogeneity to personalized treatment. *J. Clin. Investig.* **2023**, *133*, e163447. [CrossRef]
32. Ghouzlani, A.; Kandoussi, S.; Tall, M.; Reddy, K.P.; Rafii, S.; Badou, A. Immune Checkpoint Inhibitors in Human Glioma Microenvironment. *Front. Immunol.* **2021**, *12*, 679425. [CrossRef]
33. Qi, Y.; Liu, B.; Sun, Q.; Xiong, X.; Chen, Q. Immune Checkpoint Targeted Therapy in Glioma: Status and Hopes. *Front. Immunol.* **2020**, *11*, 578877. [CrossRef]
34. Croese, T.; Castellani, G.; Schwartz, M. Immune cell compartmentalization for brain surveillance and protection. *Nat. Immunol.* **2021**, *22*, 1083–1092. [CrossRef]
35. Pardoll, D.M. The blockade of immune checkpoints in cancer immunotherapy. *Nat. Rev. Cancer* **2012**, *12*, 252–264. [CrossRef]

Journal of
Personalized
Medicine

MDPI

Review

Modulation of Radiation Doses and Chimeric Antigen Receptor T Cells: A Promising New Weapon in Solid Tumors—A Narrative Review

Antonio Pontoriero [1,†], Paola Critelli [1,*,†], Federico Chillari [1], Giacomo Ferrantelli [1], Miriam Sciacca [1], Anna Brogna [2], Silvana Parisi [1] and Stefano Pergolizzi [1]

1 Radiation Oncology Unit, Department of Biomedical, Dental Science and Morphological and Functional Images, University of Messina, 98125 Messina, Italy; apontoriero@unime.it (A.P.); chillari.federico@gmail.com (F.C.); giacomo.ferrantelli@outlook.com (G.F.); miriamsciacca06@gmail.com (M.S.); silvana.parisi@unime.it (S.P.); stpergolizzi@unime.it (S.P.)
2 Radiotherapy Unit, Medical Physics Unit, A.O.U. "G. Martino", 98125 Messina, Italy; anna.brogna@polime.it
* Correspondence: paolacritelli@outlook.com
† These authors contributed equally to this work.

Abstract: Tumor behavior is determined by its interaction with the tumor microenvironment (TME). Chimeric antigen receptor (CART) cell therapy represents a new form of cellular immunotherapy (IT). Immune cells present a different sensitivity to radiation therapy (RT). RT can affect tumor cells both modifying the TME and inducing DNA damage, with different effects depending on the low and high doses delivered, and can favor the expression of CART cells. CART cells are patients' T cells genetically engineered to recognize surface structure and to eradicate cancer cells. High-dose radiation therapy (HDRT, >10–20 Gy/fractions) converts immunologically "cold" tumors into "hot" ones by inducing necrosis and massive inflammation and death. LDRT (low-dose radiation therapy, >5–10 Gy/fractions) increases the expansion of CART cells and leads to non-immunogenetic death. An innovative approach, defined as the LATTICE technique, combines a high dose in higher FDG- uptake areas and a low dose to the tumor periphery. The association of RT and immune checkpoint inhibitors increases tumor immunogenicity and immune response both in irradiated and non-irradiated sites. The aim of this narrative review is to clarify the knowledge, to date, on CART cell therapy and its possible association with radiation therapy in solid tumors.

Keywords: CART; tumor microenvironment; immunotherapy; radiotherapy; solid tumor

1. Introduction

Cancer is characterized by a high mutation rate that leads to a process of transformation from healthy cells to cancer cells [1].

The immune system can recognize malignantly transformed cells through a group of molecules found on the surface, called tumor-associated antigens (TAAs), that differentiate a tumor cell from a normal one [2]. The first TAA was identified in the 1990s in testis cancer (MAGEA1), reporting high tumor antigenicity and a promising immunotherapeutic target [3–5].

Immunotherapy is based on the ability of T cells to activate and bind cancer cells, enhancing the immune system to recognize cancer as a foreign invader.

A new therapeutic approach which aims to prevent treatment resistance, reducing the tumor burden, is represented by adoptive cellular therapy (ACT). ACT, or cellular immunotherapy, is a form of immunotherapy based on a patient's T cells, which are genetically engineered to recognize cancer cells and then reinfused back into the patient [6].

To date, there are three major modalities of ACT: tumor-infiltrating lymphocytes (TILs), genetically engineered T cell receptors (TCRs), and chimeric antigen receptor (CAR) T cells.

TILs are a polyclonal population of lymphocytes that reside in the tumor with broad antigen recognition in tumor cells [7].

TCRs are engineered T cells that recognize HLA-presented peptides derived from the proteins of all cellular compartments [8].

CART cells represent one of the most promising approaches in tumor immunotherapy, especially in treating hematological tumors [9–16].

In solid tumors, efficacies are not demonstrated yet. The first therapeutic approach in solid tumors was reported in 2006 by Rosemberg. He found that TCR-T therapy could recognize the melanocyte-differentiating antigen (MART-1) with highly positive results in the treatment [17,18]; afterward, Cartellieri et al. showed that in melanoma, CART can significantly improve survival conditions without interruption [19].

The aim of this narrative review is to clarify the knowledge, to date, on CART cell therapy and its possible association with radiation therapy in solid tumors.

2. CART: Chimeric Antigen Receptor (CAR) T Cells

In 2017, the FDA approved the first anti-CD19 CART cell product, tisagenlecleucel, for relapsed and/or refractory B-cell precursor acute lymphoblastic leukemia (B-ALL) in pediatric and young adult patients.

CART involves lymphocytes entirely engineered to recognize any cell surface structure, independently of the MHC (major histocompatibility complex) presentation, leading to stronger T cell activation, a more robust anti-tumor response in vivo, and the eradication of tumor cells [7].

2.1. CART Cell Structure

To date, four generations of CART cells are known. In the first generation of CART cells, the extracellular moiety for antigen recognition is most commonly a single-chain variable fragment of an antibody (hinge or spacer structure). This structure is anchored to a transmembrane component with an attachment, on the intracytoplasmic cell membrane, to T-cell signaling molecules. First-generation CARs only had an intracellular signaling domain of CD3ξ (cluster differentiation 3ξ) to activate T cells [20,21]. The receptors that contained single-chain variable fragments recognized antigens independently of the MHC (major histocompatibility complex) and comprised target cell surface proteins, carbohydrates, and glycolipids [22]. First-generation CARs can induce a cytotoxic antitumor response when T cells are activated. They can eliminate cancer cells effectively through secreting granzyme and expressing FasL (Fas cell surface death receptor ligand) and tumor-necrosis-factor-related apoptosis-inducing ligand (TRAIL) [23]. After repeated exposure to antigens, they do not result in T cell expansion [24]. In the second generation, Maher et al. interposed a costimulatory signaling domain 4-1BB (CD137 or tumor necrosis factor receptor superfamily 9-TNFRSF9) or CD28 costimulatory signaling domain between both the transmembrane and T-cell activating domains of a ζ chain fusion [25]. CD28, in association with co-stimulatory CD3ξ, represents the intracellular signaling domain that allows T cell activation and proliferation [23,26]. Third-generation CARs comprise three intracellular signaling domains: CD3ξ and two costimulatory domains, CD28 and 4-IBB [23]. In fourth-generation CARs, T cells are redirected to improve cytotoxicity and edit the immune system with the inducible release of a transgenic payload (TRUCKs). CAR-redirected T cells deliver a transgenic product ('payload') to the targeted tumor tissue, and it is made of a nuclear factor of activated T cell (NFAT) domain, a suicide gene, or signaling domain that induces the production and release of proinflammatory cytokines, like Interleukin-7 (IL-7), IL-18, or IL-12 [27]. IL-12 improves T cell activation, modulates the immunological and vascular TME, and recruits additional immune cells.

To date, tisagenlecleucel and axicabtagene ciloleucel are the only CD19-targeted CART cells approved, and they belong to the second generation [28].

2.2. Toxicities

Principal CART cells' side effects are related to massive T cell activation. Different grading systems are currently used for CART-cell-related toxicity (ASTCT, CARTOX, and CTCAEv5.0), with significant differences between grading systems and the potential to undertreat or overtreat symptoms [29,30].

2.2.1. On-Target On-Tumor Toxicity: Cytokine Release Syndrome

According to the American Society for Transplantation and Cellular Therapy (ASTCT), cytokine release syndrome (CRS) is defined as an excessive response following any immune therapy that determines the activation or recruitment of endogenous or infused T cells and/or other immune effector cells [31]. The syndrome is related to rapid immune reactions driven by the massive release of cytokines, such as IFN-γ, IL-6, and IL-10. It develops several days after CART-cell infusion; manifests with fever, hypotension, and tachycardia; and can potentially progress to hemodynamic instability, resulting in end-organ injury [32–34].

Effective therapeutic options are tocilizumab, an anti-IL6 receptor antibody, and corticosteroids [35–37].

2.2.2. On-Target Off-Tumor Toxicity

On-target off-tumor toxicity represents a major obstacle to successful cancer immunotherapy. It is induced by a direct attack on healthy tissue cells expressing the targeted antigen. Considering the strength of redirected T cells, toxicity in non-pathogenic tissues can be highly damaging. It is typically managed in two ways: restricting antigen choice with co-stimulation-only CARs that lead to cytotoxic activation only when they meet a tumor cell or by accepting non-tumor antigen expression and the potentially associated severe toxicities [38].

2.2.3. Off-Target Toxicity

Off-Target toxicity occurs when the transduced T cell population attacks an antigen other than the targeted one or activates themselves regardless of their specificity. The off-target recognition of cross-reactive antigens has not been detected in CART-cell trials to date [39].

2.2.4. Neurotoxicity: ICANS (Immune-Effector-Cell-Associated Neurotoxicity Syndrome)

ASTCT defined ICANS as a pathologic process involving the central nervous system following any immune therapy that is characterized by the activation or recruitment of endogenous or infused T cells and/or other immune effector cells [31].

The incidence of immune-effector-cell-related neurotoxicity syndrome is closely correlated with CRS; it is more common in patients with B-ALL than in those with other diseases that receive CD19-specific CART-cell therapy [40,41]. The median time to the beginning of neurotoxicity ranges from 4 to 10 days after CART cell infusion with a median duration of 5–14 days. Symptoms can comprise headache, lethargy, impaired attention, dysgraphia, apraxia, aphasia, agitation, tremor, encephalopathy, and seizures. Treatment for neurotoxicity consists of supportive care, with or without corticosteroids and/or cytokine-directed therapies, based on the presence of active CRS [42].

2.2.5. Immunogenicity: Anaphylaxis

The potential immunogenicity of antigens used in engineered T cells may lead to severe anaphylaxis [43,44]. It might be associated with the release of IgE (immunoglobulin E) antibodies specific to the CAR-modified T cell product or to the in vitro T cell production process. High levels of tryptase, pathognomonic mast cell activation, and cytokines, particularly IL-6, IL-10, and IL-2, were observed in a clinical study given repeated infusions of the CART cells [45].

In some cases, CART cell therapy may be characterized by limited efficacy against solid tumors. One of the principal causes of a lacking or weak response is poor T cell expansion and T cell exhaustion triggered by co-inhibitory pathways [46]. Therefore, a combination of CART cells and immune checkpoint inhibitors (ICIs) is thought to lead to strong immune responses.

3. Tumor Microenvironment (TME)

Tumors' behavior is determined by their intrinsic characteristics and by their interaction with components of the TME. The TME is a highly structured ecosystem constituted by an immune and vascular part and extracellular matrix (ECM) fraction. The immune component consists of different immune cells, such as T cells, natural killer (NK) cells, dendritic cells (DCs), myeloid-derived suppressor cells (MDSCs), and tumor-associated macrophages (TAMs). M1 macrophages are pro-inflammatory phenotypes and are able to initiate and maintain inflammatory responses, secreting pro-inflammatory cytokines, activating endothelial cells, and inducing the recruitment of other immune cells into the inflamed tissue. On the other hand, M2 macrophages promote the exhaustion of inflammation, phagocytose apoptotic cells, drive collagen deposition, ensure tissue integrity, and release anti-inflammatory mediators [47]; the vascular component comprises blood and lymphatic endothelial cells that communicate with one another and with the different cancer cells present in the TME.

The ECM fraction consists of complex collagen fibers and other glycoproteins; the ECM is formed by laminin, fibronectin, elastin, and collagen. ECM aggregates in solid tumors are more than 60% of tumor mass [48]. Cancer-associated fibroblasts (CAFs) and mesenchymal stem cells (MSCs) represent the stromal component [49–51].

The main suppressive factors of solid-tumor TME factors are MDSCs, Tregs (regulatory T cells), chemokines, and cytokines produced by immune cells that activate transcription factors such as AP-1, NFκB, and STAT3, which support malignant cell proliferation and survival [52,53]. All TME components promote inflammation, induce the formation of new blood vessels, support tumor growth, avoid destruction by the immune system, evade cell death, and induce the activation of invasion and spreading to other parts of the body. Simultaneously, they stimulate the recruitment of immune cells at the site of neoplastic processing.

Principal components of the immune response are represented by several subpopulations of T lymphocytes. Th1 (T helper 1 lymphocytes) cells producing INFγ (interferon γ) have antitumor activity, stimulate cytotoxic T lymphocytes and NK cells, and recruit macrophages for their anti-tumor activity. On the other hand, Tregs have an inhibitory effect on Th1 lymphocytes, promoting immunosuppression and tumor cell growth. Th2 and Th17 produce cytokines (e.g., IL-4, IL-5, IL-13, IL-17, IL-21, and IL-22) that contribute to enhanced tissue inflammation and boost tumor growth. Regulatory T lymphocytes (CD4, CD25) inhibit the activity of other lymphocytes, mainly T cytotoxic ones [54–56].

The amount of T cells in neoplastic tissue seems to have a prognostic value [57]. In particular, one of the prognostic factors is represented by the presence of CD8-positive cytotoxic T lymphocytes in the TME before starting treatment because it plays one of the most important roles in the immune response [58,59].

Based on the cellular composition of lymphocyte infiltration cells in the TME, solid tumors distinguish three immune profiles. The "hot" tumors, or inflammatory tumors, are strongly infiltrated by a wide variety of cells: B lymphocytes, CD4-positive and CD8-positive T cells, Treg lymphocytes, macrophages, fibroblasts, and MDSCs, with many inflammatory signals and strong leukocyte infiltration. Additionally, these tumors are characterized by the presence of intra-tumor chemokines (e.g., CXCL9, CXCL10, CCL5) [60]. They have high cell density inside the tumor regardless of cell density in the tumor periphery. The "cold" tumors, or non-inflammatory tumors, are characterized by low cell density inside and outside the tumor and inflammatory signs. The "cold tumors" can be distinguished into two types: so-called "immune desert" tumors, with the presence of macrophages, Treg lymphocytes, and MDSCs in the absence of infiltration or activation of T lymphocytes, and tumors with "immune exclusion" characterized by high immune-cell density at the periphery or inside the stromal tissue and low density in the core of the tumor [61]. The immune cells do not infiltrate the parenchyma of the tumors due to the presence of the barrier character of fibroblast cells surrounding the tumor parenchyma [62].

The main differences between hot and cold tumors are summarized in Table 1.

Table 1. Characteristics of hot and cold tumors.

	T Cell Infiltration	Mutation Burden and PD-L1 Expression	Response to Immunotherapy	Example
Hot Tumor	- High cell density inside the tumor - Many inflammatory signals	High mutation burden and high expression of PD-L1	Sensitive	Melanoma, non-small-cell lung cancer, and cancers of the bladder, head and neck, kidney, liver
Cold Tumor	- Low cell density inside and outside the tumor - Low inflammatory signs	Low mutation burden and low expression of PD-L1	Resistant	Breast, ovary, prostate, pancreas, brain glioblastoma

Many solid tumors show hyperoxygenation, resulting in areas of permanent or transient hypoxia [63,64]. Hypoxia promotes the expression of HIF-1 (Hypoxia-Inducible Factor 1), for which overexpression highly correlates with worse prognosis for several solid cancers. Hypoxia stimulates the growth of tumor cells, inducing changes in the TME. By cross-talking with the nuclear factor-kB pathway, HIF-1a (Hypoxia Inducible Factor 1 Subunit Alpha) is able to modulate principal inflammatory functions in myeloid cells; promote the proliferation of regulatory lymphocytes that inhibit the differentiation of effector T cells [65,66], cell-cycle changes, and heat stress response; and play a critical role in high radioresistance [64].

Low levels of oxygen lead cells to reprogram energy metabolism. Cancer cells exhibit repressed mitochondrial respiration and a high rate of glucose uptake even in the presence of oxygen. This metabolic process, known as both the Warburg effect and aerobic glycolysis, promotes survival and long-term maintenance for tumor cells [67–69].

In dendritic cells and macrophages, pro-inflammatory stimuli induce the shift to aerobic glycolysis. In macrophages, the glycolytic phenotype promotes polarization from anti-inflammatory/pro-resolving M2 to the classically activated pro-inflammatory M1 and the production of many inflammatory mediators.

HIF-1α activates the secretion of pro-angiogenic factors such as VEGF-A. VEGF-A inhibits the release of inter-endothelial and vascular cell adhesion molecules (ICAM-1, VCAM-1) and hinders the migration of CART cells across the vascular endothelial cell barrier into the tumor tissue [70,71].

Hypoxia is associated with a poor prognosis and resistance to chemotherapy and radiotherapy [72].

The passage and activation of CART cells depend on tumor blood vessels; therefore, when CART cells are far away from blood vessels, they cannot reach tumor tissues, resulting in therapy resistance. At the same time, in a hypoxic TME, tumor cells produce cytokines, which are recruited to immunosuppressive cells to deplete CART cells, preventing their differentiation into effector memory cells [73].

To overcome hypoxia-related resistance, recently, some authors developed a dual oxygen-sensing approach to detect cell targets in hypoxia conditions. CAR cells were fused with an oxygen-dependent degradation domain (ODD) of HIF1α (CAR-ODD) [74,75]. Afterward, the CAR was implemented, adding the CAR's promoter in the long terminal repeat (LTR) enhancer region of hypoxia-responsive elements (HREs), leading to HIF1α-mediated transcription of the CAR (HypoxiCAR). In this way, HypoxiCAR is able to detect surface antigens only in hypoxia conditions (0.1% O_2) [76].

There are several trials that investigate the use of CART cells therapy in solid tumors such as glioblastoma, prostate cancer, and pleural cancer [77–82].

4. Radiotherapy

Radiotherapy (RT) has an anti-tumor effect both, modifying the TME and inducing DNA damage [83–85]; the mutations induced by RT enhance the expression of TAA, activate and increase endogenous-target antigen-specific immune responses, and favor the survival of antigen-positive cells [86], promoting CART cell engagement and expansion and modifying the inflammatory TME with an antigen-dependent mechanism [87,88].

Therefore, the induction of target antigen expression favors the efficacy of CART cell therapy after RT [89,90]. The immune cells present different sensitivity to irreversible damage induced by RT.

RT can overcome barriers induced by immunosuppressive TME and radioresistant tumor cells [91].

In fact, RT activates immune cells, increases the density of TILs, and facilitates recognition of tumor cells by T cells with induced immune-mediated cell death through the regulation of multiple cytokine signaling, including TNF, IL-1b, IL-10, and transforming growth factor beta (TGFβ) [92,93].

Ionizing radiation leads to the impairment of vascular cells, but those remaining or surrounding the irradiated tissues produce proinflammatory change [94]. On blood vessels, RT induces an increase in the production of the integrins ICAM-1 and VCAM-1 in vascular endothelial cells and promotes the transition of CART cells across the vascular endothelium into the tumor tissue [95,96].

On the other hand, RT supports immunosuppression in the tumor immune microenvironment with increased Tregs infiltration in the irradiated tumor zone. Tregs, with high Akt (Akt serine/threonine-protein kinases) expression, are more radioresistant than other T cell subsets and hinder effector T cells and CART cells' activity [97–99].

Different fractionation radiation doses, rather than the total dose, can determine different effects on the TME [100,101].

Several studies showed that the best fractionation schedule to use for immunotherapy combinations was 8 Gy $\times$ 3 Fx [102–105].

In a randomized phase 2 clinical trial, Schoenfeld et al. and Monjazeb et al. evaluated metastatic NSCLC and colorectal cancer, respectively, two different RT schedules known to increase immune responses: patients received ICIs alone or with repeated low-dose RT (0.5 Gy twice per day) or hypo-fractionated radiotherapy 24 Gy (8 Gy $\times$ 3 Fx). In both cases, a reduction in CD8+ T cell populations into the TME following directed radiotherapy was observed, especially with higher radiation doses [104,105].

Meng et al. investigated that a large single dose (20 Gy) or at 2 Gy in 10 fractions (10 $\times$ 2 Gy) modifies the immunosuppressive TAMs phenotype, but some studies showed an opposite effect of short-course or low-dose RT on TAMs [106].

Pancreatic cancer is considered a cold tumor, with a low mutation burden and a low response to T cell infiltration, which indicates its weak response to immunotherapy. In a preclinical study, sialic acid Lewis-a (sLeA) CART-cell (sLeA)-expressing pancreatic cancer tumor-bearing mice were associated with 2 Gy single low-dose radiotherapy. In this trial, the authors reported that local radiation led to a higher sensitivity of pancreatic cancer cells to activated CAR-T cells, and that combination therapy increased the sensitivity of sLeA– and sLeA+ tumor cells [102].

Even Tregs cells' infiltration grade based on the dose delivered was observed [104–109].

High-dose radiation therapy (HDRT, >10–20 Gy/fractions) converts immunologically "cold" tumors into "hot" by determining the death of cancer cells, resulting in the release of proinflammatory mediators, such as damage-associated molecular patterns (DAMPs), high-mobility group box 1 protein (HMGB1), ATP, and calreticulin, which stimulate Toll-like receptor 4 (TLR4).

The combination of HDRT and ICIs hinders Tregs and mitigates exhaustion. In general, higher RT doses induce necrosis and massive inflammation [105,106], increase the proportion of M1-like macrophages in the TME, and reduce the proportion of immunosuppressive M2-like macrophages and MDSCs post conventionally fractionated RT

(2 Gy/fraction). MDSCs have an immunosuppressive effect and can prevent anti-tumor immune responses [110–112].

On the contrary, low-dose RT (LDRT, >5–10 Gy/fractions) can reprogram the TME, encouraging the infiltration of effector immune cells and modulating the stroma to allow tumor eradication.

Klug et al. were the first to demonstrate, in a mouse model of neuroendocrine pancreatic cancer, that radiation doses ranging from 0.5 to 2 Gy induced de novo T cell homing into immune "cold" tumors, promoting M1 macrophage transition, normalization of tumor blood vessels, and increasing infiltration of adoptively transferred T cells [103,113]. LDRT so polarizes pro-tumor M2 macrophages to the antitumor M1 phenotype, increases the infiltration of CD4+ T cells and NK cells, and downregulates TGF-β inhibitory cytokines [114].

Delivering a 1 Gy × 2 dose alone in a lung adenocarcinoma model showed control of tumor growth and extended survival. Moreover, the efficacy of ICIs was significantly improved when associated with LDRT. At the same time, LDRT decreased cancer-associated fibroblasts (CAFs) in the tumor stroma context and allowed for increased infiltration of immune cells [115].

LDRT (0.1 Gy) was found to block the transformation by inducing antioxidants and reducing ROS (reactive oxygen species) [116].

LDRT is usually used for hot tumors, HDRT for cold ones.

Even when CART cell therapy is used in association with RT, the fractionation dose should be defined [116,117].

Several studies suggested that LDRT makes the tumor more sensitive to CART and may be a better support to CART cell treatment based on the radioimmunological effects. LDRT increases the expansion of infused T cells [118,119].

Rotte et al. proved that there exists a threshold dose beyond which, despite enhancing the dose, further dose escalation is unlikely to result in better objective response rates (ORRs) of CARTs [120].

Moreover, LDRT may play an immunomodulatory effect when combined with ICIs. This effect was defined as "radscopal effects" by James Welsh and refers to the systemic antitumor effects based on the combination of HDRT to the primary tumor and LDRT to the metastatic site in patients undergoing immunotherapy [113].

4.1. LATTICE Therapy

An emerging and innovative approach, defined as the "LATTICE technique", represents a particular form of spatially fractionated radiation therapy that allows for the delivery of heterogeneous radiation doses.

In clinical studies, 30 patients were treated with the palliative "metabolism-guided" lattice technique, a therapeutic approach in which high doses are delivered to vertices ("peaks") allocated according to 18F-FDG uptake and maintaining low doses to the tumor periphery ("valleys"). This permits the mobilization of the systemic immune-mediated tumor response [121]. The LATTICE technique will be explained in the proper section (Section 4.1.1).

The effect of LATTICE radiotherapy may be increased by association with ICIs. The high doses delivered to vertices lead to the release of DAMPs with immunogenic cell death. The valleys' low doses maintain the residual blood flow and permit DAMP circulation, immune cell homing, and activation. Jiang et al. reported that only the association of RT and ICIs increases tumor immunogenicity and immune response both in irradiated and non-irradiated areas (abscopal effect) [122,123].

The effects of different radiation doses and ICIs on tumor cells are summarized in Figure 1.

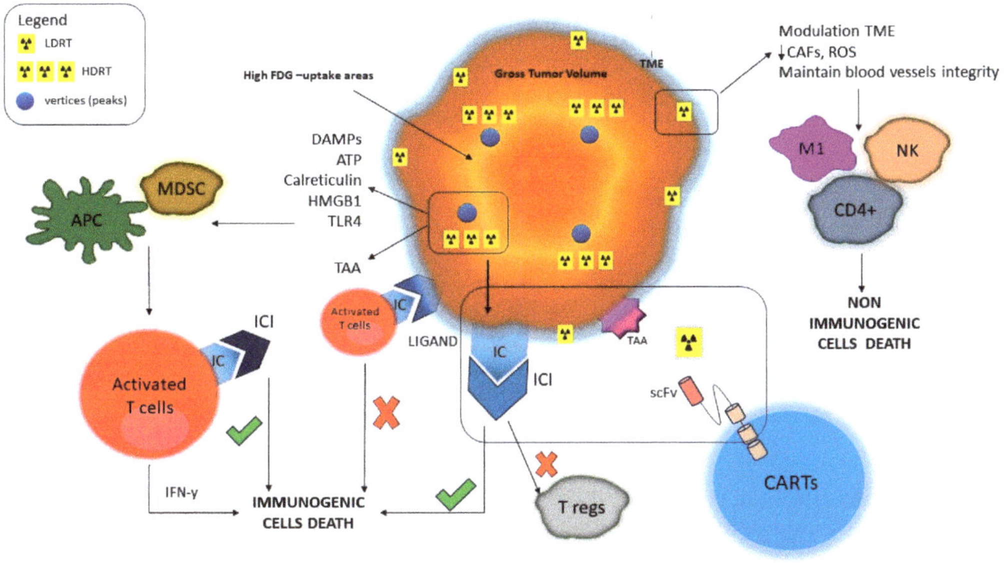

Figure 1. Effect of differentiated doses on tumor cells. High doses of radiation therapy lead to immunogenic cell death through both DAMPs, ATP, calreticulin, HMGB1, and TLR4 production, and the associated tumor antigens. This process results in the maturation of dendritic cells and the activation of T cells. Low doses of radiation therapy lead to non-immunogenic cell death through macrophage polarization (M2 → M1) and recruitment of CD4+ cells and NK cells. LDRT reduces ROS and maintains blood vessel integrity, allowing the movement of CART cells and cell effectors across the vascular endothelium into the tumor tissue. Tumor cells and activated T cells express on a surface immune checkpoint (IC). The link between the IC and the corresponding ligand inhibits T cells from killing tumor cells. The use of immune checkpoint inhibitors (ICIs) allows TC cells to kill tumor cells. The link IC–ICI blocks T reg activity. CARTs can bind antigen-associated tumors (TAAs) and induce tumor cell death. T cell exhaustion is one of the limitations of CART effects. The use of ICIs can elicit a durable response; LDRT increases the expansion of infused CART. HDRT increases immunosuppressive cells.

Because CART cell therapy is a form of immunotherapy, according to this knowledge, a heterogeneous radiation dose may be associated with CART therapy and ICIs to overcome a resistant TME.

4.1.1. LATTICE Technique

LATTICE therapy, a variant of spatially fractionated radiation therapy (SFRT), is a radiation therapy technique that allows one to deliver high lethal radiation doses to a large portion of tumor volume with OAR sparing.

The two main form of SFRT with photons are GRID radiotherapy (GRID RT, a 2-dimensional technique) and lattice radiotherapy (LRT)—a 3D configuration of GRID that allows one to deliver a high dose peak with a spherical shape within the tumor, surrounded by a lower-dose valley.

The GRID technique attempts to achieve a differential dose distribution using cerrobend blocks with holes inside, positioned into the gantry head. By alternating blocks and holes, this radiation field array generates a two-dimensional dose distribution, characterized by foci of high radiation doses (peaks) separated by low-dose areas (valleys).

With the advent of medical linear accelerators producing megavoltage (MV) photon beams and multileaf collimators (MLCs), the original GRID technique was dropped out and was replaced by the LATTICE radiotherapy technique, in which virtual grid blocks and rigid spatial dose fractionation was reproduced using treatment planning systems (TPSs) with the placement of high dose spheres, called vertices, within the tumor [124]. Usually, each vertex is about 1 to 2 cm in diameter with a distance of 2–3 cm from each other (center-to-center distance). Generally, a dose >15 Gy in a single fraction or a biological equivalent if fractionated is prescribed, since lower doses could be ineffective to achieve a satisfactory decrease in tumor volume [121].

The optimal LATTICE design is not well-defined because there is not any theory supported by evidence on this issue. In a recent study, Vertex placement did not follow a geometric pattern according to classic SFRT [125]. Because regions with different SUVs within a bulky mass could show different cell growth rates, oxygenation, and tumor microenvironments, vertices were placed in different 18F-FDG-uptake areas within the bulky disease. A "Photopenic PET Area" (PPA) showing a necrotic core and a "Super-Avid" PET Area (SAPA) with SUV > 75% SUVmax were detected. Vertices were positioned between SAPA and the remaining part of the APA ("Avid" PET Area (APA) with SUV > 2.5) [123].

Non coplanar beams or VMAT (Volumetric Modulated Arc Therapy) can be used to perform a dosimetric evaluation [126,127].

5. Conclusions

CART cells have revolutionized the treatment of several hematological malignancies, but there is little evidence on solid tumors. Based on this narrative review, promising results are also being obtained from CART cell therapy in solid tumors when combined with radiotherapy. Whereas heterogeneous radiation doses can edit the TME and enhance TAA expression, ICI therapy and CART cell therapy can determine a stronger T cell activation and a more robust anti-tumor response. Taken together, this knowledge provide the basis for a new emerging approach therapy that combines SFRT, ICIs, and CART cells.

Author Contributions: Conceptualization, A.P. and P.C.; methodology, A.B; formal analysis, P.C., A.B. and G.F; investigation, M.S. and S.P. (Silvana Parisi); resources, F.C. and G.F.; data curation, P.C. and M.S.; writing—original draft preparation, A.P and P.C.; writing—review and editing, A.P and S.P. (Stefano Pergolizzi). All authors have read and agreed to the published version of the manuscript.

Funding: This research received no external funding.

Institutional Review Board Statement: Not applicable.

Informed Consent Statement: Not applicable.

Data Availability Statement: Not applicable.

Conflicts of Interest: The authors declare no conflict of interest.

References

1. Linnemann, C.; Mezzadra, R.; Schumacher, T.N.M. TCR repertoires of intratumoral T-cell subsets. *Immunol. Rev.* **2013**, *257*, 72–82. [CrossRef] [PubMed]
2. Blattman, J.N.; Greenberg, P.D. Cancer Immunotherapy: A Treatment for the Masses. *Science* **2004**, *305*, 200–205. [CrossRef] [PubMed]
3. Pardoll, D. Does the Immune System See Tumors as Foreign or Self? *Annu. Rev. Immunol.* **2003**, *21*, 807–839. [CrossRef]
4. Traversari, C.; van der Bruggen, P.; Luescher, I.F.; Lurquin, C.; Chomez, P.; Van Pel, A.; De Plaen, E.; Amar-Costesec, A.; Boon, T. A nonapeptide encoded by human gene MAGE-1 is recognized on HLA-A1 by cytolytic T lymphocytes directed against tumor antigen MZ2-E. *J. Exp. Med.* **1992**, *176*, 1453–1457. [CrossRef] [PubMed]
5. Stone, B.; Schummer, M.; Paley, P.J.; Crawford, M.; Ford, M.; Urban, N.; Nelson, B.H. MAGE-F1, a novel ubiquitously expressed member of the MAGE superfamily. *Gene* **2001**, *267*, 173–182. [CrossRef]
6. Sharpe, M.; Mount, N. Genetically modified T cells in cancer therapy: Opportunities and challenges. *Dis. Model. Mech.* **2015**, *8*, 337–350. [CrossRef] [PubMed]
7. Kirtane, K.; Elmariah, H.; Chung, C.H.; Abate-Daga, D. Adoptive cellular therapy in solid tumor malignancies: Review of the literature and challenges ahead. *J. Immunother. Cancer* **2021**, *9*, e002723. [CrossRef]
8. Shafer, P.; Kelly, L.M.; Hoyos, V. Cancer Therapy with TCR-Engineered T Cells: Current Strategies, Challenges, and Prospects. *Front. Immunol.* **2022**, *13*, 835762. [CrossRef] [PubMed]

9. Maude, S.L.; Frey, N.; Shaw, P.A.; Aplenc, R.; Barrett, D.M.; Bunin, N.J.; Chew, A.; Gonzalez, V.E.; Zheng, Z.; Lacey, S.F.; et al. Chimeric antigen receptor T cells for sustained remissions in leukemia. *N. Engl. J. Med.* **2014**, *371*, 1507–1517. [CrossRef]
10. Lee, D.W.; Kochenderfer, J.N.; Stetler-Stevenson, M.; Cui, Y.K.; Delbrook, C.; Feldman, S.A.; Fry, T.J.; Orentas, R.; Sabatino, M.; Shah, N.N.; et al. T cells expressing CD19 chimeric antigen receptors for acute lymphoblastic leukaemia in children and young adults: A phase 1 dose-escalation trial. *Lancet* **2015**, *385*, 517–528. [CrossRef] [PubMed]
11. Davila, M.L.; Riviere, I.; Wang, X.; Bartido, S.; Park, J.; Curran, K.; Chung, S.S.; Stefanski, J.; Borquez-Ojeda, O.; Olszewska, M.; et al. Efficacy and toxicity management of 19-28z CAR T cell therapy in B cell acute lym-phoblastic leukemia. *Sci. Transl. Med.* **2014**, *6*, 224ra225. [CrossRef] [PubMed]
12. Turtle, C.J.; Hanafi, L.-A.; Berger, C.; Gooley, T.A.; Cherian, S.; Hudecek, M.; Sommermeyer, D.; Melville, K.; Pender, B.; Budiarto, T.M.; et al. CD19 CAR–T cells of defined CD4+:CD8+ composition in adult B cell ALL patients. *J. Clin. Investig.* **2016**, *126*, 2123–2138. [CrossRef]
13. Grupp, S.A.; Kalos, M.; Barrett, D.; Aplenc, R.; Porter, D.L.; Rheingold, S.R.; Teachey, D.T.; Chew, A.; Hauck, B.; Wright, J.F.; et al. Chimeric Antigen Receptor–Modified T Cells for Acute Lymphoid Leukemia. *N. Engl. J. Med.* **2013**, *368*, 1509–1518. [CrossRef] [PubMed]
14. Porter, D.L.; Hwang, W.-T.; Frey, N.V.; Lacey, S.F.; Shaw, P.A.; Loren, A.W.; Bagg, A.; Marcucci, K.T.; Shen, A.; Gonzalez, V.; et al. Chimeric antigen receptor T cells persist and induce sustained remissions in relapsed refractory chronic lymphocytic leukemia. *Sci. Transl. Med.* **2015**, *7*, 303ra139. [CrossRef] [PubMed]
15. Porter, D.L.; Levine, B.L.; Kalos, M.; Bagg, A.; June, C.H. Chimeric Antigen Receptor–Modified T Cells in Chronic Lymphoid Leukemia. *N. Engl. J. Med.* **2011**, *365*, 725–733. [CrossRef]
16. Brudno, J.N.; Somerville, R.P.; Shi, V.; Rose, J.J.; Halverson, D.C.; Fowler, D.H.; Gea-Banacloche, J.C.; Pavletic, S.Z.; Hickstein, D.D.; Lu, T.L.; et al. Allogeneic T Cells That Express an Anti-CD19 Chimeric Antigen Receptor Induce Remissions of B-Cell Malignancies That Progress after Allogeneic Hematopoietic Stem-Cell Transplantation without Causing Graft-Versus-Host Disease. *J. Clin. Oncol.* **2016**, *34*, 1112–1121. [CrossRef] [PubMed]
17. Morgan, R.A.; Dudley, M.E.; Wunderlich, J.R.; Hughes, M.S.; Yang, J.C.; Sherry, R.M.; Royal, R.E.; Topalian, S.L.; Kammula, U.S.; Restifo, N.P.; et al. Cancer Regression in Patients After Transfer of Genetically Engineered Lymphocytes. *Science* **2006**, *314*, 126–129. [CrossRef]
18. Johnson, L.A.; Heemskerk, B.; Powell, D.J.; Cohen, C.J.; Morgan, R.A.; Dudley, M.E.; Robbins, P.F.; Rosenberg, S.A. Gene Transfer of Tumor-Reactive TCR Confers Both High Avidity and Tumor Reactivity to Nonreactive Peripheral Blood Mononuclear Cells and Tumor-Infiltrating Lymphocytes. *J. Immunol.* **2006**, *177*, 6548–6559. [CrossRef]
19. Cartellieri, M.; Bachmann, M.; Feldmann, A.; Bippes, C.; Stamova, S.; Wehner, R.; Temme, A.; Schmitz, M. Chimeric Antigen Receptor-Engineered T Cells for Immunotherapy of Cancer. *J. Biomed. Biotechnol.* **2010**, *2010*, 956304. [CrossRef] [PubMed]
20. Sadelain, M.; Brentjens, R.; Rivière, I. The basic principles of chimeric antigen receptor design. *Cancer Discov.* **2013**, *3*, 388–398. [CrossRef] [PubMed]
21. Brandjes, B.D.; Davila, M.L. Adding chimeric antigen receptor induced killer cells to the medical oncology shelf. *J. Clin. Investig.* **2019**, *129*, 5077–5078. [CrossRef] [PubMed]
22. Brocker, T. Chimeric Fv-zeta or Fv-epsilon receptors are not sufficient to induce activation or cytokine production in peripheral T cells. *Blood* **2000**, *96*, 1999–2001. [CrossRef] [PubMed]
23. Huan, T.; Li, H.; Tang, B. Radiotherapy plus CAR-T cell therapy to date: A note for cautions optimism? *Front. Immunol.* **2022**, *13*, 1033512. [CrossRef] [PubMed]
24. Gong, M.C.; Latouche, J.B.; Krause, A.; Heston, W.D.; Bander, N.H.; Sadelain, M. Cancer patient T cells genetically targeted to prostate specific membrane antigen specifically lyse prostate cancer cells and release cytokines in response to prostate-specific mem-brane antigen. *Neoplasia* **1999**, *1*, 123–127. [CrossRef]
25. Maher, J.; Brentjens, R.J.; Gunset, G.; Riviere, I.; Sadelain, M. Human T-lymphocyte cytotoxicity and proliferation directed by a single chimeric TCRzeta/CD28 receptor. *Nat. Biotechnol.* **2002**, *20*, 70–75. [CrossRef]
26. Fujiwara, K.; Kitaura, M.; Tsunei, A.; Kusabuka, H.; Ogaki, E.; Okada, N. Structure of the signal transduction domain in sec-ond generation CAR regulates the input efficiency of CAR signals. *Int. J. Mol. Sci.* **2021**, *22*, 2476. [CrossRef]
27. Chmielewski, M.; Abken, H. TRUCKs: The fourth generation of CARs. *Expert Opin. Biol. Ther.* **2015**, *15*, 1145–1154. [CrossRef] [PubMed]
28. Zhao, L.; Cao, Y.J. Engineered T cell therapy for cancer in the clinic. *Front. Immunol.* **2019**, *10*, 2250. [CrossRef] [PubMed]
29. Pennisi, M.; Jain, T.; Santomasso, B.D.; Mead, E.; Wudhikarn, K.; Silverberg, M.L.; Batlevi, Y.; Shouval, R.; Devlin, S.M.; Batlevi, C.; et al. Comparing CAR T-cell toxicity grading systems: Application of the ASTCT grading system and implications for management. *Blood Adv.* **2020**, *4*, 676–686. [CrossRef] [PubMed]
30. Neelapu, S.S.; Tummala, S.; Kebriaei, P.; Wierda, W.; Gutierrez, C.; Locke, F.L.; Komanduri, K.V.; Lin, Y.; Jain, N.; Daver, N.; et al. Chimeric antigen receptor T-cell therapy—Assessment and management of toxicities. *Nat. Rev. Clin. Oncol.* **2017**, *15*, 47–62. [CrossRef]
31. Lee, D.W.; Santomasso, B.D.; Locke, F.L.; Ghobadi, A.; Turtle, C.J.; Brudno, J.N.; Maus, M.V.; Park, J.H.; Mead, E.; Pavletic, S.; et al. ASTCT Consensus Grading for Cytokine Release Syndrome and Neurologic Toxicity Associated with Immune Effector Cells. *Biol. Blood Marrow Transplant.* **2019**, *25*, 625–638. [CrossRef] [PubMed]

32. Bugelski, P.J.; Achuthanandam, R.; Capocasale, R.J.; Treacy, G.; Bouman-Thio, E. Monoclonal antibodyinduced cyto-kine-release syndrome. *Expert Rev. Clin. Immunol.* **2009**, *5*, 499–521. [CrossRef] [PubMed]
33. Lee, D.W.; Gardner, R.; Porter, D.L.; Louis, C.U.; Ahmed, N.; Jensen, M.; Grupp, S.A.; Mackall, C.L. Current concepts in the diagnosis and management of cytokine release syndrome. *Blood* **2014**, *124*, 188–195. [CrossRef] [PubMed]
34. Fitzgerald, J.C.; Weiss, S.L.M.; Maude, S.L.; Barrett, D.M.; Lacey, S.F.; Melenhorst, J.J.; Shaw, P.; Berg, R.A.; June, C.H.; Porter, D.L.; et al. Cytokine Release Syndrome after Chimeric Antigen Receptor T Cell Therapy for Acute Lymphoblastic Leukemia. *Crit. Care Med.* **2017**, *45*, e124–e131. [CrossRef]
35. Teachey, D.T.; Rheingold, S.R.; Maude, S.L.; Zugmaier, G.; Barrett, D.M.; Seif, A.E.; Nichols, K.E.; Suppa, E.K.; Kalos, M.; Berg, R.A.; et al. Cytokine release syndrome after blinatumomab treatment related to ab-normal macrophage activation and ameliorated with cytokine-directed therapy. *Blood* **2013**, *121*, 5154–5157. [CrossRef] [PubMed]
36. Maude, S.L.; Barrett, D.; Teachey, D.T.; Grupp, S.A. Managing Cytokine Release Syndrome Associated with Novel T Cell-Engaging Therapies. *Cancer J.* **2014**, *20*, 119–122. [CrossRef]
37. De Benedetti, H.; Brunner, I.; Ruperto, N.; Kenwright, A.; Wright, S.; Calvo, I.; Cuttica, R.; Ravelli, A.; Schneider, R.; Woo, P.; et al. Randomized trial of tocilizumab in systemic juvenile idiopathic arthritis. *N. Engl. J. Med.* **2012**, *367*, 2385–2395. [CrossRef]
38. Fisher, J.; Abramowski, P.; Don, N.D.W.; Flutter, B.; Capsomidis, A.; Cheung, G.W.-K.; Gustafsson, K.; Anderson, J. Avoidance of On-Target Off-Tumor Activation Using a Co-stimulation-Only Chimeric Antigen Receptor. *Mol. Ther.* **2017**, *25*, 1234–1247. [CrossRef] [PubMed]
39. Cameron, B.J.; Gerry, A.B.; Dukes, J.; Harper, J.V.; Kannan, V.; Bianchi, F.C.; Grand, F.; Brewer, J.E.; Gupta, M.; Plesa, G.; et al. Identification of a Titin-Derived HLA-A1–Presented Peptide as a Cross-Reactive Target for Engineered MAGE A3–Directed T Cells. *Sci. Transl. Med.* **2013**, *5*, 197ra103. [CrossRef]
40. Mei, H.; Jiang, H.; Wu, Y.; Guo, T.; Xia, L.; Jin, R.; Hu, Y. Neurological toxicities and coagulation disorders in the cytokine release syndrome during CAR-T therapy. *Br. J. Haematol.* **2017**, *181*, 689–692. [CrossRef]
41. Brudno, J.N.; Kochenderfer, J.N. Toxicities of chimeric antigen receptor T cells: Recognition and management. *Blood* **2016**, *127*, 3321–3330. [CrossRef] [PubMed]
42. Chou, C.K.; Turtle, C.J. Assessment and management of cytokine release syndrome and neurotoxicity following CD19 CAR-T cell therapy. *Expert Opin. Biol. Ther.* **2020**, *20*, 653–664. [CrossRef]
43. Kershaw, M.H.; Westwood, J.A.; Parker, L.L.; Wang, G.; Eshhar, Z.; Mavroukakis, S.A.; White, D.E.; Wunderlich, J.R.; Canevari, S.; Rogers-Freezer, L.; et al. A Phase I Study on Adoptive Immunotherapy Using Gene-Modified T Cells for Ovarian Cancer. *Clin. Cancer Res.* **2006**, *12*, 6106–6115. [CrossRef]
44. Jensen, M.C.; Popplewell, L.; Cooper, L.J.; DiGiusto, D.; Kalos, M.; Ostberg, J.R.; Forman, S.J. Antitransgene rejection responses contribute to attenuated persistence of adoptively transferred CD20/CD19-specific chimeric antigen receptor redirected T cells in humans. *Biol. Blood Marrow Transplant.* **2010**, *16*, 1245–1256. [CrossRef] [PubMed]
45. Maus, M.V.; Haas, A.R.; Beatty, G.L.; Albelda, S.M.; Levine, B.L.; Liu, X.; Zhao, Y.; Kalos, M.; June, C.H. T Cells Expressing Chimeric Antigen Receptors Can Cause Anaphylaxis in Humans. *Cancer Immunol. Res.* **2013**, *1*, 26–31. [CrossRef]
46. Yin, Y.; Boesteanu, A.C.; Binder, Z.A.; Xu, C.; Reid, R.A.; Rodriguez, J.L.; Cook, D.R.; Thokala, R.; Blouch, K.; McGettigan-Croce, B.; et al. Checkpoint blockade reverses anergy in IL-13Rα2 Humanized scFv-Based CAR T cells to treat murine and canine gliomas. *Mol. Ther. Oncolytics* **2018**, *11*, 20–38. [CrossRef]
47. Viola, A.; Munari, F.; Sánchez-Rodríguez, R.; Scolaro, T.; Castegna, A. The Metabolic Signature of Macrophage Responses. *Front. Immunol.* **2019**, *10*, 1462. [CrossRef]
48. Huang, J.; Zhang, L.; Wan, D.; Zhou, L.; Zheng, S.; Lin, S.; Qiao, Y. Extracellular matrix and its therapeutic potential for cancer treatment. *Signal Transduct. Target. Ther.* **2021**, *6*, 153. [CrossRef]
49. Antoñana-Vildosola, A.; Zanetti, S.R.; Palazon, A. Enabling CAR-T cells for solid tumors: Rage against the suppressive tumor microenvironment. *Int. Rev. Cell Mol. Biol.* **2022**, *37*, 123–147. [CrossRef]
50. Kroemer, G.; Galluzzi, L.; Kepp, O.; Zitvogel, L. Immunogenic Cell Death in Cancer Therapy. *Annu. Rev. Immunol.* **2013**, *31*, 51–72. [CrossRef] [PubMed]
51. Bejarano, L.; Jordao, M.J.; Joyce, J.A. Therapeutic Targeting of the Tumor Microenvironment. *Cancer Discov.* **2021**, *11*, 933–959. [CrossRef] [PubMed]
52. Babar, Q.; Saeed, A.; Tabish, T.A.; Sarwar, M.; Thorat, N.D. Targeting the tumor microenvironment: Potential strategy for cancer therapeutics. *Biochim. Biophys. Acta (BBA)—Mol. Basis Dis.* **2023**, *1869*, 166746. [CrossRef] [PubMed]
53. Guha, P.; Heatherton, K.R.; O'Connell, K.P.; Alexander, I.S.; Katz, S.C. Assessing the Future of Solid Tumor Immunotherapy. *Biomedicines* **2022**, *10*, 655. [CrossRef]
54. Grivennikov, S.I.; Greten, F.R.; Karin, M. Immunity, inflammation, and cancer. *Cell* **2010**, *140*, 883–899. [CrossRef] [PubMed]
55. Bożyk, A.; Wojas-Krawczyk, K.; Krawczyk, P.; Milanowski, J. Tumor Microenvironment—A Short Review of Cellular and Interaction Diversity. *Biology* **2022**, *11*, 929. [CrossRef]
56. Rossi, M.; Altomare, E.; Botta, C.; Cantafio, M.E.G.; Sarvide, S.; Caracciolo, D.; Riillo, C.; Gaspari, M.; Taverna, D.; Conforti, F.; et al. miR-21 antagonism abrogates Th17 tumor promoting functions in multiple myeloma. *Leukemia* **2020**, *35*, 823–834. [CrossRef]
57. Galli, F.; Aguilera, J.V.; Palermo, B.; Markovic, S.N.; Nisticò, P.; Signore, A. Relevance of immune cell and tumor microenvironment imaging in the new era of immunotherapy. *J. Exp. Clin. Cancer Res.* **2020**, *39*, 89. [CrossRef]

58. Lee, J.; Lozano-Ruiz, B.; Yang, F.M.; Fan, D.D.; Shen, L.; González-Navajas, J.M. The Multifaceted Role of Th1, Th9, and Th17 Cells in Immune Checkpoint Inhibition Therapy. *Front. Immunol.* **2021**, *12*, 625667. [CrossRef]
59. Jeske, S.S.; Weissinger, S.E.; Veit, J.A.; Brunner, C.; Huber, U.; Theodoraki, M.N.; Hoffmann, T.K.; Schuler, P.J.; Doescher, J. Treatment-induced changes of lymphocyte subsets in patients with adenoid cystic carcinoma of the head and neck. *Eur. Arch. Oto-Rhino-Laryngol.* **2019**, *276*, 1465–1473. [CrossRef]
60. De Guillebon, E.; Dardenne, A.; Saldmann, A.; Séguier, S.; Tran, T.; Paolini, L.; Lebbe, C.; Tartour, E. Beyond the concept of cold and hot tumors for the development of novel predictive biomarkers and the rational design of immunotherapy combination. *Int. J. Cancer* **2020**, *147*, 1509–1518. [CrossRef]
61. Chen, D.S.; Mellman, I. Elements of cancer immunity and the cancer-immune set point. *Nature* **2017**, *541*, 321–330. [CrossRef] [PubMed]
62. van der Woude, L.L.; Gorris, M.; Halilovic, A.; Figdor, C.G.; de Vries, I.J.M. Migrating into the Tumor: A Roadmap for T Cells. *Trends Cancer* **2017**, *3*, 797–808. [CrossRef] [PubMed]
63. Forster, J.C.; Marcu, L.G.; Bezak, E. Approaches to combat hypoxia in cancer therapy and the potential for in silico models in their evaluation. *Phys. Medica* **2019**, *64*, 145–156. [CrossRef]
64. Xie, G.; Liu, Y.; Yao, Q.; Zheng, R.; Zhang, L.; Lin, J.; Guo, Z.; Du, S.; Ren, C.; Yuan, Q.; et al. Hypoxia-induced angiotensin II by the lactate-chymase-dependent mechanism mediates radioresistance of hypoxic tumor cells. *Sci. Rep.* **2017**, *7*, 42396. [CrossRef]
65. Farc, O.; Cristea, V. An overview of the tumor microenvironment, from cells to complex networks (Review). *Exp. Ther. Med.* **2020**, *21*, 96. [CrossRef]
66. Petrova, V.; Annicchiarico-Petruzzelli, M.; Melino, G.; Amelio, I. The hypoxic tumour microenvironment. *Oncogenesis* **2018**, *7*, 10. [CrossRef]
67. Luo, W.; Semenza, G.L. Emerging roles of PKM2 in cell metabolism and cancer progression. *Trends Endocrinol. Metab.* **2012**, *23*, 560–566. [CrossRef]
68. Iacobini, C.; Vitale, M.; Pugliese, G.; Menini, S. The "sweet" path to cancer: Focus on cellular glucose metabolism. *Front. Oncol.* **2023**, *13*, 1202093. [CrossRef]
69. Liberti, M.V.; Locasale, J.W. The Warburg Effect: How Does it Benefit Cancer Cells? *Trends Biochem. Sci.* **2016**, *41*, 211–218. [CrossRef]
70. Majidpoor, J.; Mortezaee, K. Angiogenesis as a hallmark of solid tumors clinical perspectives. *Cell Oncol.* **2021**, *44*, 715–737. [CrossRef] [PubMed]
71. He, H.; Liao, Q.; Zhao, C.; Zhu, C.; Feng, M.; Liu, Z.; Jiang, L.; Zhang, L.; Ding, X.; Yuan, M.; et al. Conditioned CAR T cells by hypoxia inducible transcription amplification (HiTA) system significantly enhances systemic safety and retains anti-tumor efficacy. *J. Immunother. Cancer* **2021**, *9*, e002755. [CrossRef]
72. Overgaard, J. Hypoxic modification of radiotherapy in squamous cell carcinoma of the head and neck—A systematic review and meta-analysis. *Radiother. Oncol.* **2011**, *100*, 22–32. [CrossRef]
73. Rodriguez Garcia, A.; Palazon, A.; Noguera Ortega, E.; Powell, D.J.; Guedan, S. CAR T cells Hit the tumor mi-croenvironment: Strategies to overcome tumor escape. *Front. Immunol.* **2020**, *11*, 1109. [CrossRef]
74. Berahovich, R.; Liu, X.; Zhou, H.; Tsadik, E.; Xu, S.; Golubovskaya, V.; Wu, L. Hypoxia Selectively Impairs CAR-T Cells In Vitro. *Cancers* **2019**, *11*, 602. [CrossRef] [PubMed]
75. Juillerat, A.; Marechal, A.; Filhol, J.M.; Valogne, Y.; Valton, J.; Duclert, A.; Duchateau, P.; Poirot, L. An oxygen sensitive self-decision making engineered CAR T-cell. *Sci. Rep.* **2017**, *7*, srep39833. [CrossRef]
76. Huang, L.E.; Gu, J.; Schau, M.; Bunn, H.F. Regulation of hypoxia-inducible factor 1alpha is mediated by an O_2-dependent degradation domain via the ubiquitin-proteasome pathway. *Proc. Natl. Acad. Sci. USA* **1998**, *95*, 7987–7992. [CrossRef]
77. Brown, C.E.; Alizadeh, D.; Starr, R.; Weng, L.; Wagner, J.R.; Naranjo, A.; Ostberg, J.R.; Blanchard, M.S.; Kilpatrick, J.; Simpson, J.; et al. Regression of Glioblastoma after Chimeric Antigen Receptor T-Cell Therapy. *N. Engl. J. Med.* **2016**, *375*, 2561–2569. [CrossRef] [PubMed]
78. Ahmed, N.; Brawley, V.; Hegde, M.; Bielamowicz, K.; Kalra, M.; Landi, D.; Robertson, C.; Gray, T.L.; Diouf, O.; Wakefield, A.; et al. HER2-Specific Chimeric Antigen Receptor–Modified Virus-Specific T Cells for Progressive Glioblastoma: A Phase 1 Dose-Escalation Trial. *JAMA Oncol.* **2017**, *3*, 1094–1101. [CrossRef] [PubMed]
79. Narayan, V.; Gladney, W.; Plesa, G.; Vapiwala, N.; Carpenter, E.; Maude, S.L.; Lal, P.; Lacey, S.F.; Melenhorst, J.J.; Sebro, R.; et al. A phase I clinical trial of PSMA-directed/TGFβ-insensitive CAR-T cells in metastatic castration-resistant prostate cancer. *J. Clin. Oncol.* **2019**, *37*, TPS347. [CrossRef]
80. Dorff, T.B.; Blanchard, S.; Carruth, P.; Wagner, J.; Kuhn, P.; Chaudhry, A.; Adkins, L.; Thomas, S.; Martirosyan, H.; Chu, P.; et al. A phase I study to evaluate PSCA-targeting chimeric antigen receptor (CAR)-T cells for patients with PSCA+ metastatic castration-resistant prostate cancer (mCRPC). *J. Clin. Oncol.* **2020**, *38*, TPS250. [CrossRef]
81. Adusumilli, P.S.; Zauderer, M.G.; Rusch, V.W.; O'Cearbhaill, R.; Zhu, A.; Ngai, D.; McGee, E.; Chintala, N.; Messinger, J.; Cheema, W.; et al. Regional delivery of mesothelin-targeted CAR T cells for pleural cancers: Safety and preliminary efficacy in combination with anti-PD-1 agent. *J. Clin. Oncol.* **2019**, *37*, 2511. [CrossRef]
82. Kosti, P.; Opzoomer, J.W.; Larios-Martinez, K.I.; Henley-Smith, R.; Scudamore, C.L.; Okesola, M.; Taher, M.Y.; Davies, D.M.; Muliaditan, T.; Larcombe-Young, D.; et al. Hypoxia-sensing CAR T cells provide safety and efficacy in treating solid tumors. *Cell Rep. Med.* **2021**, *2*, 100227. [CrossRef]

83. Pai, S.I.; Cesano, A. Tumor Microenvironment. In *Physiology & Behavior*; Lee, P.P., Marincola, F.M., Eds.; Springer International Publishing: Cham, Switzerland, 2020; Volume 180, pp. 139–148.
84. Touat, M.; Li, Y.Y.; Boynton, A.N.; Spurr, L.F.; Iorgulescu, J.B.; Bohrson, C.L.; Cortes-Ciriano, I.; Birzu, C.; Geduldig, J.E.; Pelton, K.; et al. Mechanisms and therapeutic implications of hypermutation in gliomas. *Nature* **2020**, *580*, 517–523. [CrossRef]
85. Wang, Z.; Cao, Y.J. Adoptive Cell Therapy Targeting Neoantigens: A Frontier for Cancer Research. *Front. Immunol.* **2020**, *11*, 176. [CrossRef]
86. Seyedin, S.N.; Schoenhals, J.E.; Lee, D.A.; Cortez, M.A.; Wang, X.; Niknam, S.; Tang, C.; Hong, D.S.; Naing, A.; Sharma, P.; et al. Strategies for combining immunotherapy with radiation for anticancer therapy. *Immunotherapy* **2015**, *7*, 967–980. [CrossRef]
87. Liu, Z.; Zhao, Q.; Zheng, Z.; Liu, S.; Meng, L.; Dong, L.; Jiang, X. Vascular normalization in immunotherapy: A promising mecha nisms combined with radiotherapy. *Biomed. Pharmacother.* **2021**, *139*, 111607. [CrossRef] [PubMed]
88. Hauth, F.; Ho, A.Y.; Ferrone, S.; Duda, D.G. Radiotherapy to enhance chimeric antigen receptor T cell therapeutic efficacy in solid tumors: A narrative review. *JAMA Oncol.* **2021**, *7*, 1051–1059. [CrossRef] [PubMed]
89. Chruściel, E.; Urban-Wójciuk, Z.; Arcimowicz, Ł.; Kurkowiak, M.; Kowalski, J.; Gliwiński, M.; Marjański, T.; Rzyman, W.; Biernat, W.; Dziadziuszko, R.; et al. Adoptive cell therapy—Harnessing antigen-specific t cells to target solid tumours. *Cancers* **2020**, *12*, 683. [CrossRef] [PubMed]
90. Lhuillier, C.; Rudqvist, N.-P.; Elemento, O.; Formenti, S.C.; Demaria, S. Radiation therapy and anti-tumor immunity: Exposing immunogenic mutations to the immune system. *Genome Med.* **2019**, *11*, 40. [CrossRef]
91. Walle, T.; Monge, R.M.; Cerwenka, A.; Ajona, D.; Melero, I.; Lecanda, F. Radiation effects on antitumor immune responses: Current perspectives and challenges. *Ther. Adv. Med. Oncol.* **2018**, *10*, 1–27. [CrossRef]
92. Barker, H.E.; Paget, J.T.E.; Khan, A.A.; Harrington, K.J. The tumour microenvironment after radiotherapy: Mechanisms of resistance and recurrence. *Nat. Rev. Cancer* **2015**, *15*, 409–425. [CrossRef] [PubMed]
93. Li, M.O.; Sanjabi, S.; Flavell, R.A. Transforming Growth Factor-β Controls Development, Homeostasis, and Tolerance of T Cells by Regulatory T Cell-Dependent and -Independent Mechanisms. *Immunity* **2006**, *25*, 455–471. [CrossRef]
94. Demaria, S.; Golden, E.B.; Formenti, S.C. Role of Local Radiation Therapy in Cancer Immunotherapy. *JAMA Oncol.* **2015**, *1*, 1325–1332. [CrossRef]
95. Singh, A.K.; McGuirk, J.P. CAR T cells: Continuation in a revolution of immunotherapy. *Lancet Oncol.* **2020**, *21*, e168–e178. [CrossRef] [PubMed]
96. Rodriguez Ruiz, M.E.; Garasa, S.; Rodriguez, I.; Solorzano, J.L.; Barbes, B.; Yanguas, A.; Teijeira, A.; Etxeberria, I.; Aristu, J.J.; Halin, C.; et al. Intercellular adhesion Molecule 1 and vascular cell adhesion molecule are induced by ionizing radiation on lymphatic endo-thelium. *Int. J. Radiat. Oncol. Biol. Phys.* **2017**, *97*, 389–400. [CrossRef] [PubMed]
97. Karin, N. The multiple faces of CXCL12 (SDF 1alpha) in the regulation of immunity during health and disease. *J. Leukoc. Biol.* **2010**, *88*, 463–473. [CrossRef]
98. Li, C.G.; He, M.R.; Wu, F.L.; Li, Y.J.; Sun, A.M. Akt promotes irradiation induced regulatory T cell survival in hepatocellular car-cinoma. *Am. J. Med. Sci.* **2013**, *346*, 123–127. [CrossRef]
99. Park, H.-R.; Jung, U. Depletion of NK Cells Resistant to Ionizing Radiation Increases Mutations in Mice after Whole-body Irradiation. *In Vivo* **2021**, *35*, 1507–1513. [CrossRef] [PubMed]
100. Pontoriero, A.; Critelli, P.; Conti, A.; Cardali, S.; Angileri, F.F.; Germanò, A.; Lillo, S.; Carretta, A.; Brogna, A.; Santacaterina, A.; et al. The "Combo" radiotherapy treatment for high-risk grade 2 meningiomas: Dose escalation and initial safety and efficacy analysis. *J. Neuro-Oncol.* **2022**, *161*, 203–214. [CrossRef]
101. Parisi, S.; Ferini, G.; Cacciola, A.; Lillo, S.; Tamburella, C.; Santacaterina, A.; Bottari, A.; Brogna, A.; Ferrantelli, G.; Pontoriero, A.; et al. A non-surgical COMBO-therapy approach for locally advanced unresectable pancreatic adenocarcinoma: Preliminary results of a prospective study. *Radiol. Medica* **2022**, *127*, 214–219. [CrossRef]
102. DeSelm, C.; Palomba, M.L.; Yahalom, J.; Hamieh, M.; Eyquem, J.; Rajasekhar, V.K.; Sadelain, M. Low dose radiation conditioning enables CAR T cells to mitigate antigen escape. *Mol. Ther.* **2018**, *26*, 2542–2552. [CrossRef]
103. Klug, F.; Prakash, H.; Huber, P.E.; Seibel, T.; Bender, N.; Halama, N.; Pfirschke, C.; Voss, R.H.; Timke, C.; Umansky, L.; et al. Low dose irradiation programs macrophage differentiation to an iNOS+/M1 phenotype that orchestrates effective T cell immunotherapy. *Cancer Cell* **2013**, *24*, 589–602. [CrossRef] [PubMed]
104. Schoenfeld, J.D.; Giobbie-Hurder, A.; Ranasinghe, S.; Kao, K.Z.; Lako, A.; Tsuji, J.; Liu, Y.; Brennick, R.C.; Gentzler, R.D.; Lee, C.; et al. Durvalumab plus tremelimumab alone or in combination with low-dose or hypofractionated radiotherapy in metastatic non-small-cell lung cancer refractory to previous PD(L)-1 therapy: An open-label, multicentre, randomised, phase 2 trial. *Lancet Oncol.* **2022**, *23*, 279–291. [CrossRef]
105. Monjazeb, A.M.; Giobbie-Hurder, A.; Lako, A.; Thrash, E.M.; Brennick, R.C.; Kao, K.Z.; Manuszak, C.; Gentzler, R.D.; Tesfaye, A.; Jabbour, S.K.; et al. A Randomized Trial of Combined PD-L1 and CTLA-4 Inhibition with Tar-geted Low-Dose or Hypofractionated Radiation for Patients with Metastatic Colorectal Cancer. *Clin. Cancer Res. Off. J. Am. Assoc. Cancer Res.* **2021**, *27*, 2470–2480. [CrossRef]
106. Meng, Y.; Beckett, M.A.; Liang, H.; Mauceri, H.J.; van Rooijen, N.; Cohen, K.S.; Weichselbaum, R.R. Blockade of Tumor Necrosis Factor α Signaling in Tumor-Associated Macrophages as a Radiosensitizing Strategy. *Cancer Res.* **2010**, *70*, 1534–1543. [CrossRef]

107. Zammarchi, F.; Havenith, K.; Bertelli, F.; Vijayakrishnan, B.; Chivers, S.; van Berkel, P.H. CD25 targeted antibody drug conjugate depletes regulatory T cells and eliminates established syngeneic tumors via antitumor immunity. *J. Immunother. Cancer* **2020**, *8*, e000860. [CrossRef] [PubMed]
108. Sia, J.; Hagekyriakou, J.; Chindris, I.; Albarakati, H.; Leong, T.; Schlenker, R.; Keam, S.P.; Williams, S.G.; Neeson, P.J.; Johnstone, R.W.; et al. Regulatory T cells shape the differential impact of radiation dose fractionation schedules on host innate and adaptive antitumor immune defenses. *Int. J. Radiat. Oncol. Biol. Phys.* **2021**, *111*, 502–514. [CrossRef] [PubMed]
109. Laurent, P.A.; Morel, D.; Meziani, L.; Depil, S.; Deutsch, E. Radiotherapy as a means to increase the efficacy of T cell therapy in solid tumors. *Oncoimmunology* **2023**, *12*, 2158013. [CrossRef] [PubMed]
110. Prasanna, A.; Ahmed, M.M.; Mohiuddin, M.; Coleman, C.N. Exploiting sensitization windows of opportunity in hyper and hypo-fractionated radiation therapy. *J. Thorac. Dis.* **2014**, *6*, 287–302. [CrossRef]
111. Morisada, M.; Clavijo, P.E.; Moore, E.; Sun, L.; Chamberlin, M.; Van Waes, C.; Hodge, J.W.; Mitchell, J.B.; Friedman, J.; Allen, C.T. PD-1 blockade reverses adaptive immune resistance induced by high-dose hypofractionated but not low-dose daily fractionated radiation. *OncoImmunology* **2018**, *7*, e1395996. [CrossRef]
112. Navarro-Martín, A.; Galiana, I.L.; Frances, M.A.B.; Cacicedo, J.; Cortés, R.C.; Anton, S.C.; Sánchez, S.P.; Cuevas, S.B.; Parry, R.; Edo, F.G. Preliminary Study of the Effect of Stereotactic Body Radiotherapy (SBRT) on the Immune System in Lung Cancer Patients Unfit for Surgery: Immunophenotyping Analysis. *Int. J. Mol. Sci.* **2018**, *19*, 3963. [CrossRef]
113. Vanpouille-Box, C.; Alard, A.; Aryankalayil, M.J.; Sarfraz, Y.; Diamond, J.M.; Schneider, R.J.; Inghirami, G.; Coleman, C.N.; Formenti, S.C.; Demaria, S. DNA exonuclease Trex1 regulates radiotherapy-induced tumour immunogenicity. *Nat. Commun.* **2017**, *8*, 15618. [CrossRef]
114. Barsoumian, H.B.; Ramapriyan, R.; Younes, A.I.; Caetano, M.S.; Menon, H.; Comeaux, N.I.; Cushman, T.R.; Schoenhals, J.E.; Cadena, A.P.; Reilly, T.P.; et al. Low-dose radiation treatment enhances systemic antitumor immune responses by overcoming the inhibitory stroma. *J. Immunother. Cancer* **2020**, *8*, e000537. [CrossRef] [PubMed]
115. Patel, R.R.; Barsoumian, H.; Verma, V.; Cortez, M.A.; Welsh, J.W. Low-Dose Radiation Decreases Cancer-Associated Fibro-blasts and May Increase T-Cell Trafficking into Tumors. *Int. J. Radiat. Oncol. Biol. Phys.* **2020**, *108*, e530–e531. [CrossRef]
116. Kim, R.-K.; Kim, M.-J.; Seong, K.M.; Kaushik, N.; Suh, Y.; Yoo, K.-C.; Cui, Y.-H.; Jin, Y.W.; Nam, S.Y.; Lee, S.-J. Beneficial effects of low dose radiation in response to the oncogenic KRAS induced cellular transformation. *Sci. Rep.* **2015**, *5*, 15809. [CrossRef]
117. Donlon, N.E.; Power, R.; Hayes, C.; Reynolds, J.V.; Lysaght, J. Radiotherapy, immunotherapy, and the tumour microenvi-ron ment: Turning an immunosuppressive milieu into a therapeutic opportunity. *Cancer Lett.* **2021**, *502*, 84–96. [CrossRef] [PubMed]
118. Ratnayake, G.; Reinwald, S.; Edwards, J.; Wong, N.; Yu, D.; Ward, R.; Smith, R.; Haydon, A.; Au, P.M.; van Zelm, M.C.; et al. Blood T cell profiling in metastatic melanoma patients as a marker for response to immune checkpoint inhibitors combined with radio therapy. *Radiother. Oncol.* **2022**, *173*, 299–305. [CrossRef]
119. Morris, E.C.; Neelapu, S.S.; Giavridis, T.; Sadelain, M. Cytokine release syndrome and associated neurotoxicity in cancer im-mu notherapy. *Nat. Rev. Immunol.* **2022**, *22*, 85–96. [CrossRef]
120. Rotte, A.; Frigault, M.J.; Ansari, A.; Gliner, B.; Heery, C.; Shah, B. Dose–response correlation for CAR-T cells: A systematic review of clinical studies. *J. Immunother. Cancer* **2022**, *10*, e005678. [CrossRef]
121. Ferini, G.; Parisi, S.; Lillo, S.; Viola, A.; Minutoli, F.; Critelli, P.; Valenti, V.; Illari, S.I.; Brogna, A.; Umana, G.E.; et al. Impressive Results after "Metabolism-Guided" Lattice Irradiation in Patients Submitted to Palliative Radiation Therapy: Preliminary Results of LATTICE_01 Multicenter Study. *Cancers* **2022**, *14*, 3909. [CrossRef] [PubMed]
122. Jiang, L.; Li, X.; Zhang, J.; Li, W.; Dong, F.; Chen, C.; Lin, Q.; Zhang, C.; Zheng, F.; Yan, W.; et al. Combined High-Dose LATTICE Radiation Therapy and Immune Checkpoint Blockade for Advanced Bulky Tumors: The Concept and a Case Report. *Front. Oncol.* **2021**, *10*, 548132. [CrossRef]
123. Ferini, G.; Valenti, V.; Tripoli, A.; Illari, S.I.; Molino, L.; Parisi, S.; Cacciola, A.; Lillo, S.; Giuffrida, D.; Pergolizzi, S. Lattice or Oxygen-Guided Radiotherapy: What If They Converge? Possible Future Directions in the Era of Immunotherapy. *Cancers* **2021**, *13*, 3290. [CrossRef]
124. Duriseti, S.; Kavanaugh, J.; Goddu, S.; Price, A.; Knutson, N.; Reynoso, F.; Michalski, J.; Mutic, S.; Robinson, C.; Spraker, M.B. Spatially fractionated stereotactic body radiation therapy (Lattice) for large tumors. *Adv. Radiat. Oncol.* **2021**, *6*, 100639. [CrossRef] [PubMed]
125. Wu, X.; Perez, N.C.; Zheng, Y.; Li, X.; Jiang, L.; Amendola, B.E.; Xu, B.; Mayr, N.A.; Lu, J.J.; Hatoum, G.F.; et al. The Technical and Clinical Implementation of LATTICE Radiation Therapy (LRT). *Radiat. Res.* **2020**, *194*, 737–746. [CrossRef] [PubMed]
126. Blanco Suarez, J.M.; Amendola, B.E.; Perez, N.; Amendola, M.; Wu, X. The use of Lattice radiation therapy (LRT) in the treatment of bulky tumors: A case report of a large metastatic mixed mullerian ovarian tumor. *Cureus* **2015**, *7*, e389. [CrossRef] [PubMed]
127. Ertan, F.; Yeginer, M.; Zorlu, F. Dosimetric Performance Evaluation of MLC-based and Cone-based 3D Spatially Fractionated LATTICE Radiotherapy. *Radiat. Res.* **2023**, *199*, 161–169. [CrossRef]

Journal of *Personalized Medicine*

MDPI

Review

The Role of Radiotherapy in the Management of Vaginal Melanoma: A Literature Review with a Focus on the Potential Synergistic Role of Immunotherapy

Francesco Cuccia [1,*], Salvatore D'Alessandro [1,2], Livio Blasi [3], Vito Chiantera [4] and Giuseppe Ferrera [1]

1 Radiotherapy Unit, Radiation Oncology, ARNAS Civico Hospital, 90100 Palermo, Italy; titodales@gmail.com (S.D.); giuseppe.ferrera@arnascivico.it (G.F.)
2 Radiation Oncology School, University of Palermo, 90100 Palermo, Italy
3 Medical Oncology, ARNAS Civico Hospital, 90100 Palermo, Italy; livio.blasi@arnascivico.it
4 Gynecological Oncology, ARNAS Civico Hospital, 90100 Palermo, Italy; vito.chiantera@arnascivico.it
* Correspondence: francesco.cuccia@arnascivico.it

Abstract: Among the mucosal melanomas, vaginal melanomas are very rare tumors, accounting for less than 20% of melanomas arising from the female genital tract. They occur most frequently in women in post-menopausal age, but younger patients may also experience this neoplasm, mainly located in the lower third of the vagina or the anterior wall. The optimal management of this tumor remains controversial, with surgery reported as the most frequently adopted approach. However, a clear benefit of surgical treatment in terms of survival has not yet been demonstrated. Conversely, radiotherapy may represent an attractive non-invasive alternative, and there are several favorable reports of the role of radiation therapy, either delivered with photons, brachytherapy, or hadrontherapy. A wide range of techniques and fractionation regimens are reported with substantially good tolerance to the treatment, and acute G3 or higher toxicities are reported only in the case of concurrent immunotherapy. Of note, due to the rarity of the disease, there is a lack of high-level evidence for the optimal therapeutic option. In this scenario, recent studies theorize the possibility of developing combinatorial approaches of radiotherapy with immunotherapy based on cutaneous melanomas reports. In this review, we aim to summarize the evidence available in the literature supporting the role of definitive radiotherapy for vaginal melanomas, with a focus on the combination of RT with immunotherapy, in terms of optimal timing and biological rationale.

Keywords: vaginal melanoma; radiotherapy; immunotherapy

1. Introduction

Vaginal melanomas (VM) are a rare entity among the mucosal melanomas, accounting for less than 20% of melanomas located in the female genital tract. Clinical staging of VM is derived from cutaneous disease, and tumor size and lymph-nodal metastases are related to a poorer prognosis, with an overall survival rate of 5 years ranging between 5% and 25% [1].

It more commonly affects women in the post-menopausal period between 60 and 70 years of age, but sometimes it might also be observed in younger patients. The preferred site of presentation is usually the lower third of the vagina or the anterior vaginal wall. Melanocytic presentation is the most common occurrence, although very rare cases of non-melanocytic diseases are reported in the literature. Disease staging is based on the International Federation of Gynecology and Obstetrics(FIGO) classification for vaginal cancer, although TNM classification is also widely adopted, and the depth of invasion is considered an important risk factor, such as for cutaneous melanomas.

Due to the rarity of the disease, optimal management remains a matter of debate. Unlike non-melanoma vaginal cancer, where surgery has a limited role in very early stages or advanced stage IV disease with healthy structures invasion, for vaginal melanomas, surgical resection is the preferred approach, although with a debated survival benefit and a wide spectrum of complications, such as infection, bladder or urethral damage, fistulas, or hemorrhages [2].

Furthermore, diagnosis occurs more frequently in the advanced stages of the disease, with a reduced probability of surgical radicality and a higher risk of severe sequelae. However, combined approaches with adjuvant radiotherapy have resulted in very poor outcomes due to the high rates of local and distant recurrences [3].

Systemic therapy options for mucosal melanoma are limited, given the reduced response to conventional cytotoxic drugs. Also, BRAF mutations are rarely present in mucosal melanomas, compared to cutaneous disease, while, KIT mutations are more frequently reported [4].

In this scenario, immunotherapy has recently been introduced with a sensitive improvement in clinical outcomes, reporting objective response rates ranging between 20% and 75%, with durable responses reported in the literature [5].

Although response rates to immunotherapy are lower for mucosal melanomas compared to cutaneous melanomas, the possibility of combining radiotherapy with immunotherapy is an attractive treatment option in this setting [6,7].

Melanoma is traditionally considered a radio-resistant tumor with a natural capacity to repair damages caused by low-dose radiotherapy. These features of the disease have led clinicians to explore alternatives to conventional external beam radiotherapy (EBRT), such as brachytherapy or hadrontherapy, both of which can deliver higher doses to the target with limited exposure to organs at risk.

In recent years, based on the radiobiological characteristics of VM, the use of stereotactic body radiotherapy (SBRT) has also been increasingly reported, not only as a therapeutic option able to overcome the intrinsic radio-resistance of melanoma but also for its potential effect on enhanced immunogenicity [8].

SBRT allows clinicians to deliver very high doses to small volumes, with a steep dose gradient and a reduced low-dose bath of healthy nearby structures [9].

Some studies have favorably reported the combination of high-dose radiotherapy with immunotherapy, with improved clinical outcomes in comparison with patients treated with immunotherapy alone [10–13].

As surgery remains the preferred treatment option for the management of VM, radiotherapy may represent an effective alternative for patients unfit for surgical excision, with a further potential benefit provided by immunotherapy.

In this literature review, we aim to collect the available evidence in support of the use of radiotherapy for VM, with a focus on the potential synergistic use of immunotherapy.

2. Methods

A review of the literature was performed in May 2023 to select articles reporting on the safety and efficacy of definitive radiotherapy for vaginal melanoma. Publications reporting the synergistic use of radiotherapy and immunotherapy were also considered for the purpose of this study. Adjuvant or neoadjuvant radiotherapy cases were not considered for the purpose of this study. We searched the PubMed, Scopus, and Embase databases to retrieve papers containing combinations (by AND/OR) of the following search terms: "vagina", "melanoma", "radiotherapy", "stereotactic radiotherapy", and "radiation therapy". Only the articles published between January 1995 and April 2023 were considered eligible for the present study. All the studies selected as potentially eligible for this review were screened by two authors (FC and SDA), with a third author (GF) involved in the case of disagreement between the first two.

Due to the rarity of the disease, case reports were considered eligible for the purpose of the present study. Non-English publications, reviews, and studies involving patients treated with surgery were excluded.

The following data were extracted from all the selected publications: first author and year of publication, number of patients treated, median age, study design, intent and radiotherapy fractionation, radiotherapy technique, any concurrent systemic therapies, clinical outcomes (local control, LC; overall survival, OS), and grades and incidence rates of adverse events. Median follow-up was calculated starting from the end of radiotherapy; LC was defined as the interval between the end of treatment and the last follow-up known or the occurrence of a disease relapse within the radiotherapy field; OS was defined as the interval between the end of treatment and the last follow-up known or the occurrence of death by any cause.

3. Results

Eighty-five studies were initially identified from the literature research. Based on the abovementioned criteria of inclusion/exclusion, a total of 11 studies were considered relevant for the present literature review. Seven studies were case reports and four were reports on the outcomes of retrospective series; no prospective studies were found [7,14–23] (Table 1).

The synergistic use of immunotherapy is reported in six publications [6,16,17,19–21]. A total of 36 patients were treated with definitive radiotherapy for vaginal melanoma, consisting of conventional external beam radiotherapy in 5 cases, stereotactic radiotherapy in 5 cases, hadrontherapy in 25 cases, and brachytherapy in 1 case. The median patient age was 70 years (range, 55–80 years) and tumor size ranged between 7 mm and 80 mm.

3.1. Imaging Modalities and Diagnostic Process

Physical examination and disease biopsy were performed in all the cases treated. The preferred imaging modality for local staging was contrast-enhanced pelvic magnetic resonance imaging (MRI) in all studies, whereas positron emission tomography (PET) with fluorodeoxyglucose was performed in seven studies for local and global staging.

3.2. Radiotherapy Techniques

A wide range of radiotherapy techniques and treatment schedules is reported, with hadrontherapy being the most frequently applied approach, followed by EBRT delivered with either 3D conformal radiotherapy or intensity-modulated radiotherapy. Conventional doses ranged between 45 Gy and 70 Gy using 2 Gy per fraction regimens; stereotactic radiotherapy was reported in five patients with doses ranging between 24 Gy and 30 Gy in 3–5 fractions. Treatment was generally delivered on consecutive days, and several techniques are reported. An exception is reported in the study by Parisi et al., in which SBRT was delivered once weekly on days 0, 7, and 21 [20].

Brachytherapy (BRT) is reported in a single study, with ^{103}Palladium BRT implant as a boost after conventional EBRT.

Hadrontherapy with carbon ion RT is reported in three studies for a total of 25 patients, with a median dose of 38.7 Gy_{RBE} plus a boost of up to 63 Gy in a median number of 16 fractions.

3.3. Combination with Immunotherapy or Other Systemic Treatments

Combination with immunotherapy is reported in six studies, including a case report of a metastatic patient treated at all the disease sites with dual immunocheckpoint inhibitors (nivolumab + ipilimumab), followed by maintenance nivolumab. In the remaining cases, immunotherapy was initiated concurrently with radiation therapy and maintained until disease progression. In all the cases reported, immunotherapy was combined with stereotactic radiotherapy, except for two patients treated with conventional EBRT, including one receiving a sequential brachytherapy boost.

Conventional chemotherapy was administered in two cases, including dacarbazine in one study, and temozolomide combined with tyrosine kinase inhibitors in another study.

One patient concurrently received interferon 2-α.

Table 1. Reports of definitive radiotherapy for vaginal melanomas.

Author (Year)	N. of Patients Treated	Age	Radiotherapy Setting	RT Technique	Radiotherapy Schedule	Concurrent or Sequential Systemic Treatment	G ≥ 3 Toxicity	Clinical Outcomes
Petru et al. (1998) [14]	2	73	definitive	EBRT	50 Gy/25 fx	none	none	1 local recurrence after 20 months, 1 distant progression after 2 months
Ohno et al. (2007) [15]	1	55	definitive	CIRT	57.6 Gy_{RBE}/16 fx	dacarbazine	none	Complete response after 12 months, death by disease after 18 months
McGuire et al. (2008) [16]	1	71	definitive	EBRT + BRT	46 Gy/23 fx + BRT ^{103}Pd implant 100 Gy	none	none	After 12 months local control, distant progression due to polymetastatic spread
Schiavone et al. (2016) [7]	3	61.5	definitive/neoadjuvant (2 patients received surgery about one month after RT)	EBRT (SBRT)	30 Gy/5 fx (n = 2); 60.2 Gy/28 fx (n = 1)	ipilimumab	1 acute G3 colitis; 1 acute G3 skin toxicity	2 patients NED; 1 death by disease after 16 months
Mesko et al. (2017) [18]	1	70	definitive	EBRT (photons + electrons)	45 Gy/25 fx + electron boost up to 63 Gy	ipilimumab	1 acute G3 skin toxicity	NED after 15 months of follow-up
Murata et al. (2019) [19]	22	71	definitive	CIRT	36 Gy_{RBE} + boost up to 64 Gy_{RBE}/16 fx	Interferon (n = 9); nivolumab (n = 1)	3 acute G3 skin toxicities	2 years LC = 71%; 2 years OS = 53%; 2 years DPFS = 29%
Barcellini et al. (2019) [20]	2	60.5	definitive	CIRT	38.7 Gy_{RBE}/9 fx + boost up to 68.8 Gy_{RBE}	none	none	1 patient developed distant progression after 12.6 months; 1 patient received salvage surgery after 11 months for suspected local recurrence
Parisi et al. (2020) [20]	1	80	definitive	EBRT (SBRT)	24 Gy/3 fx	pembrolizumab	none	Complete response after 12 months; NED at 18 months of follow-up
Sezen et al. (2021) [21]	1	73	palliative (metastatic patient)	EBRT (SBRT)	30 Gy/5 fx	ipilimumab + nivolumab	none	NED after 32 months from initial diagnosis (patients treated to 4 metastatic sites with SBRT in combination with immunotherapy)
Schonewolf et al. (2021) [22]	1	80	definitive	EBRT (SBRT)	30 Gy/5 fx	pembrolizumab	none	Complete local response + potential abscopal effect
Yin et al. (2022) [23]	1	55	definitive	EBRT	70 Gy/35 fx	temozolomide + anlotinib + toripalimab	none	24 months local control, distant progression after 6 months

Abbreviations: CIRT = carbon ion radiotherapy; DPFS = distant progression-free survival; EBRT = external beam radiotherapy; LC = local control; NED = no evidence of disease; OS = overall survival; RBE = relative biological effectiveness.

3.4. Clinical Outcomes

With a median follow-up of 15 months, local recurrence was observed in two cases, with patients who were candidates for surgery or systemic treatment as a second-line approach. The study by Murata et al. [18] reported 2-year LC rates of 71%. The median distant progression was 6 months (range, 2–12 months) with six patients who died of progressive disease.

Globally, radiotherapy is well tolerated, with a low incidence of G3 or higher adverse events. Six cases of acute G3 toxicity (mainly skin toxicity) were reported in patients with concurrent immunotherapy (three patients with ipilimumab, one with nivolumab, and two with interferon). Two patients received SBRT, three were treated with CIRT, and one with conventional EBRT. One patient developed acute G3 colitis when SBRT (30 Gy/5 fractions) was combined with concurrent ipilimumab.

4. Discussion

The optimal management of VM remains a matter of investigation due to the rarity of the disease. The literature reports surgery as the most frequently adopted approach. However, the extent of surgical resection may vary from wide excision to pelvic exenteration, including a more aggressive approach to the lymph nodes when compared to vulvar disease. Moreover, a clear benefit in terms of survival has not yet been demonstrated [24].

In this scenario, modern radiotherapy techniques have emerged as a potential non-invasive alternative.

Initial experiences of brachytherapy alone or in combination with EBRT are reported in the literature, suggesting the feasibility of delivering high doses to the tumor using BRT, especially as a boost after conventional EBRT [16].

Hadrontherapy has recently been reported as a potential therapeutic option for mucosal melanomas due to its higher radiobiological effect, useful in the case of radio-resistant tumor histologies, and for the peculiar dose distribution to optimally spare nearby healthy structures [25].

In addition to the major sparing of the proximal organs at risk, the higher release of energy in a single point, compared to photons, is supposed to result in a higher probability of double-strand DNA breaks, with a consequent enhanced effect of tumor cell killing [26].

All these features justify the potential of hadrontherapy for radio-resistant tumors, although the global availability of this technology is quite limited to date.

Murata et al. [18] reported the outcomes of one of the largest series of female genital tract melanomas, including 22 patients with VM, treated with CIRT. Despite referring to a series of patients with mixed primary sites, the authors reported excellent rates of complete response (about 81%) with 2-year LC, OS, and DPFS rates of 71%, 53%, and 29%, respectively. Interestingly, only three acute grade 3 skin adverse events were recorded.

Similar outcomes are reported in a smaller series by Barcellini et al. [19] including two patients with VM treated with CIRT and by Ohno et al. in a single case report [15].

Beyond the role of hadrontherapy, another topic of potential interest for the treatment of VM relies on the combination of radiotherapy with novel systemic agents.

For this purpose, an interesting case is reported by Yin et al. [23] of a 55-year-old patient with metastatic VM, who received conventional EBRT in combination with temozolomide + tyrosine kinase inhibitors, with good results in terms of local control but short-term distant progression.

In recent years, the combination of radiotherapy with immunotherapy has attracted increasing interest, as reported in other clinical settings, especially for non-small cell lung cancer, kidney cancer, cutaneous melanomas, and cutaneous squamous cell carcinoma [27,28].

Starting from pre-clinical studies that suggest a major immunogenic effect from radiotherapy when delivered using higher doses per fraction (i.e., 8 to 10 Gy for 1–3 fractions) [29], several studies highlight SBRT as a means of releasing neo-antigens capable of activating and proliferating T-cells against tumor cells. This effect favorably combines with the intrinsic activity of recruiting T-cells mediated by immunotherapy [28]. Moreover,

SBRT, compared to conventionally fractionated radiotherapy, generates higher endothelial vascular damage, which facilitates the delivery of targeted therapies to the tumor [30].

Several reports in the literature, specifically for cutaneous melanoma, support the combination of immunotherapy with high-dose SBRT, particularly for brain metastases [31,32].

On the contrary, the combination of SBRT with immunotherapy for extracranial melanoma is currently a matter of debate, with some studies reporting a detrimental impact of radiotherapy when combined with immunotherapy [33,34].

In contrast, Youland et al. [35] reported improved outcomes for extracranial melanomas when SBRT is chosen as the preferred approach, with a statistically significant impact on local control, distant progression, and overall survival in a cohort of 75 patients.

This conflicting evidence highlights the need to further investigate the optimal combination of radiotherapy with immunotherapy, not only in terms of dose and fractionation but also (and probably with more interest) for the sequencing of these two therapeutic tools [36].

A majority of the literature supports the beneficial effect of upfront SBRT followed by immunotherapy in order to enhance the response of the immune system, and other combinations are also reported in the scientific community. Fenioux et al. recently reported favorable outcomes in a cohort of 62 patients with brain metastases from melanoma when immunotherapy was delivered for a long interval (12 weeks) prior to stereotactic radiosurgery [36].

A recent literature review published by Tian et al. reported improved outcomes for brain metastases when concurrent radiotherapy and immunotherapy were delivered in terms of clinical outcomes, but at the same time, the authors focused on the need for a precise definition of "concurrent administration" in terms of time intervals. Starting from an analysis of the biological mechanisms of both SBRT and immunotherapy, the authors hypothesized a peak in the immunogenic effect of high-dose radiotherapy within 24–72 h from the end of treatment, suggesting that right after this interval, immunotherapy has a higher benefit due to the radiotherapy boost effect [37].

Of note, a major incidence of adverse events is reported in the case of concurrent SBRT with immunocheckpoint inhibitors.

Despite being referred to as cutaneous melanoma, all these data suggest the need for better design prospective studies with precise time intervals between SBRT and immunotherapy since this feature might be crucial for an optimal combinatorial response.

Nonetheless, another caveat in the combination of radiotherapy (either with conventional fractionation or SBRT) with immunotherapy is represented by the potential increased risk of severe adverse events [38].

Mesko et al. [17] reported a case of a 70-year-old patient who received conventional EBRT (45 Gy + electron boost up to 63 Gy) for a VM with concurrent ipilimumab. Despite reporting severe acute skin toxicity, the patient remained free of disease after 15 months, with a complete response on PET-FDG scan. Data on skin toxicity with concurrent radiotherapy and ipilimumab are limited, but the authors addressed this phenomenon to the high dose of the target and the size of the planning target volume (PTV).

Schiavone et al. [7] reported the outcomes of a case series including three patients with VM treated with concurrent radiotherapy and immunotherapy, with two patients treated with 30 Gy/5 fx with good tolerance. Notably, two patients in this series also received surgery after the radiotherapy treatment in order to maximize local control.

In light of the higher risk of toxicity when administered concurrently with immunocheckpoint inhibitors, SBRT appears to be a more attractive alternative, as it is usually delivered in smaller volumes compared to the larger volumes of conventional EBRT, and SBRT also offers the abovementioned potential to enhance the response to immunotherapy.

In this scenario, favorable responses are reported. Parisi et al. [20] reported a case of complete remission of VM treated with volumetric modulated arc technique (VMAT)-based SBRT (24 Gy/3 fx once a week) plus pembrolizumab in an 80-year-old patient unfit for surgical approaches. This report highlights the feasibility of stereotactic approaches in older cancer patients, suggesting the potential synergistic role of radiation therapy and immunotherapy, especially when radiotherapy is delivered at higher doses per fraction [27].

In agreement with this, Schonewolf et al. [22] reported a similar case in an 80-year-old patient unfit for surgery treated with SBRT (30 Gy/5 fx) combined with pembrolizumab, obtaining a complete metabolic response not only to the site of the primary tumor but also to locoregional metastases (not included in the RT field), suggesting a potential abscopal effect. In the same study, the authors also reported similar good outcomes in another case (not included in the present review) of a 56-year-old patient who received SBRT plus immunotherapy and subsequent surgery on the primary tumor.

Sezen et al. [21] reported the outcomes of a 73-year-old patient with upfront metastatic VM who received concurrent nivolumab and ipilimumab with palliative 30 Gy/5 fx to the primary tumor site for vaginal bleeding. The subsequent PET-FDG scan detected a complete response to the site of SBRT, and the onset of three liver metastases and one to the right groin. All these sites received SBRT treatment in combination with double immunotherapy followed by nivolumab monotherapy maintenance, with the patient reaching a complete metabolic response 32 months after the diagnosis. This study reinforces the hypothesis of high-dose radiotherapy as a sort of in-situ vaccine, able to facilitate the release of antigens enhancing the immune response to tumor cells [28,39].

Furthermore, it is also theorized that low-dose radiotherapy may have a favorable combination with immunotherapy by increasing the T-cell homing, thus evoking a systemic response with a different biological mechanism than the well-known abscopal effect [40,41].

The present literature review has some limitations. First of all, the available evidence mostly consists of case reports or retrospective series with very limited follow-ups and different doses and techniques. In order to assess the sole impact of radiotherapy in the management of VM, only curative treatments were considered for the purpose of this analysis.

We also proposed a focus on a favorable combination with immunotherapy, aiming to translate the knowledge derived from cutaneous melanoma.

Also, this field appears to have several areas to be fully explored, starting from the exact interaction between radiotherapy and immunotherapy in terms of biological mechanisms to the need to precisely identify the optimal sequencing of these two therapeutic tools [42].

In conclusion, the optimal treatment for vaginal melanoma remains a matter of debate, with surgery, radiotherapy, and immunotherapy as the three main strategies currently available. Of course, as surgery remains the most frequently preferred treatment option, radiotherapy could be considered for patients unfit for invasive approaches. In this scenario, this literature review reports the substantial feasibility of exclusive radiotherapy with or without novel systemic agents. Studies with larger sample sizes are advocated, but in light of the currently available limited evidence, multidisciplinary management of patients with VM is considered mandatory.

Funding: This research received no external funding.

Institutional Review Board Statement: Not applicable.

Informed Consent Statement: Informed consent was obtained from all subjects involved in the study.

Data Availability Statement: Data available on request.

Conflicts of Interest: The authors declare no conflict of interest.

References

1. Jamaer, E.; Liang, Z.; Stagg, B. Primary malignant melanoma of the vagina. *BMJ Case Rep.* **2020**, *13*, e232200. [CrossRef] [PubMed]
2. Terzakis, E.; Grigoriadis, C.; Decavalas, G. Vaginal primary malignant melanoma: Report of four cases and review of the literature. *Eur. J. Gynecol. Oncol.* **2011**, *32*, 122–124.
3. Wu, Y.; Li, H.; Tan, L.; Lai, Y.; Li, Z. Different clinico-pathological and prognostic features of vulvar, vaginal, and cervical melanomas. *Hum. Pathol.* **2023**, *131*, 87–97. [CrossRef] [PubMed]

4. Lotem, M.; Anteby, S.; Peretz, T.; Ingber, A.; Avinoach, I.; Prus, D. Mucosal melanoma of the female genital tract is a multifocal disorder. *Gynecol. Oncol.* **2003**, *88*, 45–50. [CrossRef] [PubMed]
5. Indini, A.; Di Guardo, L.; Cimminiello, C.; Lorusso, D.; Raspagliesi, F.; Del Vecchio, M. Investigating the role of immunotherapy in advanced/recurrent female genital tract melanoma: A preliminary experience. *J. Gynecol. Oncol.* **2019**, *30*, e94. [CrossRef]
6. Hodi, F.S.; O'Day, S.J.; McDermott, D.F.; Weber, R.W.; Sosman, J.A.; Haanen, J.B.; Gonzalez, R.; Robert, C.; Schadendorf, D.; Hassel, J.C.; et al. Improved survival with ipilimumab in patients with metastatic melanoma. *N. Engl. J. Med.* **2010**, *363*, 711–723. [CrossRef]
7. Schiavone, M.B.; Broach, V.; Shoushtari, A.N.; Carvajal, R.D.; Alektiar, K.; Kollmeier, M.A.; Abu-Rustum, N.R.; Leitao, M.M., Jr. Combined immunotherapy and radiation for treatment of mucosal melanomas of the lower genital tract. *Gynecol. Oncol. Rep.* **2016**, *16*, 42–46. [CrossRef]
8. Kim, H.J.; Chang, J.S.; Roh, M.R.; Oh, B.H.; Chung, K.Y.; Shin, S.J.; Koom, W.S. Effect of radiotherapy combined with pembrolizumab on local tumor control in mucosal melanoma patients. *Front. Oncol.* **2019**, *9*, 835. [CrossRef]
9. Stinauer, M.A.; Kavanagh, B.D.; Schefter, T.E.; Gonzalez, R.; Flaig, T.; Lewis, K.; Robinson, W.; Chidel, M.; Glode, M.; Raben, D. Stereotactic body radiation therapy for melanoma and renal cell carcinoma: Impact of single fraction equivalent dose on local control. *Radiat. Oncol.* **2011**, *6*, 34. [CrossRef]
10. Luke, J.J.; Lemons, J.M.; Karrison, T.G.; Pitroda, S.P.; Melotek, J.M.; Zha, Y.; Al-Hallaq, H.A.; Arina, A.; Khodarev, N.N.; Janisch, L.; et al. Safety and clinical activity of pembrolizumab and multisite stereotactic body radiotherapy in patients with advanced solid tumors. *J. Clin. Oncol.* **2018**, *36*, 1611–1618. [CrossRef]
11. Postow, M.A.; Knox, S.J.; Goldman, D.A.; Elhanati, Y.; Mavinkurve, V.; Wong, P.; Halpenny, D.; Reddy, S.K.; Vado, K.; McCabe, D.; et al. A prospective, phase 1 trial of nivolumab, ipilimumab, and radiotherapy in patients with advanced melanoma. *Clin. Cancer Res.* **2020**, *26*, 3193–3201. [CrossRef] [PubMed]
12. Twyman-Saint Victor, C.; Rech, A.J.; Maity, A.; Rengan, R.; Pauken, K.E.; Stelekati, E.; Benci, J.L.; Xu, B.; Dada, H.; Odorizzi, P.M.; et al. Radiation and dual checkpoint blockade activate non-redundant immune mechanisms in cancer. *Nature* **2015**, *520*, 373–377. [CrossRef] [PubMed]
13. Cushman, T.R.; Gomez, D.; Kumar, R.; Likacheva, A.; Chang, J.Y.; Cadena, A.P.; Paris, S.; Welsh, J.W. Combining radiation plus immunotherapy to improve systemic immune response. *J. Thorac. Dis.* **2018**, *10* (Suppl. 3), S468–S479. [CrossRef]
14. Petru, E.; Nagele, F.; Czerwenka, K.; Graf, A.H.; Lax, S.; Bauer, M.; Pehamberger, H.; Vavra, N. Primary malignant melanoma of the vagina: Long-term remission following radiation therapy. *Gynecol. Oncol.* **1998**, *70*, 23–26. [CrossRef] [PubMed]
15. Ohno, T.; Kato, S.; Sasaki, E.; Mizutani, K.; Tsujii, H. Carbon ion radiotherapy for vaginal malignant melanoma: A case report. *Int. J. Gynecol. Cancer* **2007**, *17*, 1163–1166. [CrossRef] [PubMed]
16. McGuire, S.E.; Frank, S.J.; Eifel, P.J. Treatment of recurrent vaginal melanoma with external beam radiation therapy and palladium-103 brachytherapy. *Brachytherapy* **2008**, *7*, 359–363. [CrossRef]
17. Mesko, S.; Konecny, G.E.; Tumeh, P.C.; Kamrava, M. Enhanced skin toxicity with concurrent ipilimumab and radiation in vaginal/vulvar melanoma: A case report and literature review. *BJR Case Rep.* **2017**, *2*, 20160002. [CrossRef]
18. Murata, H.; Okonogi, N.; Wakatsuki, M.; Kato, S.; Kiyohara, H.; Karasawa, K.; Ohno, T.; Nakano, T.; Kamada, T.; Shozu, M.; et al. Long-Term Outcomes of Carbon-Ion Radiotherapy for Malignant Gynecological Melanoma. *Cancers* **2019**, *11*, 482. [CrossRef]
19. Barcellini, A.; Vitolo, V.; Facoetti, A.; Fossati, P.; Preda, L.; Fiore, M.R.; Vischioni, B.; Iannalfi, A.; Bonora, M.; Ronchi, S.; et al. Feasibility of Carbon Ion Radiotherapy in the Treatment of Gynecological Melanoma. *In Vivo* **2019**, *33*, 473–476. [CrossRef]
20. Parisi, S.; Lillo, S.; Cacciola, A.; Santacaterina, A.; Palazzolo, C.; Platania, A.; Settineri, N.; Franchina, T.; Tamburella, C.; Pergolizzi, S. Vaginal Mucosal Melanoma: A Complete Remission after Immunotherapy and '0-7-21' Radiotherapy Regimen (24 Gy/3 fractions/21 days). *Folia Med.* **2020**, *62*, 605–609. [CrossRef]
21. Sezen, D.; Patel, R.R.; Tang, C.; Onstad, M.; Nagarajan, P.; Patel, S.P.; Welsh, J.W.; Lin, L.L. Immunotherapy combined with high- and low-dose radiation to all sites leads to complete clearance of disease in a patient with metastatic vaginal melanoma. *Gynecol. Oncol.* **2021**, *161*, 645–652. [CrossRef]
22. Schonewolf, C.A.; Jaworski, E.M.; Allen, S.G.; McLean, K.; Lao, C.D.; Schuchter, L.M.; Tanyi, J.; Taunk, N.K. Complete Response After Stereotactic Body Radiation Therapy with Concurrent Immunotherapy for Vaginal Melanoma. *Adv. Radiat. Oncol.* **2021**, *7*, 100839. [CrossRef] [PubMed]
23. Yin, P.; Ma, X.; Zhang, Y.; Song, Y.; Wang, Y.; Lu, Z. Primary vaginal malignant melanoma successfully treated with combination therapy: A case report. *Oncol. Lett.* **2022**, *24*, 430. [CrossRef] [PubMed]
24. Miner, T.J.; Delgado, R.; Zeisler, J.; Busam, K.; Alektiar, K.; Barakat, R.; Poynor, E. Primary vaginal melanoma: A critical analysis of therapy. *Ann. Surg. Oncol.* **2004**, *11*, 34–39. [CrossRef] [PubMed]
25. Cuccia, F.; Fiore, M.R.; Barcellini, A.; Iannalfi, A.; Vischioni, B.; Ronchi, S.; Bonora, M.; Riva, G.; Vai, A.; Facoetti, A.; et al. Outcome and Toxicity of Carbon Ion Radiotherapy for Axial Bone and Soft Tissue Sarcomas. *Anticancer Res.* **2020**, *40*, 2853–2859. [CrossRef]
26. Barcellini, A.; Vitolo, V.; Cobianchi, L.; Peloso, A.; Vanoli, A.; Mirandola, A.; Facoetti, A.; Fiore, M.R.; Iannalfi, A.; Vischioni, B.; et al. Re-irradiation with Carbon Ion Radiotherapy for Pelvic Rectal Cancer Recurrences in Patients Previously Irradiated to the Pelvis. *In Vivo* **2020**, *34*, 1547–1553. [CrossRef]
27. Mazzola, R.; Jereczek-Fossa, B.A.; Franceschini, D.; Tubin, S.; Filippi, A.R.; Tolia, M.; Lancia, A.; Minniti, G.; Corradini, S.; Arcangeli, S.; et al. Oligometastasis and local ablation in the era of systemic targeted and immunotherapy. *Radiat. Oncol.* **2020**, *15*, 92. [CrossRef]

28. Ferini, G.; Castorina, P.; Valenti, V.; Illari, S.I.; Sachpazidis, I.; Castorina, L.; Marrale, M.; Pergolizzi, S. A Novel Radiotherapeutic Approach to Treat Bulky Metastases Even From Cutaneous Squamous Cell Carcinoma: Its Rationale and a Look at the Reliability of the Linear-Quadratic Model to Explain Its Radiobiological Effects. *Front. Oncol.* **2022**, *12*, 809279. [CrossRef]
29. Buchwald, Z.S.; Wynne, J.; Nasti, T.H.; Zhu, S.; Mourad, W.F.; Yan, W.; Gupta, S.; Khleif, S.N.; Khan, M.K. Radiation, immune checkpoint blockade and the Abscopal effect: A critical review on timing. Dose and Fractionation. *Front. Oncol.* **2018**, *8*, 612. [CrossRef]
30. Park, H.J.; Griffin, R.J.; Hui, S.; Levitt, S.H.; Song, C.W. Radiation-induced vascular damage in tumors: Implications of vascular damage in ablative hypofractionated radiotherapy (SBRT and SRS). *Radiat. Res.* **2012**, *177*, 311–327. [CrossRef]
31. Diao, K.; Bian, S.X.; Routman, D.M.; Yu, C.; Ye, J.C.; Wagle, N.A.; Wong, M.K.; Zada, G.; Chang, E.L. Stereotactic radiosurgery and ipilimumab for patients with melanoma brain metastases: Clinical outcomes and toxicity. *J. Neuro-Oncol.* **2018**, *139*, 421–429. [CrossRef] [PubMed]
32. Anderson, E.S.; Postow, M.A.; Wolchok, J.D.; Young, R.J.; Ballangrud, Å.; Chan, T.A.; Yamada, Y.; Beal, K. Melanoma brain metastases treated with stereotactic radiosurgery and concurrent pembrolizumab display marked regression; efficacy and safety of combined treatment. *J. Immunother. Cancer* **2017**, *5*, 76. [CrossRef] [PubMed]
33. Gabani, P.; Robinson, C.G.; Ansstas, G.; Johanns, T.M.; Huang, J. Use of extracranial radiation therapy in metastatic melanoma patients receiving immunotherapy. *Radiother. Oncol.* **2018**, *127*, 310–317. [CrossRef] [PubMed]
34. Cuccia, F.; Mazzola, R.; Pastorello, E.; Figlia, V.; Giaj-Levra, N.; Nicosia, L.; Ricchetti, F.; Rigo, M.; Attinà, G.; Vitale, C.; et al. SBRT for elderly oligometastatic patients as a feasible, safe and effective treatment opportunity. *Clin. Exp. Metastasis* **2021**, *38*, 475–481. [CrossRef]
35. Youland, R.S.; Blanchard, M.L.; Dronca, R.; Kottschade, L.; Markovic, S.N.; Olivier, K.R.; Park, S.S. Role of radiotherapy in extracranial metastatic malignant melanoma in the modern era. *Clin. Transl. Radiat. Oncol.* **2017**, *6*, 25–30. [CrossRef] [PubMed]
36. Stoian, A.R.; Rahnea-Nita, G.; Ciuhu, A.N.; Gales, L.; Anghel, R.M.; Rebegea, L.F.; Rahnea-Nita, R.A.; Andronache, L.F.; Soare, I.; Stoleriu, G. The Benefits and Challenges of the Multimodal Treatment in Advanced/Metastatic Malignant Melanoma. *Diagnostics* **2023**, *13*, 1635. [CrossRef]
37. Tian, W.; Chu, X.; Tanzhu, G.; Zhou, R. Optimal timing and sequence of combining stereotactic radiosurgery with immune checkpoint inhibitors in treating brain metastases: Clinical evidence and mechanistic basis. *J. Transl. Med.* **2023**, *21*, 244. [CrossRef]
38. Parisi, S.; Napoli, I.; Lillo, S.; Cacciola, A.; Ferini, G.; Iatì, G.; Pontoriero, A.; Tamburella, C.; Davì, V.; Pergolizzi, S. Spine eburnation in a metastatic lung cancer patient treated with immunotherapy and radiotherapy. The first case report of bystander effect on bone. *J. Oncol. Pharm. Pract.* **2022**, *28*, 237–241. [CrossRef]
39. Ridolfi, L.; de Rosa, F.; Ridolfi, R.; Gentili, G.; Valmorri, L.; Scarpi, E.; Parisi, E.; Romeo, A.; Guidoboni, M. Radiotherapy as an immunological booster in patients with metastatic melanoma or renal cell carcinoma treated with high-dose Interleukin-2: Evaluation of biomarkers of immunologic therapeutic response. *J. Transl. Med.* **2014**, *12*, 262. [CrossRef]
40. Menon, H.; Chen, D.; Ramapriyan, R.; Verma, V.; Barsoumian, H.B.; Cushman, T.R.; Younes, A.I.; Cortez, M.A.; Erasmus, J.J.; de Groot, P.; et al. Influence of low-dose radiation on abscopal responses in patients receiving high-dose radiation immunotherapy. *J. Immunother. Cancer* **2019**, *7*, 237. [CrossRef]
41. Welsh, J.M.; de Groot, P.; Naing, A.; Hess, K.R.; Heymach, J.V.; Papadimitrakopoulou, V.A.; Cushman, T.R.; Subbiah, V.; Chang, J.Y. Phase II trial of Ipilimumab with stereotactic radiation therapy for metastatic disease: Outcomes, toxicities, and low-dose radiation-related abscopal responses. *Cancer Immunol. Res.* **2019**, *7*, 1903–1909. [CrossRef] [PubMed]
42. Zhang, Z.; Liu, X.; Chen, D.; Yu, J. Radiotherapy combined with immunotherapy: The dawn of cancer treatment. *Signal Transduct. Target. Ther.* **2022**, *7*, 258. [CrossRef] [PubMed]

Journal of *Personalized Medicine*

MDPI

Communication

Introducing Radiotherapy in Metastatic Merkel Cell Carcinoma Patients with Limited Progression on Avelumab: An Effective Step against Primary and Secondary Immune Resistance?

Gianluca Ferini [1,*], Valentina Zagardo [1], Paola Critelli [2], Anna Santacaterina [3], Serena Sava [4], Mandara Muralidhar Harikar [5], Tejas Venkataram [5], Giuseppe Emmanuele Umana [5], Anna Viola [4], Vito Valenti [1] and Stefano Forte [4]

1 REM Radioterapia srl, Via Penninazzo 11, 95029 Viagrande, Italy; valentina.zagardo@gmail.com (V.Z.); vito.valenti@grupposamed.com (V.V.)
2 Department of Biomedical, Dental Science and Morphological and Functional Images, University of Messina, 98122 Messina, Italy; paola.critelli@unime.it
3 Radiation Oncology Unit, Papardo Teaching Hospital, 98158 Messina, Italy; anna.santacaterina@virgilio.it
4 Istituto Oncologico del Mediterraneo, 95029 Viagrande, Italy; serena.sava@grupposamed.com (S.S.); anna.viola@fondazioneiom.it (A.V.); stefano.forte@grupposamed.com (S.F.)
5 Department of Neurosurgery, Trauma Center, Gamma Knife Center, Cannizzaro Hospital, 95126 Catania, Italy; mandara.harikar@gmail.com (M.M.H.); tejas.venkataram@gmail.com (T.V.); umana.nch@gmail.com (G.E.U.)
* Correspondence: gianluca.ferini@grupposamed.com; Tel.: +39-095-789-9569

Abstract: Purpose: To investigate the ability of radiotherapy (RT) to prolong progression-free survival (PFS) and to report treatment-related toxicities among oligoprogressive metastatic Merkel cell carcinoma (mMCC) patients on avelumab. Methods: We retrospectively collected clinical data on mMCC patients who underwent radiotherapy for limited progression on avelumab. Patients were categorized as primary or secondary immune refractory depending on the time of onset of resistance to immunotherapy (at the first or subsequent follow-up visits after avelumab initiation). Pre- and post-RT PFS were calculated. Overall survival (OS) from the first progression treated with RT was also reported. Radiological responses and toxicities were evaluated according to the irRECIST criteria and RTOG scoring system, respectively. Results: Eight patients, including five females, with a median age of 75 years, met our inclusion criteria. The median gross tumor and clinical target volumes at first progression on avelumab were 29.85 cc and 236.7 cc, respectively. The treatment sites included lymph node, skin, brain, and spine metastases. Four patients received more than one course of RT. Most patients were treated with palliative radiation doses (mainly 30 Gy in 3 Gy/day fractions). Two patients were treated with stereotactic RT. Five/eight patients were primary immune refractory. The objective response rate at the first post-RT assessment was 75%, whereas no local failure was reported. The median pre-RT PFS was 3 months. The pre-RT PFS was 37.5% at 6 months and 12.5% at 1 year. The median post-RT PFS was not reached. The post-RT PFS was 60% at 6 months and 1 year. The post-RT OS was 85.7% at 1 year and 64.3% at 2 years. No relevant treatment-related toxicity was observed. After a median follow-up of 18.5 months, 6/8 patients are still alive and continuing on avelumab therapy. Conclusions: Adding radiotherapy to mMCC patients with limited progression on avelumab seems to be safe and effective in prolonging the successful use of immunotherapy, regardless of the type of immune refractoriness.

Keywords: Merkel cell carcinoma; oligometastasis; oligoprogressive; radiotherapy; stereotactic radiotherapy; immunotherapy; immune resistance

1. Introduction

Merkel cell carcinoma (MCC) is a rare aggressive neuroendocrine skin tumor with a marked propensity for metastatic progression [1]. This occurrence translates into a dismal prognosis reaching a 1-year survival rate of about 38% [2]. The recent advent of immunotherapy, especially avelumab, has improved the prognosis of metastatic MCC (mMCC) [3]. In this stage, radiotherapy (RT) was mainly used for symptom palliation of painful metastases (either affecting the bones or not) or skin-ulcerating nodules or bulky mediastinal masses stenosing bronchi or great vessels [4]. In the JAVELIN trial, the avelumab arm reported 1-year progression-free and overall survival (OS) rates of 30% and 52%, which are significantly better than historical controls, although still not satisfactory [5]. Unlike platinum-based chemotherapy, avelumab produces more sustained responses after the first year of treatment [6]. The prolongation of PFS with immunotherapy raises some questions on the correct management of MCC patients with limited progressive disease, to whom the concepts of oligoprogression or oligorecurrence may be attributed. The latter refer to an intermediate disease extent between locoregional and polymetastatic ones, comprising up to five metastases, and is relatively novel for MCC, given its typical rapid progression in the previous chemotherapy era [7]. RT has proven to be effective in prolonging PFS in oligometastic tumors other than MCC [8]. Regarding this skin cancer, no reports are still available. In MCC patients with limited disease progression, RT might have a crucial role in reversing incoming refractoriness to immunotherapy, particularly in such a setting devoid of further effective systemic treatments. This use of RT has also been cautiously endorsed by a recent Delphi consensus, although no clinical validation exists [9].

Herein we describe a small series of patients with mMCC who had oligo-progression or -recurrence during avelumab treatment and then were treated with RT. We also provide a comprehensive overview of the literature on the subject.

2. Methods

We queried our mono-institutional database for mMCC patients undergoing RT from 2017 (approval date of avelumab for MCC in Italy) to 28 February 2023. Inclusion criteria were progression on avelumab and RT to all progressive disease sites, regardless of their extent and the RT technique used. Considering the peculiar biological behavior of the MCC, we did not screen the patients according to the concept of oligoprogression as commonly intended. Consequently, no restrictions on the number and size of irradiated metastases were applied. All fractionation schemes and RT techniques were welcome. Patients could have received cytotoxic chemotherapy prior to avelumab treatment or switched to it upon the completion of RT after immunotherapy failure. Exclusion criteria were radiotherapy delivered as adjuvant treatment for locoregional disease extent (stages I-III) or without at least one response assessment after avelumab initiation. No other immune checkpoint inhibitors were possible since avelumab is the only one approved for MCC in our country.

Regarding the RT target delineation, the gross tumor volume (GTV) was the progressive macroscopic disease as detected on the computed tomography (CT) simulation with the support of 18F-FDG positron emission tomography (PET), if any. GTV was included in a larger volume accounting for the probable subclinical spread of tumor cells, namely the clinical target volume (CTV), e.g., the entire inguinal lymph node basin in case of an isolated metastasis located therein. Given the lack of precise instructions to delineate the CTV within the context of the study, a certain arbitrariness was allowed. In cases of stereotactic radiosurgery (SRS) for brain metastases, only the GTV and planning target volume (PTV) were contoured. When stereotactic body radiation therapy (SBRT) was used for extracranial targets, the CTV delineation was at the discretion of the treating physician, unless otherwise stated by any consensus papers [10].

Patients were categorized as primary or secondary immune-refractory depending on the time of onset of resistance to avelumab: progressive disease (PD) at the first follow-up visit after avelumab initiation (requiring per-protocol confirmation as specified below) vs. PD at any other follow-up. These visits were scheduled every three months and included both physical and instrumental exams (CT and/or PET).

A series of demographic and treatment data was collected, including ECOG performance status, baseline immune status (immunocompetent vs. immunosuppressed), total radiation dose and fractionation, biologically effective dose (BED) using an α/β value of 10 Gy for tumor, number of RT courses, RT treatment site, GTV and CTV size, number of treated metastases, RT technique, further systemic treatments (before or after avelumab therapy), immune sensitivity at the time of RT (primary vs. secondary refractory), survival state at the date of the last follow-up (alive or not on 28 February 2023). The presence of the Merkel cell polyomavirus in the tumor genome as well as the PD-L1 status were not routinely investigated according to our standard clinical practice and should be considered unknown for all patients.

The study endpoints were the post-RT assessment of local control (LC), progression-free survival (at any site), overall survival, and the objective response rate (ORR). Radiological responses were defined as complete response (CR), partial response (PR), stable disease (SD), and progressive disease (PD), and assessed as per irRECIST criteria, according to which any first progression must be confirmed by repeating the instrumental evaluation at least four weeks later [11]. We also reported pre-RT PFS, which is the time interval between avelumab initiation and subsequent RT-treated progression. Toxicities were graded according to RTOG [12].

Univariate probabilities of post-RT OS and PFS were calculated using the Kaplan–Meier method [13]. The analyses were performed using R V.4.1.1 (R package survival).

3. Results

Our final cohort comprised eight patients (three males, five females) whose age ranged from 61 to 86 (median 75, interquartile range 16.25). No patients were immunosuppressed as none had immunodeficiency disease or received immunosuppressive drugs for any autoimmune conditions. The median total radiation dose was 30 Gy (range 19.5–36) in 10 fractions (range 3–12), corresponding to a median BED of 39 Gy (range 32.2–59.5). The number of RT courses was one for four patients, two in the other three, and four in one patient. The treatment sites included lymph node, skin, brain and spine metastases. The median GTV and CTV sizes at the first RT course were 29.85 cc (range 10–209) and 236.7 cc (range 37–516), respectively, encompassing a median of one metastasis (range 1–4). Overall, GTV and CTV ranged from 10 to 209 cc (median 29.35 cc) and from 25 to 3744 cc (median 236.7 cc), respectively, while the number of metastases treated simultaneously was 15 in the fourth course of one patient. Volumetric modulated arc therapy was used in six patients, while SRS and SBRT were used in the other two. Avelumab was first-line treatment in all but two patients who had previously been treated with cisplatin-based chemotherapy. Five/eight patients were to be considered as primary immune refractory. Six/eight were alive at the last follow-up. The above information is summarized in Table 1.

ORR (PR + CR) at the first post-RT assessment was 75%. Only two patients had SD. No patient exhibited in-field failure (LC equal to 100%).

The highest acute toxicity was a self-limiting G1 skin erythema in one patient. No treatment-related chronic toxicities were reported.

Starting from the date of the first RT, the median follow-up was 18.5 months (range 4–63). The median pre-RT PFS was 3 months as a result of having more than half of the patients with primary immune resistance. The pre-RT PFS was 37.5% at 6 months and 12.5% at 1 year. The median post-RT PFS was not reached as only four patients experienced further progression after RT administration. The post-RT PFS was 60% at 6 months and 1 year. The post-RT OS was 85.7% at 1 year and 64.3% at 2 years. The survival curves are in Figures 1–3. The disease course of each patient is graphically displayed in Figure 4. Given the small sample size, no CTV or GTV thresholds can be detected to predict any association with survival outcomes.

Table 1. Patients' characteristics. RT, radiotherapy; GTV, gross tumor volume; CTV, clinical target volume; VMAT, volumetric modulated arc therapy; SRS, stereotactic radiosurgery; SBRT, stereotactic body radiation therapy.

	Patients % (*n*)
Age, median (range) years	75 (61–86)
Sex	
Male	37.5 (3/8)
Female	62.5 (5/8)
Median Total Radiation Dose	30 (19.5–36)
Number of RT courses	
1	50 (4/8)
2	37.5 (3/8)
4	12.5 (1/8)
Type of treatment	
VMAT	75 (6/8)
SRS and SBRT	25 (2/8)
Treatment before Avelumab	
None	75 (6/8)
Cisplatin-based chemotherapy	25 (2/8)
Treatment after Avelumab	
None	75 (6/8)
Cisplatin-based chemotherapy	25 (2/8)
Primary immune refractory patients	62.5 (5/8)
Patients alive at last follow-up	75 (6/8)
Patients who had local control	100 (8/8)
	Median (range)
Median GTV at the first RT course, cc	29.85 (10–209)
Median CTV at the first RT course, cc	236.7 (37–516)
Median overall GTV, cc	29.35 (10–209)
Median overall CTV, cc	236.7 (25–3744)
Median number of simultaneously RT-treated metastases	1 (1–15)

Avelumab therapy was successfully maintained and is still ongoing in all but two patients who briefly switched to cytotoxic chemotherapy at the third and fifth progression, respectively, ultimately dying of the disease.

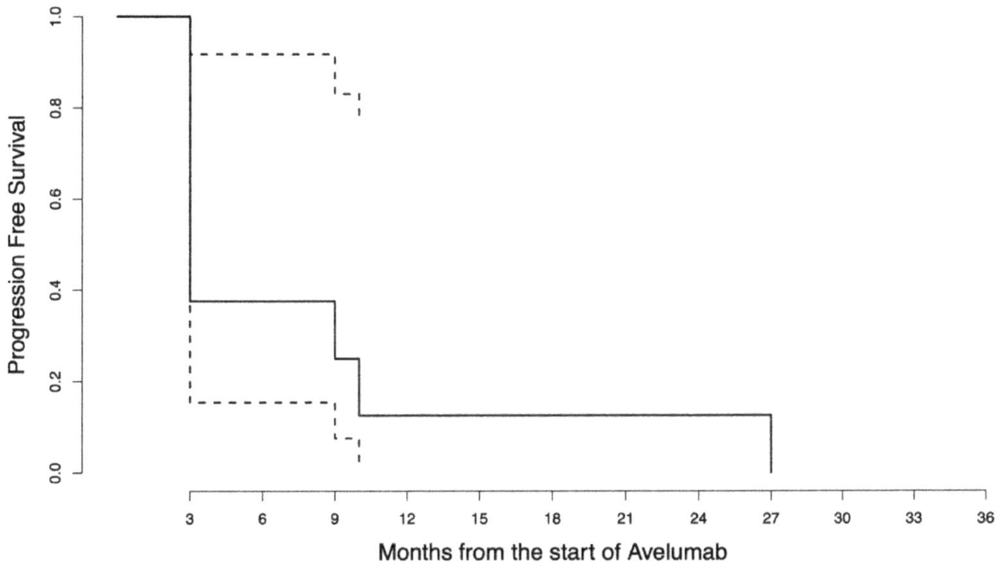

Figure 1. Pre-radiotherapy progression-free survival curve. The survival function is represented by the solid line, where the steps represent the events that have occurred (first disease progression after avelumab initiation). The dashed lines represent the 95% confidence interval.

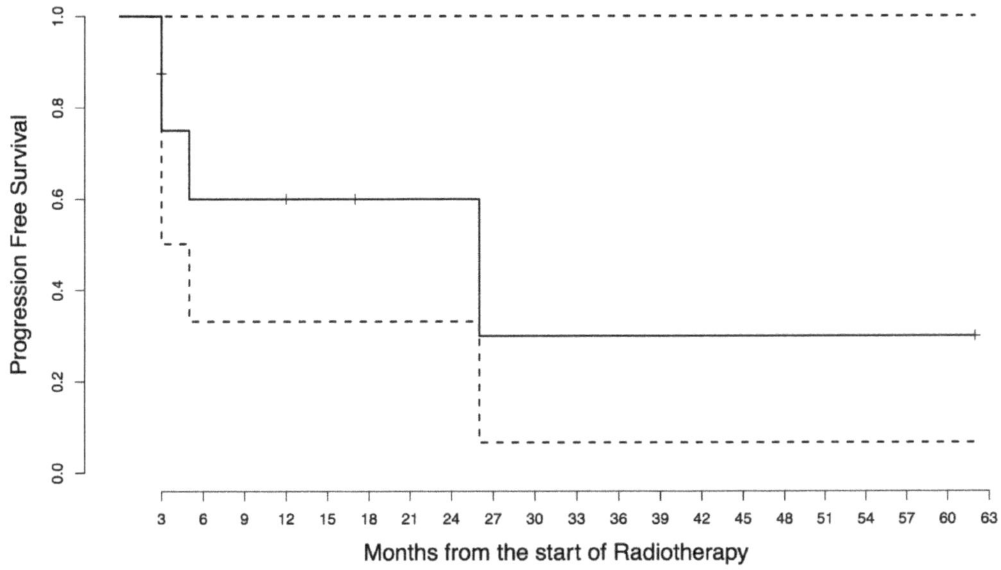

Figure 2. Post-radiotherapy progression-free survival curve. The survival function is represented by the solid line, where the steps represent the events that have occurred (first disease progression after radiotherapy) while the vertical bars represent the censored patients. The dashed lines represent the 95% confidence interval.

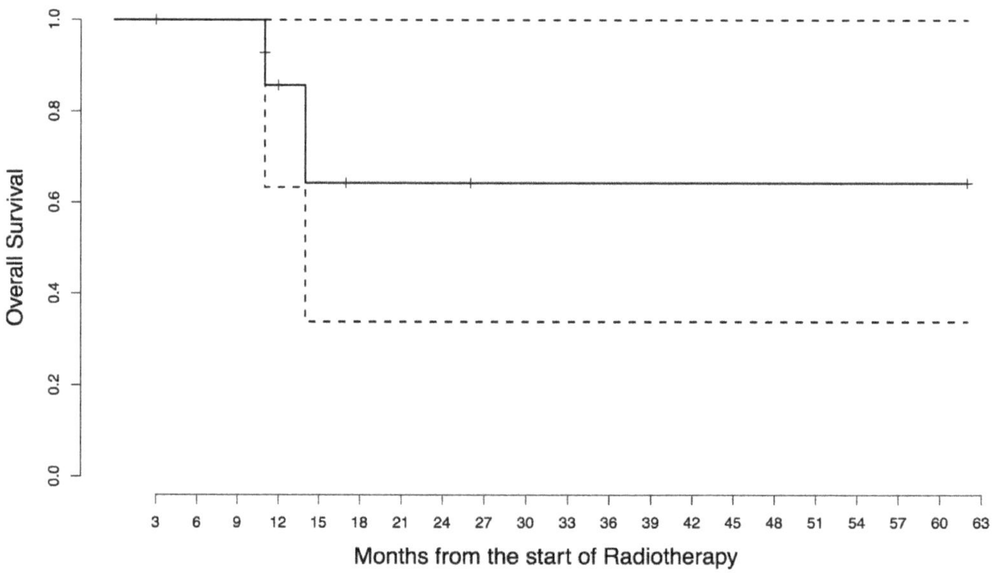

Figure 3. Post-radiotherapy overall survival curve. The survival function is represented by the solid line, where the steps represent the events that have occurred (death) while the vertical bars represent the censored patients. The dashed lines represent the 95% confidence interval.

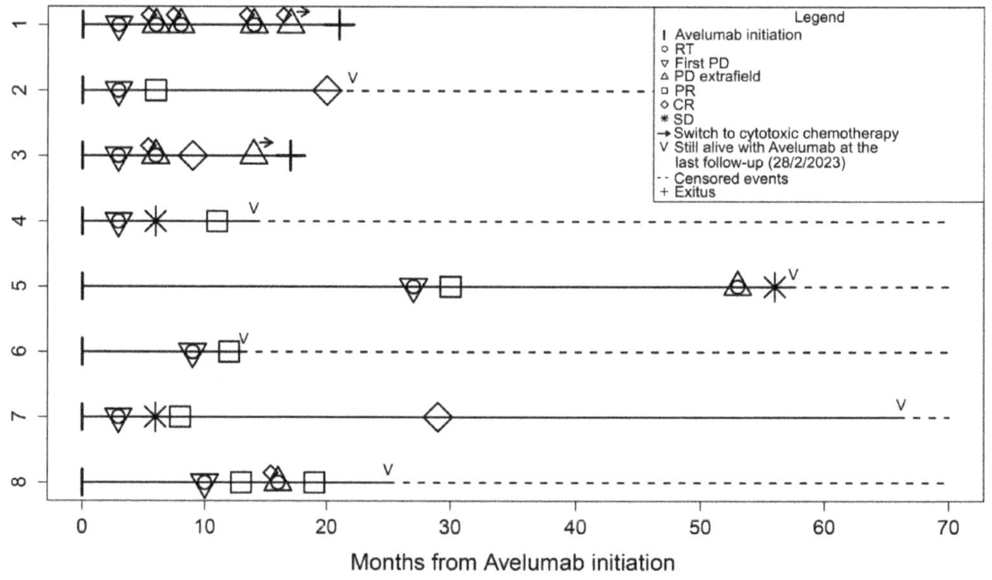

Figure 4. Timeline of all patients included with the explanation of the events in the legend. RT, radiotherapy; PD, progressive disease; PR, partial response; CR, complete response; SD, stable disease. For patients 5 and 8, two cycles of SBRT each were used; the others were treated with palliative RT schemes (the circles stand for RT courses, as explained in the figure legend).

4. Discussion

To our knowledge, this is the first short report describing the integration of radiotherapy in the setting of MCC patients progressing during avelumab treatment. We reported promising results in terms of LC and PFS and no significant toxicities. To date, oligometastatic status for MCC has been only conceptualized, being still clinically unproven. Indeed, in the SABR-COMET trials, this condition has been described for the most common solid malignancies including, above all, breast, prostate, colorectal and lung cancers [8]. A recent trial is expanding this concept even to other tumors [14]; among these, the only skin-derived cancer was melanoma, already included in other similarly conceived studies [15,16]. Case reports hypothesized the oligometastatic stage also for cutaneous squamous cell carcinoma [17], which has mostly local aggressiveness like the basal cell one [18,19].

While oligometastatic disease generally refers to a condition starting with few metastases ($\leq$5) diagnosed synchronously to the primary tumor uncontrolled, oligoprogression and oligorecurrence are characterized by a low tumor burden refractory to ongoing therapies (metachronous metastases). These disease stages are still amenable to metastases-directed local therapies, which allow the need for switching the ongoing systemic treatment to be postponed [20]. This is particularly important in the scenario investigated here, since the PD-1/PD-L1 blockade represents the last line of treatment, given the limited and transient effectiveness of classic cytotoxic chemotherapies. In our case series, 6/8 patients continued an effective use of avelumab after radiotherapy.

Oligometastatic status is generally linked to the use of stereotactic body radiation therapy (SBRT) to control with ablative radiation doses in a few daily fractions ($\leq$5) no more than five metastases, usually not exceeding 5 cm in diameter [21]. We have chosen not to strictly adhere to this rigid definition for several reasons: (1) MCC is a greatly radiosensitive tumor responding also to radiation doses much lower than those used in SBRT; (2) MCC may progress along a wide skin area developing more than five nodules or a lymph node basin producing bulky masses greater than 5 cm, but still amenable to radiotherapy; (3) MCC has a typical subclinical spread between contiguous metastases, which often justifies the irradiation of a CTV much larger than the GTV. These facts make the classic dimensional and numerical criteria inadequate in defining the oligometastatic status for MCC, which likely needs ad hoc considerations. Our GTVs ranged from 10 to 209 cc, while CTVs from 25 to 3744 cc. The largest CTV refers to the whole skin of the left lower limb of a patient in whom previous three RT courses had failed to prolong PFS, as described in [22]. Palliative doses were the most common, having been used in 6/8 patients: by delivering a 3 Gy/day fraction, a total dose of 30 Gy was administered to 5 patients and 36 Gy to another one. Among these, local tumor regression was observed in all patients. The decision to subject two patients to SBRT rather than to the classic palliative radiotherapy treatments depended on the location (one brain, one vertebra, and two skin nodules) and on the small size of the metastases. Intriguingly, one of these two patients exhibited no objective response at the second course. Overall, four patients had further progressions treated with RT after the first course: in two patients, disease control was effectively restored, whereas, in the other two, RT was unable to stop a rapidly evolving systemic progression, ultimately culminating in death despite a last-ditch attempt to switch from avelumab to cisplatin-based chemotherapy (Figure 4).

Concerning the efficacy of low-dose palliative radiation, our results agree with those of Iyer et al. [23], who reported a durable objective response in 94% of patients with mMCC (including 45% of CR) treated with 8 Gy-single-fraction RT. Even these authors claimed a convenient synergy between RT and the host immune system (when not suppressed due to comorbidities). Both low (2–4 Gy per fraction) and high (>5 Gy per fraction) radiation doses may work as immune stimulants, the former by upregulating the major histocompatibility complex, the latter by increasing antigen release and priming T cells into the tumor (as well as directly inducing cell death by apoptosis or necrosis) [24–26]. Furthermore, very low doses (0.5–1 Gy per fraction) counteract the tumor immune desertification by mobilizing T cells from draining lymph nodes, thus enhancing tumor responsiveness to combined immunotherapy (IT) [25]. Irradiating a CTV significantly larger than GTV, as in most of our cases, could have a dual function: 1) to sterilize any microscopic tumor deposits in the area surrounding the GTV; 2) to extend the off-target volume receiving the immunoactivating low doses. The latter antitumor effect might be weakened by radiation-induced lymphopenia, thus requiring caution in delineating CTV and using dose-scattering intensity-modulated radiotherapy (IMRT) techniques [27]. The small size of our sample prevented us from providing recommendations on CTV delineation. According to our report, classic palliative RT schemes appear sufficient and adequate to achieve durable tumor control, making the use of time-consuming and costly SBRT unnecessary. It should be noted that none of our patients was treated with 8 Gy single-fraction RT: although Iyer et al. reported excellent results with this dosage, other authors doubt its adequacy and suggest tripling its administration to obtain better outcomes [23,28]. In our clinical practice, when the patient's life expectancy is longer than six months, multi-fraction palliative schemes are preferred over the 8 Gy single fraction as the latter carries a higher risk of need for re-treatment [29].

Most of our patients had limited disease progression (median GTV < 30 cc) on IT. The mechanism underlying this acquired immune resistance probably involves localized defects in tumor antigen presentation and recognition by the host immune system [30]. RT may ablate the refractory focus, prolonging tumor response to IT [31]. This happened in most of our patients. Our preliminary results introduce MCC among oligoprogressive cancer histologies benefitting from RT to reverse incoming immunologically cold tumor subpopulations [32,33].

A series of interesting findings emerges from reviewing the pertinent literature. In cases of limited brain metastases, SRS, as characterized by less cognitive deteriorating effects than whole-brain RT, might be preferred over this [34]. In the pre-avelumab era, Jacob et al. reported a successful use of SRS for two metachronous brain metastases in an MCC patient who subsequently died of leptomeningeal spread [35]. Stereotactic RT showed excellent local control in another patient with limited brain metastases from a primary parotid Merkel-type small cell neuroendocrine carcinoma, which is indistinguishable from classic MCC [36]. In the latter case, avelumab would have been initiated as a salvage treatment, given the failure of chemotherapy and the limited efficacy of RT in significantly prolonging the patient's PFS. Regarding intracranial oligoprogression during avelumab treatment, a brief report by Fife et al. promotes the addition of SRS to IT: avelumab's effects on intracranial metastases were transient or even null in all four patients, while two of them actually benefitted from brain SRS [37]. The outcome of our single case of intracranial metastasis, together with all the above, further supports the use of brain SRS.

Concerning the management of extracranial oligo-progression or -recurrence from MCC, there are few reports with both SBRT and non-stereotactic schemes. SBRT was effectively used at a dose of 25 Gy (with a hotspot of 33.57 Gy) in 5 fractions every other day for a challenging intracardiac MCC metastasis, which arose after a durable complete response to avelumab, lasting 2 years and 5 months. The subsequent treatment success allowed safely resuming of IT, which ensured excellent systemic disease control until the last documented follow-up (almost 1 year after SBRT delivery) [38]. A similar course was observed in an HIV-positive patient, who, while switching to avelumab, received SBRT at a dose of 30 Gy in six daily fractions to a para-cardiac lymph node metastasis progressing on pembrolizumab therapy and was still progression-free 8 months later [39]. Large doses in a few fractions can also be particularly useful in some extremely palliative settings that require rapid and sustained relief of symptoms and a reduction in daily visits to the oncological center, such as in medically frail or elderly patients [18,40]. On the other side, conventionally fractionated radiotherapy was able to restore sensitivity to IT in two MCC patients, whose metastases had become late refractory to pembrolizumab and avelumab, respectively. At the last follow-up after RT, both patients were alive, achieving an exceptionally long PFS (20 months and 2.5 years, respectively) [41,42].

RT is known to synergize with the antitumor effects of PD1/PD-L1 axis blockade [43,44]. This probably underlies some tumor responses that extend beyond the radiation field, as in the case series by Xu et al. These authors reported the impressive outcomes of two patients with mMCC progressing on PD-1 inhibitor therapy and then treated with 8 Gy-single-fraction palliative radiotherapy to some portion of the tumor masses: surprisingly, both patients rapidly experienced a marked reduction until disappearance not only of the irradiated tumor portion, but also of the distant out-of-field tumor sites [45]. In fact, the abscopal effect has been rarely reported, and no way is yet available to systematically engage it to enhance systemic tumor control, being able to be elicited even in the absence of IT [46]. In the NCT03071406 trial, SBRT delivery to a tumor site did not produce a significant response in non-irradiated ones among mMCC patients treated with ipilimumab plus nivolumab, ultimately resulting in no ORR difference compared to IT alone [47]. This is why we decided to focus on those patients for whom it was possible to irradiate all macroscopic disease sites.

On the other hand, i.e., from the point of view of toxicity, it is well-known that combining RT with IT, as well as with other drugs, may give rise to unexpected events, such as the bystander effect, radiation recall phenomena, or even life-threatening autoimmune paraneoplastic disorders [48–50]. In our small cohort, we did not report any significant higher-than-expected toxicity.

A very interesting finding of our investigation concerns the proven ability of RT to reverse both primary and secondary immune resistance. Indeed, three out of five patients with primary immune resistance showed sustained PFS following RT to the immune-refractory tumor sites detected at the first follow-up after avelumab initiation. Furthermore, RT was able to effectively prolong PFS even in those three patients who had secondarily developed immune resistance to avelumab. Notably, RT was delivered a second time in two of these patients, allowing them to successfully continue avelumab therapy. These results are of outstanding importance if we consider that a short report from the ADOREG registry showed an ORR of 50% (7/14) in avelumab-refractory mMCC patients later treated with ipilimumab plus nivolumab and immune-related toxicities requiring treatment discontinuation in 21% (3/14) of them [51]. Our findings mean that the possible positive interactions between RT and IT in mMCC patients deserve further attention from clinicians and researchers.

Successful interactions between RT and IT have been recently reviewed by Yi et al., but their summary does not include MCC histology [52]. Furthermore, some preclinical models could clarify whether personalization of stereotactic radiotherapy in combination with IT is needed [53]. Several lines of evidence advocate the use of RT for MCC, but none in the context explored here [54,55].

The main limitations of our study are the small number of patients and the heterogeneity of the target size and dose fractionation, which did not make it possible to draw clear conclusions about the most suitable RT approach. However, based on the favorable benefit–risk ratio, adding radiotherapy for rescuing mMCC patients with limited progression on avelumab might be a compelling strategy. The encouraging findings reported here should not be ignored and warrant further investigation in large prospective trials, possibly of the multicenter type to overcome the patient recruitment difficulties linked to the tumor rarity.

MCC is rare and the oligoprogression brought to the attention of radiation oncologists is even more so. Our retrospective observations from a single institution would translate into a prospective recruitment rate of approximately 1.33 patients per year. The latter, considering avelumab's well-proven efficacy and its recent approval as factors limiting the development of the disease stage investigated here, may be in line with the all-stage rate reported by Wang et al. over forty years, equal to about 13 patients per year [56]. Spreading awareness of our preliminary results among medical oncologists could lead to an increase in our low recruitment rate. Meanwhile, our findings aim to serve as a hypothesis-generating and -testing proof-of-concept study.

5. Conclusions

Radiotherapy seems to be well tolerated and effective in prolonging progression-free survival in mMCC patients with limited progression on avelumab, thus allowing its continuation. In achieving that goal, low radiation doses, such as those used in palliative schemes, might be as equally effective as high ablative ones, with even fewer concerns about treatment tolerance. However, the suggestive data presented here need to be validated in large prospective trials, pending new drugs that will hopefully extend the therapeutic algorithm for the metastatic stage of such aggressive cancer.

Author Contributions: Conceptualization, G.F. and V.Z.; methodology, G.F.; software, S.F.; validation, G.F., V.Z. and S.F.; formal analysis, S.F.; investigation, V.Z.; resources, G.F.; data curation, V.Z.; writing—original draft preparation, G.F.; writing—review and editing, G.F.; visualization, G.F., V.Z., P.C., A.S., S.S., M.M.H., T.V., G.E.U., A.V., V.V. and S.F.; supervision, G.F.; project administration, G.F. All authors have read and agreed to the published version of the manuscript.

Funding: This research received no external funding.

Institutional Review Board Statement: All procedures performed in studies involving human participants were in accordance with the ethical standards of the institutional and/or national research committee and with the 1964 Helsinki Declaration and its later amendments or comparable ethical standards. Ethical approval was waived by the local Ethics Committee in view of the retrospective nature of the study and because all the procedures being performed were part of routine care.

Informed Consent Statement: Patients signed informed consent regarding publishing their data.

Data Availability Statement: All the generated data are available upon request to the corresponding author.

Conflicts of Interest: The authors declare no conflict of interest.

Abbreviations

RT	radiotherapy
PFS	progression-free survival
MCC	merkel cell carcinoma
mMCC	metastatic Merkel cell carcinoma
OS	overall survival
irRECIST	immune-related Response Evaluation Criteria in Solid Tumours
RTOG	Radiation Therapy Oncology Group
GTV	gross tumor volume
CTV	clinical target volume
PTV	planning target volume
SBRT	stereotactic body radiation therapy
SRS	stereotactic radiosurgery
VMAT	volumetric modulated arc therapy
IMRT	intensity-modulated radiotherapy
BED	biologically effective dose
ECOG	Eastern Cooperative Oncology Group
IT	immunotherapy
ORR	objective response rate
CR	complete response
PR	partial response
SD	stable disease
PD	progressive disease
LC	local control
PD1	Programmed cell death protein 1
PD-L1	programmed cell death ligand 1
18F-FDG	$[^{18}F]$Fluorodeoxyglucose
PET	positron emission tomography
CT	computed tomography

References

1. Tello, T.L.; Coggshall, K.; Yom, S.S.; Yu, S.S. Merkel cell carcinoma: An update and review: Current and future therapy. *J. Am. Acad. Dermatol.* **2018**, *78*, 445–454. [CrossRef] [PubMed]
2. Gonzalez, M.R.; Bryce-Alberti, M.; Portmann-Baracco, A.; Castillo-Flores, S.; Pretell-Mazzini, J. Treatment and survival outcomes in metastatic Merkel cell carcinoma: Analysis of 2010 patients from the SEER database. *Cancer Treat. Res. Commun.* **2022**, *33*, 100665. [CrossRef] [PubMed]
3. D'Angelo, S.P.; Bhatia, S.; Brohl, A.S.; Hamid, O.; Mehnert, J.M.; Terheyden, P.; Shih, K.C.; Brownell, I.; Lebbé, C.; Lewis, K.D.; et al. Avelumab in patients with previously treated metastatic Merkel cell carcinoma (JAVELIN Merkel 200): Updated overall survival data after >5 years of follow-up. *ESMO Open* **2021**, *6*, 100290. [CrossRef]
4. Khan, L.; Barnes, E.A. Radiotherapy for metastatic merkel cell carcinoma: A review of the literature. *J. Skin Cancer* **2012**, *2012*, 654981. [CrossRef]
5. Kaufman, H.L.; Russell, J.S.; Hamid, O.; Bhatia, S.; Terheyden, P.; D'Angelo, S.P.; Shih, K.C.; Lebbé, C.; Milella, M.; Brownell, I.; et al. Updated efficacy of avelumab in patients with previously treated metastatic Merkel cell carcinoma after $\geq$1 year of follow-up: JAVELIN Merkel 200, a phase 2 clinical trial. *J. Immunother. Cancer* **2018**, *6*, 7. [CrossRef] [PubMed]
6. Iyer, J.G.; Blom, A.; Doumani, R.; Lewis, C.; Tarabadkar, E.S.; Anderson, A.; Ma, C.; Bestick, A.; Parvathaneni, U.; Bhatia, S.; et al. Response rates and durability of chemotherapy among 62 patients with metastatic Merkel cell carcinoma. *Cancer Med.* **2016**, *5*, 2294–2301. [CrossRef]
7. Pacifico, P.; Colciago, R.R.; De Felice, F.; Boldrini, L.; Salvestrini, V.; Nardone, V.; Desideri, I.; Greco, C.; Arcangeli, S. A critical review on oligometastatic disease: A radiation oncologist's perspective. *Med. Oncol.* **2022**, *39*, 181. [CrossRef]
8. Palma, D.A.; Olson, R.; Harrow, S.; Gaede, S.; Louie, A.V.; Haasbeek, C.; Mulroy, L.; Lock, M.; Rodrigues, G.B.; Yaremko, B.P.; et al. Stereotactic Ablative Radiotherapy for the Comprehensive Treatment of Oligometastatic Cancers: Long-Term Results of the SABR-COMET Phase II Randomized Trial. *J. Clin. Oncol.* **2020**, *38*, 2830–2838. [CrossRef]
9. Spada, F.; Bossi, P.; Caracò, C.; Sileni, V.C.; Dei Tos, A.P.; Fazio, N.; Grignani, G.; Maio, M.; Quaglino, P.; Queirolo, P.; et al. Nationwide multidisciplinary consensus on the clinical management of Merkel cell carcinoma: A Delphi panel. *J. Immunother. Cancer* **2022**, *10*, e004742. [CrossRef]
10. Cox, B.W.; Spratt, D.E.; Lovelock, M.; Bilsky, M.H.; Lis, E.; Ryu, S.; Sheehan, J.; Gerszten, P.C.; Chang, E.; Gibbs, I.; et al. International Spine Radiosurgery Consortium consensus guidelines for target volume definition in spinal stereotactic radiosurgery. *Int. J. Radiat. Oncol. Biol. Phys.* **2012**, *83*, e597–e605. [CrossRef]
11. Borcoman, E.; Nandikolla, A.; Long, G.; Goel, S.; Le Tourneau, C. Patterns of Response and Progression to Immunotherapy. *Am. Soc. Clin. Oncol. Educ Book* **2018**, *38*, 169–178. [CrossRef] [PubMed]
12. Cox, J.D.; Stetz, J.; Pajak, T.F. Toxicity criteria of the Radiation Therapy Oncology Group (RTOG) and the European Organization for Research and Treatment of Cancer (EORTC). *Int. J. Radiat. Oncol. Biol. Phys.* **1995**, *31*, 1341–1346. [CrossRef] [PubMed]
13. Kaplan, E.L.; Meier, P. Nonparametric Estimation from Incomplete Observations. *J. Am. Stat. Assoc.* **1958**, *53*, 457–481. [CrossRef]
14. Sherry, A.D.; Bathala, T.K.; Liu, S.; Fellman, B.M.; Chun, S.G.; Jasani, N.; Guadagnolo, B.A.; Jhingran, A.; Reddy, J.P.; Corn, P.G.; et al. Definitive Local Consolidative Therapy for Oligometastatic Solid Tumors: Results From the Lead-in Phase of the Randomized Basket Trial EXTEND. *Int. J. Radiat. Oncol. Biol. Phys.* **2022**, *114*, 910–918. [CrossRef]
15. Urbanski, A.; Minnemann, J.; Mauch, C.; Schmidt, T.; Kreuzberg, N.; Schlaak, M.; Bruns, C.J.; Stippel, D.L.; Wahba, R. Oligometastatic disease and visceral resections in advanced malignant melanoma: A propensity-matched analysis. *Langenbecks. Arch. Surg.* **2023**, *408*, 53. [CrossRef]
16. Bates, J.E.; Youn, P.; Usuki, K.Y.; Walter, K.A.; Huggins, C.F.; Okunieff, P.; Milano, M.T. Brain metastasis from melanoma: The prognostic value of varying sites of extracranial disease. *J. Neurooncol.* **2015**, *125*, 411–418. [CrossRef]
17. Ferini, G.; Castorina, P.; Valenti, V.; Illari, S.I.; Sachpazidis, I.; Castorina, L.; Marrale, M.; Pergolizzi, S. A Novel Radiotherapeutic Approach to Treat Bulky Metastases Even From Cutaneous Squamous Cell Carcinoma: Its Rationale and a Look at the Reliability of the Linear-Quadratic Model to Explain Its Radiobiological Effects. *Front. Oncol.* **2022**, *12*, 809279. [CrossRef]
18. Ferini, G.; Molino, L.; Bottalico, L.; De Lucia, P.; Garofalo, F. A small case series about safety and effectiveness of a hypofractionated electron beam radiotherapy schedule in five fractions for facial non melanoma skin cancer among frail and elderly patients. *Rep. Pract. Oncol. Radiother.* **2021**, *26*, 66–72. [CrossRef]
19. Ferini, G.; Palmisciano, P.; Forte, S.; Viola, A.; Martorana, E.; Parisi, S.; Valenti, V.; Fichera, C.; Umana, G.E.; Pergolizzi, S. Advanced or Metastatic Cutaneous Squamous Cell Carcinoma: The Current and Future Role of Radiation Therapy in the Era of Immunotherapy. *Cancers* **2022**, *14*, 1871. [CrossRef]
20. Mazzola, R.; Jereczek-Fossa, B.A.; Franceschini, D.; Tubin, S.; Filippi, A.R.; Tolia, M.; Lancia, A.; Minniti, G.; Corradini, S.; Arcangeli, S.; et al. Oligometastasis and local ablation in the era of systemic targeted and immunotherapy. *Radiat. Oncol.* **2020**, *15*, 92. [CrossRef]
21. Cacciola, A.; Parisi, S.; Tamburella, C.; Lillo, S.; Ferini, G.; Molino, L.; Iatì, G.; Pontoriero, A.; Bottari, A.; Mazziotti, S.; et al. Stereotactic body radiation therapy and radiofrequency ablation for the treatment of liver metastases: How and when? *Rep. Pract. Oncol. Radiother.* **2020**, *25*, 299–306. [CrossRef]

22. Ferini, G.; Valenti, V.; Puliafito, I.; Illari, S.I.; Marchese, V.A.; Borzì, G.R. Volumetric Modulated Arc Therapy Capabilities for Treating Lower-Extremity Skin Affected by Several Merkel Cell Carcinoma Nodules: When Technological Advances Effectively Achieve the Palliative Therapeutic Goal while Minimising the Risk of Potential Toxicities. *Medicina* **2021**, *57*, 1379. [CrossRef] [PubMed]
23. Iyer, J.G.; Parvathaneni, U.; Gooley, T.; Miller, N.J.; Markowitz, E.; Blom, A.; Lewis, C.W.; Doumani, R.F.; Parvathaneni, K.; Anderson, A.; et al. Single-fraction radiation therapy in patients with metastatic Merkel cell carcinoma. *Cancer Med.* **2015**, *4*, 1161–1170. [CrossRef] [PubMed]
24. Kwilas, A.R.; Donahue, R.N.; Bernstein, M.B.; Hodge, J.W. In the field: Exploiting the untapped potential of immunogenic modulation by radiation in combination with immunotherapy for the treatment of cancer. *Front. Oncol.* **2012**, *2*, 104. [CrossRef] [PubMed]
25. Herrera, F.G.; Ronet, C.; Ochoa de Olza, M.; Barras, D.; Crespo, I.; Andreatta, M.; Corria-Osorio, J.; Spill, A.; Benedetti, F.; Genolet, R.; et al. Low-Dose Radiotherapy Reverses Tumor Immune Desertification and Resistance to Immunotherapy. *Cancer Discov.* **2022**, *12*, 108–133. [CrossRef] [PubMed]
26. Ferini, G.; Valenti, V.; Tripoli, A.; Illari, S.I.; Molino, L.; Parisi, S.; Cacciola, A.; Lillo, S.; Giuffrida, D.; Pergolizzi, S. Lattice or Oxygen-Guided Radiotherapy: What If They Converge? Possible Future Directions in the Era of Immunotherapy. *Cancers* **2021**, *13*, 3290. [CrossRef] [PubMed]
27. Mirestean, C.C.; Iancu, R.I.; Iancu, D.T. Immunotherapy and radiotherapy-a future partnership Focus on radiation induced lymphopenia (RIL) implications. *Bratisl. Lek. Listy* **2023**, *124*, 70–73. [CrossRef]
28. Cimbak, N.; Barker, C.A. Short-Course Radiation Therapy for Merkel Cell Carcinoma: Relative Effectiveness in a "Radiosensitive" Tumor. *Int. J. Radiat. Oncol.* **2016**, *96*, S160. [CrossRef]
29. Pergolizzi, S.; Cacciola, A.; Parisi, S.; Lillo, S.; Tamburella, C.; Santacaterina, A.; Ferini, G.; Cellini, F.; Draghini, L.; Trippa, F.; et al. An Italian survey on "palliative intent" radiotherapy. *Rep. Pract. Oncol. Radiother.* **2022**, *27*, 419–427. [CrossRef]
30. Bang, A.; Schoenfeld, J.D. Immunotherapy and radiotherapy for metastatic cancers. *Ann. Palliat. Med.* **2019**, *8*, 312–325. [CrossRef]
31. Salkeni, M.A.; Shin, J.Y.; Gulley, J.L. Resistance to Immunotherapy: Mechanisms and Means for Overcoming. In *Immunotherapy. Advances in Experimental Medicine and Biology*; Naing, A., Hajjar, J., Eds.; Springer: Cham, Switzerland, 2021; Volume 1342. [CrossRef]
32. Mahmood, U.; Huynh, M.A.; Killoran, J.H.; Qian, J.M.; Bent, E.H.; Aizer, A.A.; Mak, R.H.; Mamon, H.J.; Balboni, T.A.; Gunasti, L.; et al. Retrospective Review of Outcomes After Radiation Therapy for Oligoprogressive Disease on Immune Checkpoint Blockade. *Int. J. Radiat. Oncol. Biol. Phys.* **2022**, *114*, 666–675. [CrossRef] [PubMed]
33. Gettinger, S.N.; Wurtz, A.; Goldberg, S.B.; Rimm, D.; Schalper, K.; Kaech, S.; Kavathas, P.; Chiang, A.; Lilenbaum, R.; Zelterman, D.; et al. Clinical Features and Management of Acquired Resistance to PD-1 Axis Inhibitors in 26 Patients With Advanced Non-Small Cell Lung Cancer. *J. Thorac. Oncol.* **2018**, *13*, 831–839. [CrossRef]
34. Ferini, G.; Viola, A.; Valenti, V.; Tripoli, A.; Molino, L.; Marchese, V.A.; Illari, S.I.; Rita Borzì, G.; Prestifilippo, A.; Umana, G.E.; et al. Whole Brain Irradiation or Stereotactic RadioSurgery for five or more brain metastases (WHOBI-STER): A prospective comparative study of neurocognitive outcomes, level of autonomy in daily activities and quality of life. *Clin. Transl. Radiat. Oncol.* **2021**, *32*, 52–58. [CrossRef] [PubMed]
35. Jacob, A.T.; Alexandru-Abrams, D.; Abrams, E.M.; Lee, J.Y. Stereotactic radiosurgery for merkel cell carcinoma brain metastases. *J. Clin. Neurosci.* **2015**, *22*, 1499–1502. [CrossRef] [PubMed]
36. Young, S.; Oh, J.; Bukhari, H.; Ng, T.; Chau, N.; Tran, E. Primary Parotid Merkel Type Small Cell Neuroendocrine Carcinoma with Oligometastasis to the Brain and Adrenal Gland: Case Report and Review of Literature. *Head. Neck. Pathol.* **2021**, *15*, 311–318. [CrossRef]
37. Fife, K.; Tétu, P.; Prabhakaran, J.; Lebbé, C.; Grignani, G. Case Report: Clinical Experience With Avelumab in Patients With Metastatic Merkel Cell Carcinoma and Brain Metastases Treated in Europe. *Front. Oncol.* **2021**, *11*, 672021. [CrossRef]
38. Shi, D.D.; Liu, K.X.; Hacker, F.; Hanna, G.J.; Kwong, R.Y.; Cagney, D.N.; Mak, R.H.; Singer, L. Development and Implementation of an Online Adaptive Stereotactic Body Radiation Therapy Workflow for Treatment of Intracardiac Metastasis. *Pract. Radiat. Oncol.* **2021**, *11*, e395–e401. [CrossRef]
39. Linge, A.; Rauschenberg, R.; Blum, S.; Spornraft-Ragaller, P.; Meier, F.; Troost, E.G.C. Successful immunotherapy and irradiation in a HIV-positive patient with metastatic Merkel cell carcinoma. *Clin. Transl. Radiat. Oncol.* **2018**, *15*, 42–45. [CrossRef]
40. Zhu, J.W.; Doerwald-Munoz, L.; Lee, J.W. Medically inoperable Merkel cell carcinoma of the head and neck treated with stereotactic body radiation therapy: A case report. *Ann. Palliat. Med.* **2021**, *10*, 2354–2358. [CrossRef]
41. Bloom, B.C.; Augustyn, A.; Pezzi, T.A.; Menon, H.; Mayo, L.L.; Shah, S.J.; Schwartz, D.L.; Chmura, S.J.; Johnson, F.M.; Welsh, J.W.; et al. Rescue of Immunotherapy-Refractory Metastatic Merkel Cell Carcinoma With Conventionally Fractionated Radiotherapy and Concurrent Pembrolizumab. *Front. Oncol.* **2019**, *9*, 223. [CrossRef]
42. Leão, I.; Marinho, J.; Costa, T. Long-term response to avelumab and management of oligoprogression in Merkel cell carcinoma: A case report. *World J. Clin. Cases* **2021**, *9*, 4829–4836. [CrossRef] [PubMed]
43. Gill, S.; Nowak, A.K.; Bowyer, S.; Endersby, R.; Ebert, M.A.; Cook, A. Clinical evidence for synergy between immunotherapy and radiotherapy (SITAR). *J. Med. Imaging Radiat. Oncol.* **2022**, *66*, 881–895. [CrossRef]
44. Gong, J.; Le, T.Q.; Massarelli, E.; Hendifar, A.E.; Tuli, R. Radiation therapy and PD-1/PD-L1 blockade: The clinical development of an evolving anticancer combination. *J. Immunother. Cancer* **2018**, *6*, 46. [CrossRef] [PubMed]

45. Xu, M.J.; Wu, S.; Daud, A.I.; Yu, S.S.; Yom, S.S. In-field and abscopal response after short-course radiation therapy in patients with metastatic Merkel cell carcinoma progressing on PD-1 checkpoint blockade: A case series. *J. Immunother. Cancer* **2018**, *6*, 43. [CrossRef]
46. Cotter, S.E.; Dunn, G.P.; Collins, K.M.; Sahni, D.; Zukotynski, K.A.; Hansen, J.L.; O'Farrell, D.A.; Ng, A.K.; Devlin, P.M.; Wang, L.C. Abscopal effect in a patient with metastatic Merkel cell carcinoma following radiation therapy: Potential role of induced antitumor immunity. *Arch. Dermatol.* **2011**, *147*, 870–872. [CrossRef] [PubMed]
47. Kim, S.; Wuthrick, E.; Blakaj, D.; Eroglu, Z.; Verschraegen, C.; Thapa, R.; Mills, M.; Dibs, K.; Liveringhouse, C.; Russell, J.; et al. Combined nivolumab and ipilimumab with or without stereotactic body radiation therapy for advanced Merkel cell carcinoma: A randomised, open label, phase 2 trial. *Lancet* **2022**, *400*, 1008–1019. [CrossRef]
48. Parisi, S.; Napoli, I.; Lillo, S.; Cacciola, A.; Ferini, G.; Iatì, G.; Pontoriero, A.; Tamburella, C.; Davì, V.; Pergolizzi, S. Spine eburnation in a metastatic lung cancer patient treated with immunotherapy and radiotherapy. The first case report of bystander effect on bone. *J. Oncol. Pharm. Pract.* **2022**, *28*, 237–241. [CrossRef]
49. Sindoni, A.; Severo, C.; Vadala', R.E.; Ferini, G.; Mazzei, M.M.; Vaccaro, M.; Iatì, G.; Pontoriero, A.; Pergolizzi, S. Levetiracetam-induced radiation recall dermatitis in a patient undergoing stereotactic radiotherapy. *J. Dermatol.* **2016**, *43*, 1440–1441. [CrossRef]
50. Sherry, A.D.; Bezzerides, M.; Khattab, M.H.; Luo, G.; Ancell, K.K.; Kirschner, A.N. An autoimmune-based, paraneoplastic neurologic syndrome following checkpoint inhibition and concurrent radiotherapy for merkel cell carcinoma: Case report. *Strahlenther. Onkol.* **2020**, *196*, 664–670. [CrossRef]
51. Glutsch, V.; Schummer, P.; Kneitz, H.; Gesierich, A.; Goebeler, M.; Klein, D.; Posch, C.; Gebhardt, C.; Haferkamp, S.; Zimmer, L.; et al. Ipilimumab plus nivolumab in avelumab-refractory Merkel cell carcinoma: A multicenter study of the prospective skin cancer registry ADOREG. *J. Immunother. Cancer* **2022**, *10*, e005930. [CrossRef]
52. Yi, M.; Zheng, X.; Niu, M.; Zhu, S.; Ge, H.; Wu, K. Combination strategies with PD-1/PD-L1 blockade: Current advances and future directions. *Mol. Cancer* **2022**, *21*, 28. [CrossRef] [PubMed]
53. Moore, C.; Hsu, C.C.; Chen, W.M.; Chen, B.P.C.; Han, C.; Story, M.; Aguilera, T.; Pop, L.M.; Hannan, R.; Fu, Y.X.; et al. Personalized Ultrafractionated Stereotactic Adaptive Radiotherapy (PULSAR) in Preclinical Models Enhances Single-Agent Immune Checkpoint Blockade. *Int. J. Radiat. Oncol. Biol. Phys.* **2021**, *110*, 1306–1316. [CrossRef] [PubMed]
54. Green, C.; Isaksson Mettävainio, M.; Kjellman, C.; Ramqvist, T.; Dalianis, T.; Israelsson, P.; Lindquist, D. Combined treatment with radiotherapy, chemotherapy and avelumab results in regression of metastatic Merkel cell carcinoma and improvement of associated Lambert-Eaton myasthenic syndrome: A case report. *Oncol. Lett.* **2022**, *24*, 393. [CrossRef] [PubMed]
55. Cassler, N.M.; Merrill, D.; Bichakjian, C.K.; Brownell, I. Merkel Cell Carcinoma Therapeutic Update. *Curr. Treat Options Oncol.* **2016**, *17*, 36. [CrossRef]
56. Wang, A.J.; McCann, B.; Soon, W.C.L.; De Ieso, P.B.; Bressel, M.; Hui, A.; Chua, M.; Kok, D.L. Merkel cell carcinoma: A forty-year experience at the Peter MacCallum Cancer Centre. *BMC Cancer* **2023**, *23*, 30. [CrossRef] [PubMed]